Clinical Assessment and Treatment of Eating Disorders

Clinical Assessment and Treatment of Eating Disorders

Editor: Lewis Humphries

AMERICAN
MEDICAL PUBLISHERS
www.americanmedicalpublishers.com

AMERICAN
MEDICAL PUBLISHERS
www.americanmedicalpublishers.com

Cataloging-in-Publication Data

Clinical assessment and treatment of eating disorders / edited by Lewis Humphries.
p. cm.
Includes bibliographical references and index.
ISBN 978-1-63927-989-0
1. Eating disorders. 2. Eating disorders--Diagnosis. 3. Eating disorders--Treatment.
4. Appetite disorders. 5. Psychology, Pathological. 6. Psychiatry. I. Humphries, Lewis.
RC552.E18 C55 2023
616.852 6--dc23

American Medical Publishers,
41 Flatbush Avenue,
1st Floor, New York,
NY 11217, USA

ISBN 978-1-63927-989-0 (Hardback)

Contents

Preface

This book was inspired by the evolution of our times; to answer the curiosity of inquisitive minds. Many developments have occurred across the globe in the recent past which has transformed the progress in the field.

An eating disorder refers to a type of mental disorder characterized by abnormal eating habits that have a negative impact on a person's mental or physical health. People suffering from eating disorders may exhibit a wide range of symptoms, including food binges, severe dietary restriction and purging actions such as over exercising or vomiting. There are various types of eating disorders, such as bulimia nervosa, pica, avoidant or restrictive food intake disorder, anorexia nervosa, binge eating disorder and rumination disorder. The risk factors associated with eating disorders include family history, psychological health, extracurricular activities, aging, excessive dieting and life transitions. Eating disorders can be diagnosed through physical and psychological assessments. The treatment plans of eating disorders are unique to each individual and include a combination of therapies. The treatment varies according to the disorder, which includes limiting excess exercising, counseling, reducing efforts to eliminate food, and dietary advice. This book seeks to provide a fair idea about eating disorders and to help develop a better understanding of the latest advances in their clinical management. It will serve as a reference to a broad spectrum of readers.

This book was developed from a mere concept to drafts to chapters and finally compiled together as a complete text to benefit the readers across all nations. To ensure the quality of the content we instilled two significant steps in our procedure. The first was to appoint an editorial team that would verify the data and statistics provided in the book and also select the most appropriate and valuable contributions from the plentiful contributions we received from authors worldwide. The next step was to appoint an expert of the topic as the Editor-in-Chief, who would head the project and finally make the necessary amendments and modifications to make the text reader-friendly. I was then commissioned to examine all the material to present the topics in the most comprehensible and productive format.

I would like to take this opportunity to thank all the contributing authors who were supportive enough to contribute their time and knowledge to this project. I also wish to convey my regards to my family who have been extremely supportive during the entire project.

Editor

A theoretical review of interpersonal emotion regulation in eating disorders: enhancing knowledge by bridging interpersonal and affective dysfunction

Kara A. Christensen[1*] and Ann F. Haynos[2]

Abstract

Individuals with eating disorders (EDs) frequently report interpersonal and affective dysfunction. A useful lens for uniting these ideas is through the framework of interpersonal emotion regulation (IER), which consists of the ways others assist a distressed individual and how this shapes his or her subsequent emotional, behavioral, and cognitive responses. In this theoretical review, we provide an overview of the rationale for exploring IER and review IER processes in this population using the framework of the Process Model of Emotion Regulation. Finally, we offer suggestions for next steps in conducting research. IER offers a parsimonious way to explore social and emotional constructs related to ED pathology and may provide potential targets for prevention and intervention in these difficult-to-treat disorders.

Keywords: Interpersonal relationships, Emotion regulation, Interpersonal emotion regulation, Eating disorders

Plain English summary

People with eating disorders frequently report difficulties in their relationships and experiencing difficult-to-control emotions. We propose that studying the different ways that people receive help with managing their emotions (i.e., interpersonal emotion regulation) is promising for better characterizing the specific problems that people with eating disorders experience. In this review paper, we discuss the current research on interpersonal emotion regulation and future directions for this field. Increased knowledge of interpersonal emotion regulation could lead to the development and/or refinement of prevention and intervention methods that specifically target maladaptive social support behaviors linked to emotional distress.

* Correspondence: christensen@ku.edu

[1]Department of Psychology, University of Kansas, 1415 Jayhawk Blvd Rm 440, Lawrence, KS 66045, USA

Full list of author information is available at the end of the article

Introduction

Individuals with eating disorders (EDs) report both interpersonal and affective dysfunction [1–3], which may be united by a growing literature exploring a construct called interpersonal emotion regulation (IER; Fig. 1). IER consists of the ways in which people intentionally engage with an individual to modify the individual's emotions and how this shapes subsequent emotional, behavioral, and cognitive responses of each member of the dyad [4–9]. Although there is a long history of interest in how different aspects of close interpersonal relationships, such as feelings of security or warmth, influence the emotional health of others (e.g., attachment theory [10, 11], interpersonal theory [12], object-relations theory [13], cognitive-interpersonal model of anorexia nervosa [14, 15]), there has been considerably less work evaluating the specific strategies that people use interpersonally to modify emotional experiences.

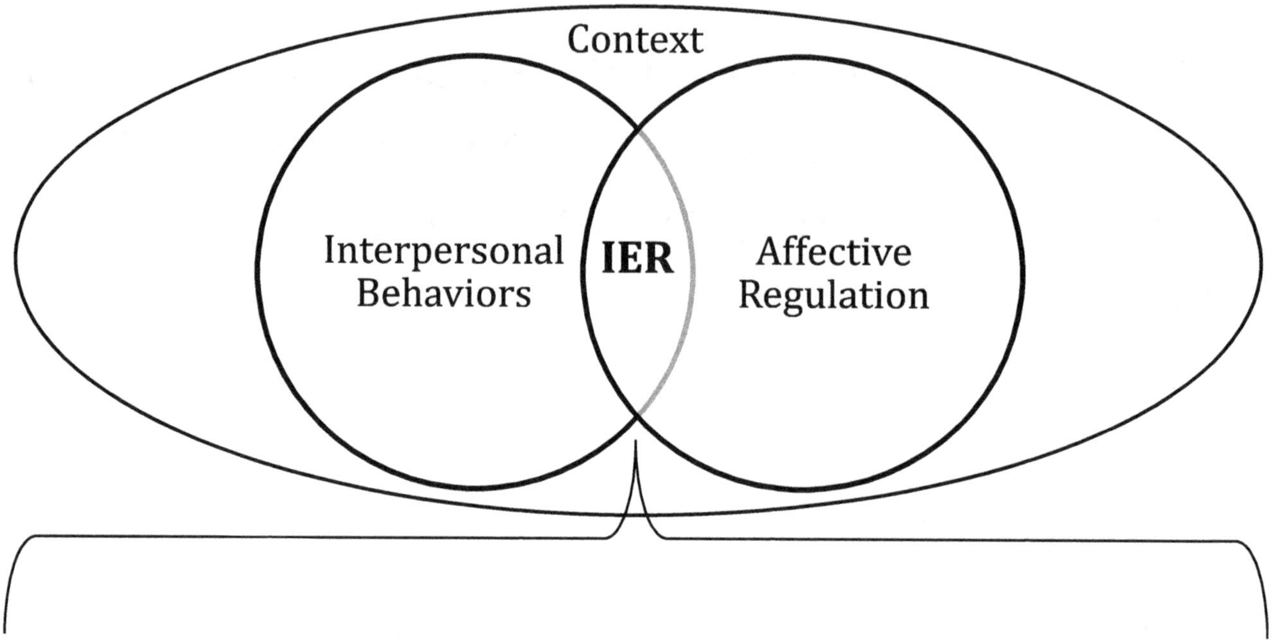

A. Situation Selection	B. Situation Modification	C. Attention Deployment	D. Cognitive Change	E. Response Modulation
- Accommodation of avoidance	- Accommodation of ED rules	- Distraction - Rumination	- Reappraisal - Reassurance-seeking	- Eating and feeding behaviors - Exercise - Substance use - Expressive suppression

Fig. 1 Process Model of Interpersonal Emotion Regulation in Eating Disorders. Interpersonal emotion regulation (IER) is at the intersection of interpersonal behaviors and affective regulation. To evaluate if interpersonal behaviors, affective regulation, and interpersonal emotion regulation are adaptive or maladaptive, one must consider contextual factors such as personal goals, culture, demographics, and stage of recovery

IER is a broad framework for understanding interpersonal emotion management dynamics that can be applied in both non-clinical and clinical contexts and is complementary to existing models of ED etiology and maintenance. Of note, IER shares similarities with other related constructs, such as attachment, social support, and emotional contagion, but differs in that it requires intentionality in trying to modify emotional response by the regulator [4]. For instance, if a person is nervous about a presentation, she may turn to a friend for reassurance, which thereby reduces her anxiety. In turn, the friend's distress caused by their friend's anxiety may also be reduced, resulting in a bidirectional, interactional process between the two members of the dyad. These types of interactions are common to many relationships and frequently benefit both members of the dyad; however, when IER is used inflexibly, inefficiently, or inappropriately, it may result in dysfunction for the individuals and their relationship. In this way, IER may serve as a risk and maintenance factor for psychopathology.

Indeed, the IER framework has been applied to explain the etiology and maintenance of psychological problems such as depression [8, 9] and anxiety disorders [8]. It has significantly expanded the understanding of potential prevention and treatment targets; however, it has yet to be applied to EDs. Studying IER may provide additional clarity in how problems in emotion regulation (ER) processes interact with interpersonal problems to promote ED behaviors. Information about IER adds explanatory value above and beyond either interpersonal or emotional problems by better capturing the dynamic ways in which people interact with each other for emotional purposes. Furthermore, information about IER may help to improve the specificity of existing models of ED etiology and maintenance by providing a framework for understanding problematic interpersonal and emotional behaviors.

In this review, we will provide evidence supporting the utility of studying IER in EDs based on interpersonal and affective dysfunction risk factors, describe the status of this area of study, and offer directions for future research. To do this, we will describe evidence for global use of IER strategies (e.g., co-rumination about general anxieties within social relationships) by individuals with EDs, as well as disorder-specific manifestations of IER (e.g., interpersonal facilitation of food avoidance to reduce anxiety).

Interpersonal problems in EDs

Individuals with EDs frequently report difficulties with social functioning [1].[1] These interpersonal difficulties may serve as both risk or maintenance factors for eating pathology, or could simply constitute interpersonal consequences of ED behavior. In terms of risk factors, at the trait level, people with EDs endorse more maladaptive interpersonal personality profiles, such as overly nurturing and accommodating, nonassertive, dependent, and socially avoidant styles [16]. People with EDs report less pleasure from social encounters and a lower interest in social interaction [17]. In prospective studies, low social support has been found to confer risk for future binge eating [18], and to interact with negative life events to predict increased bulimic symptoms [19]. Alternately, greater social support serves as a protective factor to mitigate the effects of ED risk factors [20]. ED behaviors also may produce strains on relationships that result in stressful interactions or fractures and may maintain illness. In a study of undergraduate roommate pairs, the roommates of women who endorsed higher bulimic symptoms reported lower intentions to continue living together [21]. Furthermore, carers of those with EDs tend to report high levels of psychological distress and burden [22]. Additional interpersonal problems that may be associated with EDs and affective dysfunction include, but are not limited to, social withdrawal [23, 24], perfectionism [25, 26], and interpersonal distrust [27–29].

There appears to be a bidirectional effect between interpersonal problems and ED behaviors, wherein the two may exacerbate each other, resulting in increased interpersonal dysfunction for the individual and a worsening of psychological symptoms [30, 31]. Higher levels of interpersonal problems at the onset of therapy have been associated with poorer recovery rates [32], underscoring the need to address these difficulties.

Emotion regulation difficulties in EDs

Research suggests that difficulties in emotion regulation (i.e., managing the onset, intensity, and duration of emotions) influence risk and maintenance of EDs [33, 34]. The habitual use of specific ER strategies, such as avoidance, rumination, and expressive suppression has been linked to increased ED severity, whereas the habitual use of reappraisal, problem-solving, and acceptance are associated with lower symptoms [35]. Importantly, emotional dysregulation in EDs may be both a risk and maintenance factor for eating pathology. For instance, emotion dysregulation in EDs may represent a global risk factor for psychopathology, a disorder-specific risk factor, or a combination of the two. In fact, some hypothesize that ED behaviors are secondary ER strategies that occur to manage negative affect states due to the lack of access to effective ER strategies and/or an overreliance on ineffective strategies [2, 3]. More research is needed to evaluate if emotion dysregulation in EDs is best characterized by global problems in managing affect, inappropriate ways of managing emotions (such as ED behaviors) generated by eating, shape, weight, or interpersonal stimuli, or an interaction between the two.

The literature on ER strategy usage in EDs has primarily focused on it from an *intra*personal perspective, examining how individuals with EDs manage their emotional experiences on their own (e.g., suppressing one's emotions when viewing a television program) and in *inter*personal contexts (e.g., suppressing one's facial expressions in front of a romantic partner). This approach is limited, as people frequently turn to others for assistance in managing their distress [4, 6, 7, 36, 37]. Although previous reviews have examined *intra*personal ER difficulties in EDs [2, 3, 38] and IER in healthy individuals [4, 37], there has yet to be a review that synthesizes the specific strategies that are used in interpersonally to effectively or ineffectively regulate emotions in people with EDs. Given the interpersonal and affective dysfunction associated with EDs, it is critical to construct and evaluate a comprehensive theory of IER (Fig. 1).

Process model of IER in ED populations

In this paper, we use the Process Model of Emotion Regulation [39] to describe IER in EDs. Although there are other frameworks that characterize emotion dysregulation [40], we chose the Process Model due to its large body of supporting research and use of specific strategies rather than domains of dysfunction (e.g., "lack of access to strategies"), permitting more nuanced examination of how these strategies may be used interpersonally.

According to the Process Model, ER strategies can be divided into: 1. Situation selection; 2. Situation modification; 3. Attentional deployment; 4. Cognitive change; and 5. Response modulation. Although these categories have primarily been examined as *intra*personal constructs, they can also be *inter*personal (Fig. 2). Further, as we have noted, these emotion regulation processes could directly involve ED-specific content and contexts, or could be more global in nature.

[1]In this review, we describe several interpersonal problems commonly endorsed by people with EDs to illustrate the importance of understanding interpersonal problems with this population; however, we note that this is not an exhaustive review of interpersonal problems in EDs.

	Global Intrapersonal ER	Global Interpersonal ER	ED-Specific Intrapersonal ER	ED-Specific Interpersonal ER
Situation Selection	Canceling plans to go to a restaurant to avoid being in a crowd	Selecting an uncrowded restaurant to go to with their parent	Canceling plans to go to a restaurant to avoid having to order unfamiliar food items	Selecting a restaurant for their parent that provides calorie estimates on the menu
Situation Modification	Staying in the periphery of the party to reduce anxiety about meeting new people	Going with a sibling to a party to reduce their anxiety about meeting new people	Placing food items out of view while eating	Dividing up food to make the portion appear smaller for a sibling
Attentional Deployment	Using one's phone to distract while encountering a feared object	Engaging in conversation to distract when one's partner is encountering a feared object	Using one's phone to distract while eating	Engaging in conversation to distract when one's partner is eating
Cognitive Change	Reframing thoughts about how an upcoming work presentation is an "opportunity" rather than a stressor	Helping a colleague to reframe thoughts about how an upcoming work presentation is an "opportunity" rather than a stressor	Reducing anxiety about "losing control" over eating by thinking about how one can purge afterwards	Providing a colleague with information about how a food item will not cause them to gain weight
Response Modulation	Taking a shot of alcohol to reduce distress	Offering a friend alcohol to reduce their distress	Exercising to reduce anxiety caused by unfamiliar food item	Exercising with a friend after a meal

Fig. 2 Extending the Process Model to conceptualize intrapersonal and interpersonal emotion regulation in EDs. Both intrapersonal and interpersonal ER can exist in global or ED-specific contexts

Given the wide range of potential IER behaviors, this review should not be considered exhaustive, but rather, a starting point for exploring this construct. Furthermore, strategies should not be assumed a priori to be adaptive or maladaptive; instead, context, such as personal goals, culture, demographics, and stage of recovery, guides if outcomes are adaptive (Fig. 1) [41]. We approach our model using a transdiagnostic framework, such that these processes may occur across both ED and non-ED diagnostic groups. IER has been theorized to explain emotional and interpersonal problems related to both depression [8, 9] and anxiety disorders [8], although it has yet to be applied to EDs. We believe that the IER framework, like that of intrapersonal emotion regulation describes processes that apply across all types of psychopathology; however, more research is necessary to determine if distinct strategies differentiate specific ED presentations, or ED presentations from other psychiatric concerns.

Situation selection

Situation selection refers to the ways in which individuals limit exposure to distress-eliciting stimuli. Viewed through an IER lens, situation selection could involve helping an individual avoid exposure to or removing someone from a situation that elicits an emotional response (Fig. 1a). The research on interpersonal facilitation of avoidance has primarily drawn from the literature on accommodation, which has been studied extensively in obsessive-compulsive disorder [42]. Through accommodation, the support system may maintain the illness by actively or passively allowing the person with an ED to engage in behaviors that do not promote recovery (e.g., avoiding challenging foods). In a systematic review, researchers found that accommodation of ED behaviors by caregivers was positively associated with duration of illness, suggesting the establishment of interpersonally-facilitated avoidance patterns over time [43]. Furthermore, in a study of parents of children with anorexia nervosa, accommodation had a dose-dependent effect, with poorest outcomes observed in children with two accommodating parents [44]. Overall, the research on accommodation suggests that avoidance may be an IER strategy adopted among carers of individuals with EDs that maintains illness. Other maladaptive interpersonal situation selection strategies, such as removing individuals from distress-eliciting situations, both global (e.g., school or work) and disorder-specific (e.g., going to a restaurant), have not yet been extensively investigated in EDs and warrant further research.

Situation modification

Situation modification consists of altering characteristics of an existing context in order to lower emotional response (Fig. 1b). For example, in a non-ED context, a support member could go with the person with an ED to a party, to reduce the anxiety brought up by a social situation. In a disorder-specific context, following ED rules can also be conceptualized as situation modification. Using situation modification as an IER strategy could consist of encouraging "safety" behaviors that maintain the ED (e.g., serving smaller portion sizes).

Evidence suggest that when these behaviors are undertaken, the motivation is not typically to promote the ED, but rather fear of an alliance rupture with the ill individual or to prevent more harmful behavior, such as purging or meal skipping [22].

Attentional deployment

Attentional deployment reflects how people direct attentional resources to modify the emotional impact of stimuli (Fig. 1c). Both distraction and rumination are considered to be forms of attentional deployment. The interpersonal use of distraction comprises of helping an individual to direct attention away from the stimuli towards other information, whereas interpersonal rumination is a cognitive process in which one directs the individual to focus on the causes or consequences of thoughts, feelings, or memories.

Distraction

There is little research that has examined the impact of other individuals providing distraction to those with EDs when they are experiencing negative affect; however, treatments such as dialectical-behavior therapy [45] and family-based therapy [46] suggest using this strategy to promote effective behavior (e.g., avoiding purging). Often distraction is employed in the context of the therapeutic meal; however, there is little research informing optimal strategies for meal support [47]. It is unclear whether distraction is a feasible long-term strategy or may slow food-related habituation. The employment of distraction as an IER strategy may require thoughtful consideration of the goals of usage (e.g., long-term reduction of fear vs. facilitating nutritional rehabilitation). It is probable that the utility of interpersonal distraction varies significantly by the context, such as weight status and stage of recovery. Distraction may also be used for affect that is not specifically related to the ED, such as distraction from other unpleasant emotions, such as anger at a colleague or anxiety related to a test.

Rumination

Individuals frequently engage in rumination in an attempt to exert control over emotional distress [48], although it tends to maintain negative affect [49]. Interpersonal use of rumination, also referred to as co-rumination may take two forms: mutual brooding (i.e., passively dwelling on the causes and consequences of an action) and mutual reflection (i.e., actively analyzing in order to problem-solve). Further, the content may take the form of general co-rumination (e.g., focusing on a personal problem) or ED-relevant co-rumination (e.g., engaging in "fat talk").

The general form of co-rumination has been linked to higher internalizing symptoms [50]. Although co-rumination has been associated with greater psychological difficulty concurrently and prospectively, there are no current studies examining general co-ruminative practices in individuals with EDs. Instead, the ED field has primarily focused on ED-relevant body-related co-rumination such as "fat talk", in which people interactively share and dwell on negative thoughts and feelings about their bodies [51]. Fat talk has been associated with a variety of negative consequences [52], including higher body dissatisfaction [53], negative affect [54, 55], depression [56, 57], and body checking [42], and lower self-esteem [57]. Fat talk can also be "contagious"; when people are exposed to someone engaging in fat talk, they are more likely to make disparaging comments about their own bodies and report higher negative affect and ED symptoms [43, 46, 47]. Taken together, research points to body-related co-rumination as a problematic interpersonal behavior that may amplify psychological symptoms, which makes it a promising target for intervention.

Cognitive change

Cognitive change strategies are those that are used to alter how individuals think about a situation, thereby changing its emotional impact (Fig. 1d). Interpersonal use of reappraisal and reassurance-seeking are two IER strategies that may be relevant to ED populations.

Reappraisal

Interpersonal reappraisal is a strategy whereby an individual helps another to change their cognitive interpretation of a situation to modulate affective response. Interpersonal reappraisal has been associated with better outcomes to acute stressors in a laboratory study [58]. Similarly, in young children, greater mother-child reappraisal was associated with better affective outcomes [59]. However, there is little other research examining reappraisal interpersonally; rather, previous studies have examined the broader construct of positive interpersonal behavior [60], which comprises a variety of domains including reappraisal, supportive listening, and validation.

There is no published research examining the use of reappraisal as a dyadic process in individuals with EDs. This is a significant knowledge gap, given that intrapersonal reappraisal is foundational to cognitive-behavioral approaches and therapists frequently employ thought challenging with their clients in therapy [61]. Understanding how supports or therapists can more effectively utilize reappraisal with the person with the ED when they are experiencing distress has great potential in improving treatment approaches.

Reassurance-seeking

Reassurance-seeking involves an individual repeatedly requesting information from others about a perceived threat in the environment [62]. Reassurance-seeking functions through negative reinforcement such that reassurance from others decreases anxiety and increases the likelihood of future reassurance-seeking. This behavior becomes problematic when the need for reassurance does not end when the feedback is provided; instead many individuals doubt the quality or genuineness of the provided reassurance and seek more reassurance, resulting in interpersonal strain and decreased quality of future feedback [63].

Reassurance-seeking has numerous negative emotional and interpersonal consequences. In one longitudinal study of female college students, reassurance-seeking predicted ED symptoms [64]. In another study of undergraduate students, reassurance-seeking mediated the relationship between bulimic symptoms and longitudinal interpersonal stress [21]. Finally, in a third study, those higher in reassurance seeking had a stronger positive relationship between social avoidance and ED psychopathology [57]. Of note, in these studies, reassurance-seeking was assessed by way of general tendencies to seek reassurance, rather than reassurance specifically related to ED concerns such as shape or weight. The negative interpersonal consequences of excessive reassurance-seeking may be particularly problematic for individuals with EDs, who report reduced social support [65–68].

Response modulation

Response modulation consists of strategies to alter the quality or intensity of an emotion after it has been initiated. Although there are many forms of response modulation, we have selected a couple strategies that may be of particular relevance to EDs (Fig. 1e).

Expressive suppression

Expressive suppression consists of masking facial displays of emotion. Much of the experimental and self-report research on expressive suppression has examined its use in non-social contexts (e.g., individuals suppressing facial expressions to emotion-eliciting videos). This does not capture the instances in which expressive suppression is undertaken to address perceived social concerns about the appropriateness of displaying emotions. Individuals with higher levels of ED symptoms endorse greater beliefs that emotional expression is undesirable and will lead to social rejection [69] and, consequently, are more likely to avoid expressing emotions [70]. Although it is likely that these messages have been reinforced in prior interpersonal relationships, to our knowledge there is no literature specifically examining expressive suppression as an IER strategy in EDs.

Eating disorder behaviors

Exploring how others may facilitate problematic eating patterns to regulate emotions is critical for understanding the development and maintenance of EDs. This type of behavior may begin in childhood and have consequences into adolescence and adulthood. Emotional feeding, or hedonic feeding by a caregiver to soothe negative emotions, has been associated with greater emotional eating in children [71, 72] and adolescents [73] and may continue into adulthood [74, 75]. Given that emotional eating is a risk factor for binge eating [18, 76], this IER strategy is of concern.

Although less frequently studied, exercise may also be utilized for ER to reduce negative affect and increase positive affect [77]. There is no research directly examining the link between encouraging exercise for others as an ER strategy and ED outcomes. Instead, the literature primarily focuses on facilitating exercise as a health behavior promoting physical wellness [78]; however, this represents an area warranting further research.

Discussion

There is a solid foundation to support the utility of further investigating IER in EDs; however, there are many areas where the knowledge base could be expanded. One of the primary questions that exists regarding IER in EDs is whether IER problems represent a global vulnerability to psychopathology, a disorder-specific risk factor, or an interaction between the two. Furthermore, it is unknown how IER may be shaped by the experience of EDs; for instance, if certain IER patterns develop as a result of experiencing the disorder (e.g., people engaging in fat talk then begin using more reassurance-seeking in non-ED domains). Overall, better characterizing how IER contributes to the development and maintenance of EDs could lead to improvements in our theoretical models and psychological treatments. Below we outline several research areas that would enhance the knowledge of IER processes in EDs.

Definition

Refining the definitions of IER processes is essential to providing a solid foundation for this research. Although the Process Model provides a starting place for conceptualizing IER processes, it was created as a framework for *intra*personal, not *inter*personal ER. The degree to which intrapersonal and interpersonal ER strategies align remains unknown. Therefore, more research is needed to identify the various ways in which social environments contribute to the regulation of emotions. An initial step involves qualitative and quantitative studies of the different ways that people with EDs and their social supports engage in IER. In this line of research, it would be important to differentiate strategies using to regulate general vs. ED-specific distress. It is possible that ED-specific forms of IER may exert differential (perhaps stronger) effects on affect and well-being for individuals with EDs. Alternately, ED-related IER may simply reflect broader underlying dysfunction. Future research is needed to delineate general and ED-specific IER strategies, how they interact, and how each influence ED symptoms.

Assessment

The next step in IER research involves refining assessment measures and techniques. There are existing questionnaires to examine general patterns of IER, such as the Interpersonal Emotion Regulation Questionnaire by Williams and colleagues [5] and the Interpersonal Emotion Regulation Questionnaire by Hofmann and colleagues [79], which provide information about the frequency and utility of IER, but do not provide information about the use of specific strategies. Other measures that capture IER constructs, such as the Accommodation and Enabling Scale for Eating Disorders [80], were not created for the evaluation of IER and therefore, their psychometric properties have not been assessed with these constructs in mind. Thus, there is a need to refine or develop questionnaire measures for assessing general and ED-related IER.

There also is a need to assess IER through naturalistic and experimental designs in order to circumvent memory biases inherent in self-report. Ecological momentary assessment could allow examination of IER strategies in real-time, reducing retrospective bias and permitting investigations of temporal relations between IER, and affective and behavioral outcomes. Observational studies examining how dyads interact when the individual with the ED is upset could also determine the interaction patterns associated with improved or worsening affective and behavioral responses. Examining both short- and long-term outcomes is critical, as changes in short-term affect or behavior may not map onto long-term outcomes. For instance, it may be useful to examine whether certain IER strategies (e.g., accommodating an individual's ED rule at meals) may reduce short-term negative affect, but ultimately maintain symptoms.

Context

Context is another important consideration when evaluating IER. There are a variety of factors that may influence the adaptiveness of deploying certain ER strategies [41, 81, 82], including demographics (e.g., race, gender), goals, and setting. Although meta-analyses have found that the habitual intrapersonal uses of certain strategies have positive or negative associations with psychopathology [35], not every "adaptive" strategy is appropriate in every situation and similarly, not every "maladaptive" strategy will have negative consequences [83]. Consequently, it is overly simplistic to categorize strategies as strictly adaptive or maladaptive and a thorough review of contexts and desired outcomes is necessary.

Demographic factors and culture are important contextual variables to consider when evaluating adaptation. For instance, there may be differences in the effectiveness of IER strategies when the person with an ED is a child compared to an adult and depending on the type of relationship between the dyad (e.g., parent-child, romantic partners, colleagues, acquaintances). Individual differences related to the person providing regulation may also drive the success of IER. For instance, it is possible that individuals high in expressed emotion (i.e., high in criticism, low in warmth, high in overinvolvement) may provide less effective or helpful IER to others; similarly, those low in empathy or theory of mind may be limited in their ability to recognize needs for IER and successfully execute these interpersonal behaviors. Similarly, these characteristics may alter the probability that the person with the ED solicits IER from certain individuals.

The appropriateness of IER may also vary across ED subtype and recovery status (e.g., actively ill versus remitted). For example, it is possible that IER strategies of facilitating distraction and avoidance (e.g., of feared foods) may be appropriate during nutritional rehabilitation, but function as safety behaviors once someone is in weight maintenance. Further, cultural norms may affect the consequences of different IER strategies. For example, previous research has shown that the use of intrapersonal expressive suppression is less detrimental to individuals in collectivist cultures versus more individualistic cultures [84, 85]. Future study should take these factors into account when evaluating the purpose and utility of different IER strategies.

Clinical implications

Ultimately, additional understanding of IER can have a significant impact on clinical interventions. There are many unanswered questions about the most effective ways for people to support the affected person in managing emotions with the goal of ED recovery, such as which strategies must be disrupted to reduce ED behaviors and how the supportive person can best intervene when problematic IER is occurring. This is of particular relevance to treatments such as, but not limited to, family-based therapy [46], Maudsley Model of Anorexia Nervosa Treatment for Adults (MANTRA) [86], and Uniting Couples in the treatment of Anorexia Nervosa [87–89], which utilize the relationship between the recovering individual and their caregivers, family members, or other supports to facilitate recovery. In addition, treatments utilizing the cognitive interpersonal model of anorexia nervosa have shown success targeting problematic caregiver behaviors, such as accommodation [90]. Although these treatments leverage IER processes to achieve symptom improvements, for instance by reducing accommodation or using distraction to facilitate re-feeding, they have not been systematically evaluated using this framework. Furthermore, other eating disorders treatments incorporate aspects of emotion regulation and/or interpersonal relationships, such as dialectical behavior therapy (e.g., distress tolerance, emotion regulation, and interpersonal effectiveness modules) [45] and interpersonal psychotherapy for eating disorders [91], but do not specifically look at the interactions between these constructs. Consequently, the theoretical model of IER could help treatment developers perform process and dismantling studies assessing if these treatments are correctly identifying and modifying problematic IER behaviors that may be maintaining illness. Further, this theoretical model will inform the development and/or refinement of new treatments or modules to reduce problematic IER behaviors and ruptures in relationships.

This is important as the quality of interpersonal interactions may affect outcomes for people with EDs. In one qualitative study, women recovered from AN emphasized the importance of positive support and a non-judgmental attitude from health providers and support systems [92]. Further, given that therapy relationships are typically dyadic and interactional, increased understanding of IER processes and how they impact emotional and behavioral responses could be helpful in determining helpful therapist behaviors. For the individual, a focus on IER processes may help them to more effectively utilize their support systems, thereby enhancing effective ER and reducing interpersonal difficulties.

Conclusion

Investigation of IER in EDs may yield insights into the ways in which interpersonal relationships influence how emotions are managed by individuals with EDs, and how different strategies perpetuate ED symptoms. IER represents a novel interdisciplinary field that can elucidate the unique role that other people play in guiding people with EDs through emotional distress. Ultimately, IER research holds promise to guide treatment recommendations, reduce distress and interpersonal problems in those with EDs, and empower support members to more effectively assist individuals with an ED through distress.

Abbreviations

EDs: Eating disorders; ER: Emotion regulation; IER: Interpersonal emotion regulation

Acknowledgements

Not applicable.

Authors' contributions

KAC and AFH conceptualized the paper. KAC drafted the manuscript and AFH contributed to and approved the final manuscript. The author(s) read and approved the final manuscript.

Competing interests

The authors declare that they have no competing interests.

Author details

[1]Department of Psychology, University of Kansas, 1415 Jayhawk Blvd Rm 440, Lawrence, KS 66045, USA. [2]Department of Psychiatry and Behavioral Sciences, University of Minnesota, 2450 Riverside Ave, F253, Minneapolis, MN 55454, USA.

References

1. Arcelus J, Haslam M, Farrow C, Meyer C. The role of interpersonal functioning in the maintenance of eating psychopathology: a systematic review and testable model. Clin Psychol Rev. 2013;33(1):156–67.
2. Haynos AF, Fruzzetti AE. Anorexia nervosa as a disorder of emotion Dysregulation: evidence and treatment implications. Clin Psychol Sci Pract. 2011;18(3):183–202.
3. Lavender JM, Wonderlich SA, Engel SG, Gordon KH, Kaye WH, Mitchell JE. Dimensions of emotion dysregulation in anorexia nervosa and bulimia nervosa: A conceptual review of the empirical literature. Clin Psychol Rev. 2015;40(Supplement C):111–22.
4. Zaki J, Williams WC. Interpersonal emotion regulation. Emotion. 2013;13(5): 803–10.
5. Williams WC, Morelli SA, Ong DC, Zaki J. Interpersonal emotion regulation: implications for affiliation, perceived support, relationships, and well-being. J Pers Soc Psychol. 2018;115(2):224–54.
6. Dixon-Gordon K, Bernecker S, Christensen KA. Recent innovations in the field of interpersonal emotion regulation. Curr Opin Psychol. 2015;3:36–42.
7. Rimé B. Interpersonal emotion regulation. In: Gross J, editor. Handbook of Emotion Regulation. New York: Guilford Press; 2009. p. 466–485.
8. Hofmann SG. Interpersonal emotion regulation model of mood and anxiety disorders. Cogn Ther Res. 2014;38(5):483–92.
9. Marroquín B. Interpersonal emotion regulation as a mechanism of social support in depression. Clin Psychol Rev. 2011;31(8):1276–90.
10. Bretherton I. The origins of attachment theory: John Bowlby and Mary Ainsworth. Dev Psychol. 1992;28(5):759.
11. Cassidy J, Shaver PR. Handbook of attachment: theory, research, and clinical applications. Rough Guides; 2002.
12. Sullivan HS. Interpersonal theory of personality. NY Nort 1953;.
13. Fairbairn WRD. An object-relations theory of the personality. Oxford, England: Basic Books; 1954. xi, 312. (An object-relations theory of the personality).
14. Treasure J, Schmidt U. The cognitive-interpersonal maintenance model of anorexia nervosa revisited: a summary of the evidence for cognitive, socio-emotional and interpersonal predisposing and perpetuating factors. J Eat Disord. 2013;1(1):13.
15. Treasure J, Willmott D, Ambwani S, Cardi V, Clark Bryan D, Rowlands K, et al. Cognitive interpersonal model for anorexia nervosa revisited: the perpetuating factors that contribute to the development of the severe and enduring illness. J Clin Med. 2020;9(3):630.
16. Hartmann A, Zeeck A, Barrett MS. Interpersonal problems in eating disorders. Int J Eat Disord. 2010;43(7):619–27.
17. Tchanturia K, Davies H, Harrison A, Fox JRE, Treasure J, Schmidt U. Altered social hedonic processing in eating disorders. Int J Eat Disord. 2012;45(8): 962–9.
18. Stice E, Presnell K, Spangler D. Risk factors for binge eating onset in adolescent girls: a 2-year prospective investigation. Health Psychol. 2002; 21(2):131–8.
19. Bodell LP, Smith AR, Holm-Denoma JM, Gordon KH, Joiner TE. The impact of perceived social support and negative life events on bulimic symptoms. Eat Behav. 2011;12(1):44–8.
20. Stice E. Risk and maintenance factors for eating pathology: a meta-analytic review. Psychol Bull. 2002;128(5):825–48.
21. Kwan MY, Minnich AM, Douglas V, Gordon KH, Castro Y. Bulimic symptoms and interpersonal functioning among college students. Psychiatry Res. 2017; 257:406–11.

22. Treasure J, Todd G. Interpersonal maintaining factors in eating disorder: skill sharing interventions for Carers. In: Latzer Y, stein D, editors. Bio-psycho-social contributions to understanding eating disorders. Cham: springer international publishing; 2016 [cited 2018 Sep 6]. p. 125–37. Available from: https://doi.org/10.1007/978-3-319-32742-6_9.
23. Rotenberg KJ, Bharathi C, Davies H, Finch T. Bulimic symptoms and the social withdrawal syndrome. Eat Behav. 2013;14(3):281–4.
24. Basile B. Self-disclosure in eating disorders. Eat Weight Disord - Stud Anorex Bulim Obes. 2004;9(3):217–223.
25. Bardone-Cone AM, Wonderlich SA, Frost RO, Bulik CM, Mitchell JE, Uppala S, et al. Perfectionism and eating disorders: current status and future directions. Clin Psychol Rev. 2007;27(3):384–405.
26. Dahlenburg SC, Gleaves DH, Hutchinson AD. Anorexia nervosa and perfectionism: a meta-analysis. Int J Eat Disord. 2019;52(3):219–29.
27. Olatunji BO, Levinson C, Calebs B. A network analysis of eating disorder symptoms and characteristics in an inpatient sample. Psychiatry Res. 2018; 262:270–81.
28. Solmi M, Collantoni E, Meneguzzo P, Degortes D, Tenconi E, Favaro A. Network analysis of specific psychopathology and psychiatric symptoms in patients with eating disorders. Int J Eat Disord. 2018;51(7):680–92.
29. Dingemans AE, Son GE Van, Aardoom JJ, Bruidegom K, Landt MCTS-O 't, Furth EF van. Predictors of psychological outcome in patients with eating disorders: a routine outcome monitoring study. Int J Eat Disord 2016;49(9): 863–873.
30. Rieger E, Van Buren DJ, Bishop M, Tanofsky-Kraff M, Welch R, Wilfley DE. An eating disorder-specific model of interpersonal psychotherapy (IPT-ED): causal pathways and treatment implications. Clin Psychol Rev. 2010;30(4): 400–10.
31. Treasure J, Corfield F, Cardi V. A three-phase model of the social emotional functioning in eating disorders. Eur Eat Disord Rev. 2012;20(6):431–8.
32. Jones A, Lindekilde N, Lübeck M, Clausen L. The association between interpersonal problems and treatment outcome in the eating disorders: a systematic review. Nord J Psychiatry. 2015;69(8):563–73.
33. Brockmeyer T, Skunde M, Wu M, Bresslein E, Rudofsky G, Herzog W, et al. Difficulties in emotion regulation across the spectrum of eating disorders. Compr Psychiatry. 2014;55(3):565–71.
34. Svaldi J, Griepenstroh J, Tuschen-Caffier B, Ehring T. Emotion regulation deficits in eating disorders: a marker of eating pathology or general psychopathology? Psychiatry Res. 2012;197(1–2):103–11.
35. Aldao A, Nolen-Hoeksema S, Schweizer S. Emotion-regulation strategies across psychopathology: a meta-analytic review. Clin Psychol Rev. 2010; 30(2):217–37.
36. Cole PM, Martin SE, Dennis TA. Emotion regulation as a scientific construct: methodological challenges and directions for child development research. Child Dev. 2004;75(2):317–33.
37. Grecucci A, Theuninck A, Frederickson J, Job R. Mechanisms of social emotion regulation: From neuroscience to psychotherapy. In: Emotion Regulation: Processes, Cognitive Effects, and Social Consequences. 1st ed. Nova Publishers; 2015.
38. Leehr EJ, Krohmer K, Schag K, Dresler T, Zipfel S, Giel KE. Emotion regulation model in binge eating disorder and obesity - a systematic review. Neurosci Biobehav Rev. 2015;49:125–34.
39. Gross JJ. The emerging field of emotion regulation: an integrative review. Rev Gen Psychol. 1998;2(3):271–99.
40. Gratz KL, Roemer L. Multidimensional assessment of emotion regulation and Dysregulation: development, factor structure, and initial validation of the difficulties in emotion regulation scale. J Psychopathol Behav Assess. 2004; 26(1):41–54.
41. Aldao A. The future of emotion regulation research capturing context. Perspect Psychol Sci. 2013;8(2):155–72.
42. Lebowitz ER, Panza KE, Su J, Bloch MH. Family accommodation in obsessive–compulsive disorder. Expert Rev Neurother. 2012;12(2):229–38.
43. Anastasiadou D, Medina-Pradas C, Sepulveda AR, Treasure J. A systematic review of family caregiving in eating disorders. Eat Behav. 2014;15(3):464–77.
44. Salerno L, Rhind C, Hibbs R, Micali N, Schmidt U, Gowers S, et al. An examination of the impact of care giving styles (accommodation and skilful communication and support) on the one year outcome of adolescent anorexia nervosa: testing the assumptions of the cognitive interpersonal model in anorexia nervosa. J Affect Disord. 2016;191: 230–6.
45. Chen EY, Linehan MM. Dialectical behavior therapy and eating disorders. In: Freeman A, Felgoise S, Nezu A, Nezu C, Reinecke M, editors. Encyclopedia of Cognitive Behavior Therapy. Plenum US; 2005.
46. Lock J, le Grange D. Family-based treatment of eating disorders. Int J Eat Disord. 2005;37(S1):S64–7.
47. Hage TW, Rø Ø, Moen A. To bend or not to bend? Rule adherence among staff at an eating disorder unit. Eat Disord. 2017;25(2):134–50.
48. Nolen-Hoeksema S, Wisco BE, Lyubomirsky S. Rethinking rumination. Perspect Psychol Sci. 2008;3(5):400–24.
49. Webb TL, Miles E, Sheeran P. Dealing with feeling: a meta-analysis of the effectiveness of strategies derived from the process model of emotion regulation. Psychol Bull. 2012;138(4):775–808.
50. Spendelow JS, Simonds LM, Avery RE. The relationship between co-rumination and internalizing problems: a systematic review and meta-analysis. Clin Psychol Psychother. 2017;24(2):512–27.
51. Nichter M, Vuckovic N. Fat Talk: Body Image among Adolescent Girls. Many Mirrors Body Image Soc Relat. 1994 [cited 2018 Dec 20]; Available from: https://arizona.pure.elsevier.com/en/publications/fat-talk-body-image-among-adolescent-girls.
52. Shannon A, Mills JS. Correlates, causes, and consequences of fat talk: a review. Body Image. 2015;15:158–72.
53. Sharpe H, Naumann U, Treasure J, Schmidt U. Is fat talking a causal risk factor for body dissatisfaction? A systematic review and meta-analysis. Int J Eat Disord. 2013;46(7):643–52.
54. Jones MD, Crowther JH, Ciesla JA. A naturalistic study of fat talk and its behavioral and affective consequences. Body Image. 2014;11(4):337–45.
55. Salk RH, Engeln-Maddox R. Fat talk among college women is both contagious and harmful. Sex Roles. 2012;66(9):636–45.
56. Arroyo A, Harwood J. Exploring the causes and consequences of engaging in fat talk. J Appl Commun Res. 2012;40(2):167–87.
57. Rudiger JA, Winstead BA. Body talk and body-related co-rumination: associations with body image, eating attitudes, and psychological adjustment. Body Image. 2013;10(4):462–71.
58. Lepore SJ, Fernandez-Berrocal P, Ragan J, Ramos N. It's not that bad: social challenges to emotional disclosure enhance adjustment to stress. Anxiety Stress Coping. 2004;17(4):341–61.
59. Morris AS, Silk JS, Morris MDS, Steinberg L, Aucoin KJ, Keyes AW. The influence of mother–child emotion regulation strategies on children's expression of anger and sadness. Dev Psychol. 2011;47(1):213–25.
60. Vater A, Schröder-Abe M. Explaining the link between personality and relationship satisfaction: emotion regulation and interpersonal behaviour in conflict discussions. Eur J Personal. 2015;29(2):201–15.
61. Beck AT, Rush AJ, Shaw BF, Emery G. Cognitive therapy of depression. New York: Guilford Press; 1979.
62. Joiner TE, Metalsky GI, Katz J, Beach SRH. Depression and excessive reassurance-seeking. Psychol Inq. 1999;10(3):269–78.
63. Parrish C, Radomsky A. An experimental investigation of factors involved in excessive reassurance seeking: the effects of perceived threat, responsibility and ambiguity on compulsive urges and anxiety. J Exp Psychopathol. 2011; 2(1):44–62.
64. Cooley E, Toray T, Valdez N, Tee M. Risk factors for maladaptive eating patterns in college women. Eat Weight Disord - Stud Anorex Bulim Obes. 2013;12(3):132–9.
65. Levine MP. Loneliness and eating disorders. J Psychol. 2012;146(1–2):243–57.
66. Grisset N, Norvell N. Perceived social support, social skills, and quality of relationships in bulimic women. J Consult Clin Psychol. 1992;60(2):293–9.
67. Rorty M, Yager J, Buckwalter JG, Rossotto E. Social support, social adjustment, and recovery status in bulimia nervosa. Int J Eat Disord. 1999; 26(1):1–12.
68. Tiller JM, Sloane G, Schmidt U, Troop N, Power M, Treasure JL. Social support in patients with anorexia nervosa and bulimia nervosa. Int J Eat Disord. 1997;21(1):31–8.
69. Geller J, Cockell SJ, Hewitt PL, Goldner EM, Flett GL. Inhibited expression of negative emotions and interpersonal orientation in anorexia nervosa. Int J Eat Disord. 2000;28(1):8–19.
70. Caglar-Nazali HP, Corfield F, Cardi V, Ambwani S, Leppanen J, Olabintan O, et al. A systematic review and meta-analysis of 'Systems for Social Processes' in eating disorders. Neurosci Biobehav Rev. 2014;42:55–92.
71. Braden A, Rhee K, Peterson CB, Rydell SA, Zucker N, Boutelle K. Associations between child emotional eating and general parenting style, feeding practices, and parent psychopathology. Appetite. 2014;80:35–40.

72. Rodgers RF, Paxton SJ, Massey R, Campbell KJ, Wertheim EH, Skouteris H, et al. Maternal feeding practices predict weight gain and obesogenic eating behaviors in young children: a prospective study. Int J Behav Nutr Phys Act. 2013;10(1):24.
73. Goldstein M, Tan CC, Chow CM. Maternal emotional feeding practices and adolescent daughters' emotional eating: mediating roles of avoidant and preoccupied coping. Appetite. 2017;116:339–44.
74. Hamburg ME, Finkenauer C, Schuengel C. Food for love: the role of food offering in empathic emotion regulation. Front Psychol. 2014 [cited 2018 Oct 25];5. Available from: https://www.frontiersin.org/articles/10.3389/fpsyg.2014.00032/full.
75. Christensen KA. Emotional feeding as interpersonal emotion regulation: a developmental risk factor for binge-eating behaviors. Int J Eat Disord. 2019; 52(5):515–9.
76. Allen KL, Byrne SM, La Puma M, McLean N, Davis EA. The onset and course of binge eating in 8- to 13-year-old healthy weight, overweight and obese children. Eat Behav. 2008;9(4):438–46.
77. Aldao A, Dixon-Gordon KL. Broadening the scope of research on emotion regulation strategies and psychopathology. Cogn Behav Ther. 2014;43(1):22–33.
78. Umberson D. Gender, marital status and the social control of health behavior. Soc Sci Med. 1992;34(8):907–17.
79. Hofmann SG, Carpenter JK, Curtiss J. Interpersonal emotion regulation questionnaire (IERQ): scale development and psychometric characteristics. Cogn Ther Res. 2016;30:1–16.
80. Sepulveda AR, Kyriacou O, Treasure J. Development and validation of the accommodation and enabling scale for eating disorders (AESED) for caregivers in eating disorders. BMC Health Serv Res. 2009;9(1):171.
81. Aldao A, Christensen KA. Linking the expanded process model of emotion regulation to psychopathology by focusing on behavioral outcomes of regulation. Psychol Inq. 2015;26(1):27–36.
82. Christensen KA, Aldao A. Tipping points for adapation: connecting emotion regulation, motivated behavior, and psychopathology. Curr Opin Psychol. 2015;3:70–4.
83. Troy AS, Shallcross AJ, Mauss IB. A person-by-situation approach to emotion regulation cognitive reappraisal can either help or hurt, Depending on the Context. Psychol Sci. 2013;24(12):2505–14.
84. Soto JA, Perez CR, Kim Y-H, Lee EA, Minnick MR. Is expressive suppression always associated with poorer psychological functioning? A cross-cultural comparison between European Americans and Hong Kong Chinese. Emotion. 2011;11(6):1450.
85. Su JC, Lee RM, Oishi S. The role of culture and self-construal in the link between expressive suppression and depressive symptoms. J Cross-Cult Psychol. 2013;44(2):316–31.
86. Schmidt U, Wade TD, Treasure J. The Maudsley model of anorexia nervosa treatment for adults (MANTRA): development, key features, and preliminary evidence. J Cogn Psychother. 2014;28(1):48–71.
87. Kirby JS, Runfola CD, Fischer MS, Baucom DH, Bulik CM. Couple-based interventions for adults with eating disorders. Eat Disord. 2015;23(4):356–65.
88. Runfola CD, Kirby JS, Baucom DH, Fischer MS, Baucom BRW, Matherne CE, et al. A pilot open trial of UNITE-BED: A couple-based intervention for binge-eating disorder. Int J Eat Disord. [cited 2018 Sep 12];0(0). Available from: https://onlinelibrary.wiley.com/doi/abs/10.1002/eat.22919.
89. Baucom DH, Kirby JS, Fischer MS, Baucom BR, Hamer R, Bulik CM. Findings from a couple-based open trial for adult anorexia nervosa. J Fam Psychol. 2017;31(5):584–91.
90. Goddard E, Macdonald P, Sepulveda AR, Naumann U, Landau S, Schmidt U, et al. Cognitive interpersonal maintenance model of eating disorders: intervention for carers. Br J Psychiatry. 2011;199(3):225–31.
91. Brownell KD, Fairburn CG. Eating Disorders and Obesity: A Comprehensive Handbook. Third Edition. New York: Guildford Press; 2002.
92. Linville D, Brown T, Sturm K, McDougal T. Eating disorders and social support: perspectives of recovered individuals. Eat Disord. 2012;20(3):216–31.

2

Eating disorders among patients with borderline personality disorder: understanding the prevalence and psychopathology

Mohsen Khosravi

Abstract

Background: Treatment protocols can be bolstered and etiological and maintenance factors can be recognized more easily by a superior understanding of emotions and emotion regulation in the comorbidity of borderline personality disorder (BPD) and feeding and eating disorders (FEDs). Therefore, the present study aimed at investigating the prevalence and psychopathology of FEDs in patients with BPD.

Methods: In this cross-sectional study, 220 participants were examined in three groups, namely BPD ($n = 38$), BPD + FEDs ($n = 72$), and healthy controls ($n = 110$), from August 2018 to November 2019. The participants were selected by systematic random sampling among the patients who referred to Baharan psychiatric hospital in Zahedan, Iran, with the sampling interval of 3. The subjects were evaluated by 28-item General Health Questionnaire (GHQ-28), Borderline Personality Inventory (BPI), Structured Clinical Interview for DSM-5 Personality Disorders (SCID-5-PD), Structured Clinical Interviews for DSM-5: Research Version (SCID-5-RV), the 26-item Eating Attitudes Test (EAT-26), 20-item Toronto Alexithymia Scale (TAS-20), Beck Anxiety Inventory (BAI), and Beck Depression Inventory-II (BDI-II).

Results: The results showed a 65.4% ($n = 72$) prevalence of FEDs in patients with BPD. Also, the highest and lowest prevalence rates were reported for other specified feeding and eating disorders (51.3%) and bulimia nervosa (6.9%), respectively. Although the highest mean score of TAS-20 was related to anorexia nervosa, there was no significant difference between the scores of various types of FEDs. The mediation analysis showed that anxiety and depression would play a mediating role in the relationship between alexithymia and eating-disordered behaviors.

Conclusions: The results have suggested that alexithymia, anxiety, and depression should receive clinical attention as potential therapeutic targets in the comorbidity of BPD and FEDs. The clinical implications of the research have been conducted to date, and directions for future research have been discussed.

Keywords: Alexithymia, Anxiety, Borderline personality disorder, Depression, Feeding and eating disorders, Psychopathology

Correspondence: dr_khosravi2016@yahoo.com
Department of Psychiatry and Clinical Psychology, Baharan Psychiatric Hospital, Zahedan University of Medical Sciences, Zahedan 9813913777, Iran

Plain English summary

Feeding and eating disorders (FEDs) and borderline personality disorder (BPD) are relatively common psychiatric problems amongst populations. Many people suffering from these disorders also have difficulties dealing with their emotions: they struggle to recognize and talk about their emotions (a psychological characteristic called "alexithymia") and regulate their emotions appropriately. Common comorbidity and shared psychopathology in BPD and FEDs conceptualize the relationship between eating-disordered behaviors, alexithymia, depression, and anxiety. An improved understanding of the role of emotions in the comorbidity of BPD and FEDs can help screening, enhance treatment protocols, and provide a better understanding of the etiological and maintenance factors involved in this comorbidity. Accordingly, it seems necessary to investigate the relationship between alexithymia, anxiety, depression, and eating-disordered behaviors in more detail. Therefore, the present study aimed at investigating the prevalence and psychopathology of FEDs in patients with BPD.

Background

Borderline personality disorder (BPD) is a chronic and disabling disorder, imposing many costs on societies through severe functional impairments, high risk of suicide, negative effect on the course of depressive disorders, and extensive use of treatments [1]. Clinical experience suggests that disordered-eating behavior and actual feeding and eating disorders (FEDs) are relatively common among patients with BPD such that the rate of this comorbidity has been reported at 14–53% in different studies [2–4]. Thus, this question is raised: "Is this high comorbidity an indicator of a partially causal relationship?" [5].

Despite expanded studies, the question is still unanswered [2]. In 2001, Dolan et al. [6] proposed a useful framework for developing different theoretical models to investigate the comorbidity of psychiatric disorders. For instance, the spectrum/subclinical model supposed that BPD and FEDs are similar concerning etiologies and action mechanisms [2, 6]. Based on this assumption, it can be inferred that the use of emotion regulation strategies, including rumination, suppression, and avoidance by BPD and FEDs patients, may highlight the important role of emotion regulation (as a transdiagnostic construct) in the evolution of these disorders [7].

In this respect, researchers have indicated that alexithymia (i.e., inability to recognize and express the emotions) can be involved in many types of psychopathologies, such as BPD and FEDs, by preventing the regulation of negative emotions [8, 9]. For example, Zlotnick et al. [10] and Wolff et al. [11] indicated that patients with BPD could not usually recognize emotions and their causes. Moreover, Nowakowski et al. [12] demonstrated that individuals with FEDs consistently reported higher levels of alexithymia on the 20-item Toronto Alexithymia Scale (TAS-20) compared to healthy controls. Accordingly, they suggested that patients used eating-disordered behaviors to control their emotional state.

Although there is evidence for the alexithymia effect on emotion regulation, little information has been obtained about this process so far [13]. Nevertheless, recent studies have suggested that unawareness of emotions results in the inability to regulate emotions successfully and, in turn, autonomic arousal is chronically increased [14]. Pandey and Mandal [15] suggested that the relationship between alexithymia and overestimated perceived arousal is due to the association of alexithymia with anxiety. Later, following the introduction of these issues, several authors considered alexithymia a personality trait that can give rise to anxiety and depression by causing problems in the management of emotions, anxiety, and depression [16]. Furthermore, the results of several studies suggested that, compared with the normal population, both anxiety and depression are significantly more prevalent among patients with comorbidity of BPD and FEDs, which can be mainly attributed to high levels of alexithymia in these patients [12, 13, 16]. In this regard, alexithymia could enhance anxiety and depression due to low self-esteem and insecurity. These secondary emotions increase the patients' distress and reduce their coping abilities, thereby leading to engagement in eating-disordered behaviors (e.g., bingeing, purging, and dietary restriction) in an effort to avoid or cope with the emotions [12, 16, 17].

Thus, given that FEDs is a subtype of emotional disorders, deficits in emotional processing observed in FEDs should be fully mediated by anxiety and depression. In other words, if FEDs do not constitute a distinct pathology from emotional disturbances, only anxiety and depression must mediate the relationship between alexithymia and eating-disordered behaviors [18, 19]. Consistent with the complete mediation hypothesis, Eizaguirre et al. [16] revealed that anxiety and depression can mediate the relationship between alexithymia and eating-disordered behaviors.

Moreover, an improved understanding of the role of emotions in the comorbidity of BPD and FEDs can help screening, enhance treatment protocols, and provide a better understanding of the involved etiological and maintenance factors. Therefore, it seems necessary to investigate the relationship between alexithymia, anxiety, depression, and eating-disordered behaviors in further detail. For this purpose, the present research pursues three goals, including (1) comparing the mean scores of Beck Anxiety Inventory (BAI), Beck Depression Inventory-II (BDI-II), TAS-20, the 26-item Eating

Attitudes Test (EAT-26), and 28-item General Health Questionnaire (GHQ-28) for the three study groups (including BPD, BPD + FEDs, and healthy controls); (2) comparing the mean scores of TAS-20 in terms of different FEDs subtypes in BPD + FEDs patients; (3) investigating the mediating role of anxiety and depression in the relationship between alexithymia and eating-disordered behaviors in both BPD only and BPD + FEDs groups.

Methods

Participants

This cross-sectional study was performed from August 2018 to November 2019. In this study, 110 patients with BPD and 110 healthy people were selected. The sample size was calculated based on the study performed by Eizaguirre et al. [16]. Power calculations for 80% power to detect and effect size of r = 0.3 at alpha = 0.5 yielded a necessary sample of $N = 220$ [20]. The patients with BPD were selected by systematic random sampling among the persons who referred to Baharan psychiatric hospital in Zahedan, Iran, with the sampling interval of 3. Also, the healthy people were selected out of their relatives through one-to-n matching (i.e., one case dedicated to one control). The inclusion criteria were as follows: (1) getting a score above 10 in Borderline Personality Inventory (BPI) and approved diagnosis of the disorder based on Structured Clinical Interview for DSM-5 Personality Disorders (SCID-5-PD) by a psychiatrist; (2) age range of 18–35 years; (3) ability to read and write alongside reading comprehension; (4) for healthy people, getting a score of <21 in GHQ-28 and approved mental health based on Structured Clinical Interviews for DSM-5: Research Version (SCID-5-RV) and SCID-5-PD by the psychiatrist. The exclusion criteria included the followings: (1) severe and acute physical illness; (2) brain traumatic injury; (3) comorbidity of schizophrenia and other psychotic disorders; (4) epileptic disorder; (5) intellectual disability; (6) mixed personality disorder; (7) taking any drug or substance that causes anorexia and bulimia; (8) failing to fill the questionnaires properly.

In this study, 220 participants were evaluated in three groups, namely BPD ($n = 38$), BPD + FEDs ($n = 72$), and healthy controls ($n = 110$). Table 1 presents the participants' sociodemographic information. According to the table, there was no significant difference in sociodemographic factors between the study groups.

Procedures

After the approval of the research project by the ethics committee of the Medical Faculty of the Zahedan University of Medical Sciences (IR.ZAUMS.REC.1398.212), the informed consent forms were distributed among the participants. In order to follow the Declaration of Helsinki, participation in the study was optional, and the participants could leave the study for any reason. After obtaining informed consent from the participants, GHQ-28, EAT-26, TAS-20, BAI, and BDI-II were distributed among them. Next, the psychiatrist evaluated all of the participants using SCID-5-PD and SCID-5-RV to identify the three study groups (including BPD, BPD + FEDs, and healthy controls). The questionnaires were anonymous to keep the participants' information private.

Measures

The following measures were used in this study (in general, the Cronbach's alpha values of 0.70 or higher indicate acceptable internal consistency) [21]:

TAS-20

Alexithymia was assessed with the Persian version of the TAS-20, a 20-item self-report questionnaire scored based on a five-point (1–5) Likert scale. The minimum and maximum scores are 20 and 100, respectively, and scores of ≥61 represent alexithymia [22]. In this study, the Cronbach's alpha coefficients for the TAS-20 subscales of difficulty identifying feelings, difficulty describing feelings, and externally oriented thinking were 0.85, 0.82, and 0.75, respectively, while it was 0.72 for the total scale.

BAI

Anxiety symptoms were assessed with the Persian version of the BAI, a self-report 21-item questionnaire scored based on a four-point (0–3) Likert scale. The minimum and maximum scores are 0 and 63, respectively [23]. In this study, the Cronbach's alpha coefficient for the BAI was 0.90.

BDI-II

Depressive symptoms were assessed with the Persian version of the BDI-II, a self-report 21-item questionnaire scored based on a four-point (0–3) Likert scale. The minimum and maximum scores are 0 and 63, respectively [24]. In this study, the Cronbach's alpha coefficient for the BDI-II was 0.88.

EAT-26

Eating-disordered behaviors were assessed with the Persian version of the EAT-26. In this 26-item questionnaire, the minimum and maximum scores are equal to 0 and 78, respectively. A score above 20 stands for the probability of being affected by FEDs [25]. In this study, the Cronbach's alpha coefficients for the EAT-26 subscales were as follows: drive for thinness = 0.90, restrained eating = 0.77, perceived social pressure to eat = 0.87, food preoccupation and oral control = 0.75 and bulimia = 0.71.

Table 1 Comparisons of the socio-demographic factors, BAI, BDI-II, TAS-20, EAT-26, and GHQ-28 among the three study groups ($N = 220$)

Variables	Subvariables	Healthy Controls (n = 110)	BPD (n = 38)	BPD + FEDs (n = 72)		
		n (%)	n (%)	n (%)	χ^2 (2)	
		37 (33.6)	10 (26.3)	23 (31.9)	0.71	
Age	18–23					
	24–29	43 (39.1)	16 (42.1)	26 (36.1)		
	30–35	30 (27.3)	12 (31.6)	23 (31.9)		
Gender	Male	28 (25.5)	17 (44.7)	26 (36.1)	5.26	
	Female	82 (74.5)	21 (55.3)	46 (63.9)		
Marital status	Never married	57 (51.8)	22 (57.9)	34 (47.2)	17.71	
	Married	28 (25.5)	16 (42.1)	18 (25.0)		
	Cohabiting	5 (4.5)	0 (0)	2 (2.8)		
	Widowed	2 (1.8)	0 (0)	5 (6.9)		
	Divorced	13 (11.8)	0 (0)	8 (11.1)		
	Separated	5 (4.5)	0 (0)	5 (6.9)		
Education level	Non-degree	45 (40.9)	9 (23.7)	28 (38.9)	1.84	
	High school diploma	38 (34.5)	4 (10.5)	23 (31.9)		
	Academic degree	27 (24.5)	25 (65.8)	21 (29.2)		
Income	< 10,000,000 Rials	73 (66.4)	23 (60.5)	44 (61.1)	0.70	
	≥ 10,000,000 Rials	37 (33.6)	15 (39.5)	28 (38.9)		
		M (SD)	M (SD)	M (SD)	F (2, 217)	Scheffé post-hoc test
BAI		7.94 (6.20)	50.65 (8.91)	62.30 (2.86)	2005.08***	BPD + FEDs > BPD > Healthy Controls
BDI-II		3.53 (5.62)	26.07 (4.46)	38.90 (6.40)	866.85***	BPD + FEDs > BPD > Healthy Controls
TAS-20		28.10 (7.18)	53.94 (12.95)	79.00 (9.60)	671.54***	BPD + FEDs > BPD > Healthy Controls
EAT-26		1.32 (2.11)	8.55 (5.19)	28.08 (8.45)	521.03***	BPD + FEDs > BPD > Healthy Controls
GHQ-28		10.10 (5.48)	36.73 (7.09)	58.70 (11.30)	797.78***	BPD + FEDs > BPD > Healthy Controls

Note. *BAI* Beck Anxiety Inventory, *BDI-II* Beck Depression Inventory-II, *BPD* Borderline personality disorder, *EAT-26* 26-item Eating Attitudes Test, *FEDs* Feeding and eating disorders, *TAS-20* 20-item Toronto Alexithymia Scale.
*$p < 0.05$; **$p < 0.01$; ***$p < 0.001$.

BPI

In this 53-item questionnaire (answered by yes or no), if the person's score for the 20 items of the cutoff score is above 10, the person is most likely to be affected by BPD [26]. In this study, the Cronbach's alpha coefficients for the BPI subscales of identity diffusion, primitive defense mechanisms, reality testing, and fear of closeness were 0.78, 0.82, 0.74, and 0.77, respectively, while it was 0.80 for the total scale.

SCID-5-PD

SCID-5-PD is a semi-structured clinical interview used by researchers and clinicians, which evaluates DSM-5 personality disorders under three clusters of A, B, and C, and other specific personality disorders. Several studies have reported acceptable reliability and validity of SCID-5-PD [27].

SCID-5-RV

SCID-5-RV is a semi-structured interview for major DSM-5 diagnoses, which is performed by a trained clinician or health expert familiar with the diagnostic criteria and classification of disorders in DSM-5. Several studies have reported acceptable reliability and validity of SCID-5-RV [28].

GHQ-28

GHQ-28 is a 28-item questionnaire in which items are scored in the range of 0–3. The overall score ranges between 0 and 84. A score of <21 indicates a person's mental health [29]. In this study, the Cronbach's alpha coefficients for the GHQ-28 subscales of somatic symptoms, anxiety and insomnia, social dysfunction, and severe depression were 0.76, 0.84, 0.71, and 0.88, respectively, while it was 0.90 for the total scale.

Data analysis

Statistical analysis was performed using descriptive statistics, including mean and standard deviation. Chi square test and Kruskal-Wallis test were conducted for a sociodemographic comparison of the three study groups. Also, an analysis of variance (ANOVA) was used to compare the mean scores of BAI, BDI-II, TAS-20, EAT-26, and GHQ-28. In ANOVA, the Scheffé test was applied to the post-hoc analysis. Subsequently, in BPD + FEDs group, the Pearson correlation coefficient was used to evaluate the correlation between the study variables. Also, in this group, the mediation analysis was conducted to investigate the mediating effect of anxiety and depression on the relationship between alexithymia and eating-disordered behaviors using the Hayes' PROCESS macro for SPSS [30]. As outlined in Preacher and Hayes [31], mediation emerges when the indirect effect is significant and the confidence intervals do not contain zero. Furthermore, given the relationship of sociodemographic factors (including age, gender, marital status, education level, and income) with anxiety, depression [32–35], and FEDs [36, 37] obtained in previous studies, the above-mentioned factors were considered as covariates in the mediation analysis. Meanwhile, data analysis was performed by SPSS 25, and the significance level was set at $P < 0.05$.

Results

Preliminary analysis

According to Table 1, there was a significant difference between the scores of BAI, BDI-II, TAS-20, EAT-26, and GHQ-28 among the three study groups. Based on Scheffé post-hoc test, the highest scores of BAI, BDI-II, TAS-20, EAT-26, and GHQ-28 were reported for BPD + EFD group, and the lowest scores were reported for healthy controls.

The results of the SCID-5-RV interview indicated a 65.4% current prevalence of FEDs in patients with BPD. The highest and lowest frequencies were reported for other specified feeding and eating disorders (51.3%) and bulimia nervosa (6.9%), respectively (Fig. 1). No FEDs case was observed in the BPD only group through clinical interviewing. Although the mean scores of TAS-20 in the BPD + FEDs group were significantly higher than those of the BPD only group, this difference was not significant in terms of different types of FEDs (Fig. 2).

Associations of study variables

The results of correlation in both the BPD only and BPD + FEDs groups suggested a significant positive correlation between the scores of EAT-26 and BAI (r = 0.58; $p < 0.01$), BDI-II (r = 0.52; $p < 0.01$), and TAS-20 (r = 0.59; $p < 0.01$). Furthermore, there was a significant positive correlation between the scores of TAS-20 and BAI (r = 0.67; $p < 0.01$) and BDI-II (r = 0.52; $p < 0.01$) (see Table 2).

Mediation analysis

The mediation analysis was performed using Hayes' PROCESS tool in SPSS (Model = 4, Bootstrap

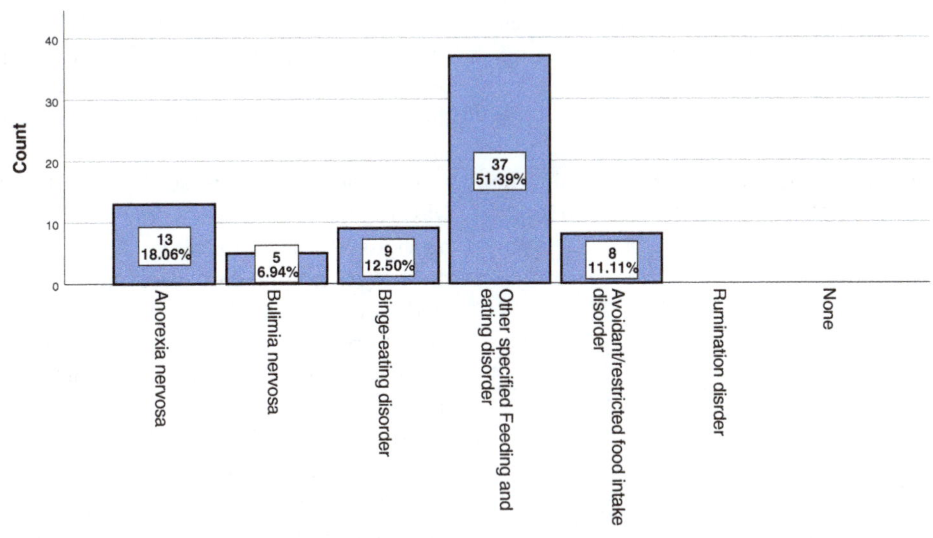

Fig. 1 The prevalence of different types of FEDs in BPD + FEDs group (*n* = 72). *Note.* BPD: borderline personality disorder; FEDs: Feeding and eating disorders

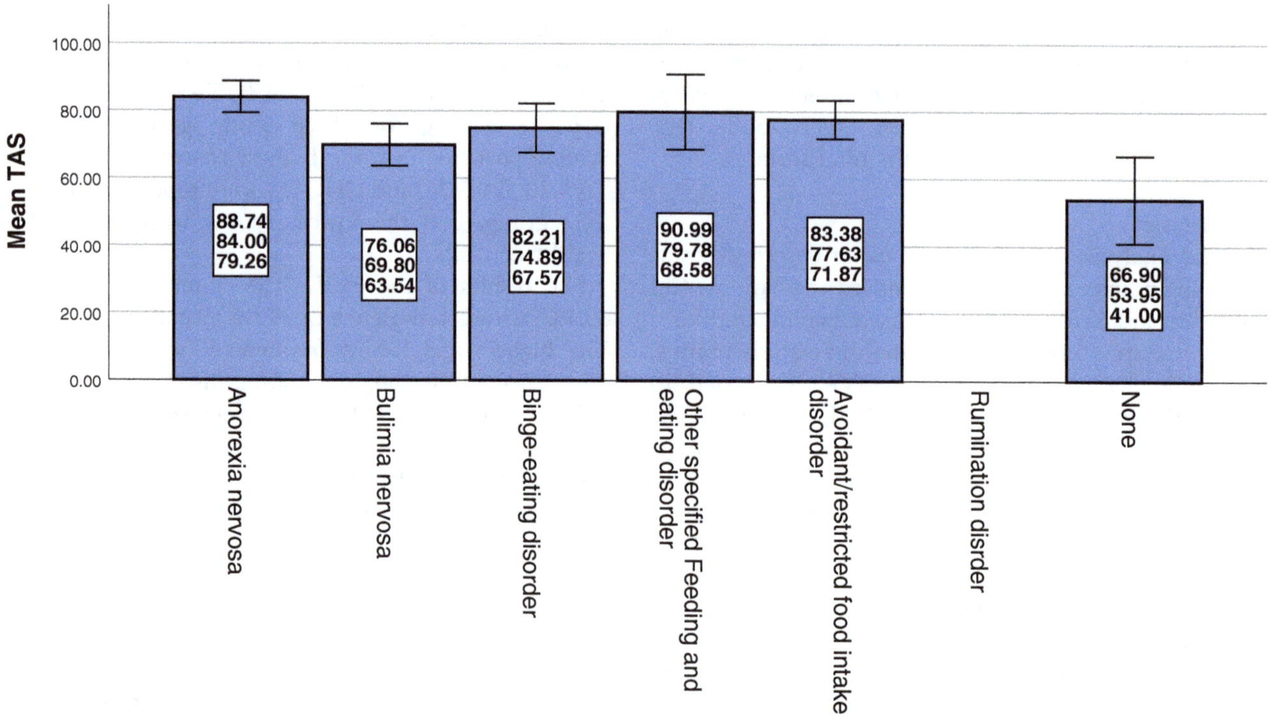

Fig. 2 Total alexithymia scores (TAS) by different types of FEDs (Error bars: 95% CI, ± 1 SD) (n = 110). *Note.* ANOVA: $F(5, 104) = 43.65$, $p < 0.001$; Scheffé post-hoc test: Anorexia nervosa, Bulimia nervosa, Binge-eating disorder, Other specified feeding and eating disorders, Avoidant/restricted food intake disorder > None

Samples = 5000). As hypothesized, a significant indirect effect of Alexithymia was direst observed on eating-disordered behaviors through anxiety and depression ($\beta = 0.12$, 95% CI: 0.005, 0.26; $\beta = 0.10$, 95% CI: 0.004, 0.18, respectively). The mediators (i.e., anxiety and depression) could account for roughly 54% ($P_M = 0.54$) and 45% ($P_M = 0.45$) of the total effect of alexithymia on EAT-26 total score, respectively. Hence, the overall hypothesis that anxiety and depression mediate the effect of alexithymia on eating-disordered behaviors was supported (Fig. 3).

Discussion

In this study, there was a significant difference in the scores of BAI, BDI-II, TAS-20, EAT-26, and GHQ-28 among the three study groups. The highest scores were reported for the BPD + FEDs group, and the lowest scores were obtained for healthy controls. These findings were consistent with the results of the study performed by Eizaguirre et al. [16], Nowakowski et al. [12], and Gilboa-Schechtman et al. [18] who showed that the scores of TAS-20, BAI, and BDI-II in the BPD + FEDs group are higher than those of healthy controls. These results indicated that the BPD + FEDs patients had more difficulties in identifying and describing their emotions than BPD only patients and healthy controls potentially due to a greater degree of distress and less effective coping styles [12, 16].

Table 2 Correlations between BAI, BDI-II, TAS-20, and EAT-26 in BPD + FEDs group ($n = 72$)

Variables	M (SD)	1	2	3	4
1. BAI	58.69 (7.59)	1			
2. BDI-II	34.76 (8.35)	0.53^{**}	1		
3. TAS-20	71.06 (15.31)	0.67^{**}	0.52^{**}	1	
4. EAT-26	22.71 (12.03)	0.58^{**}	0.52^{**}	0.59^{**}	1

Note. *BAI* Beck Anxiety Inventory, *BDI-II* Beck Depression Inventory-II, *EAT-26* 26-item Eating Attitudes Test, *TAS-20* 20-item Toronto Alexithymia Scale
$^{*}p < 0.05$; $^{**}p < 0.01$; $^{***}p < 0.001$

Additionally, in this study, a higher FEDs prevalence was reported among patients with BPD compared to previous studies (65.4% vs. 14–53%). The highest and the lowest frequencies were reported for other specified feeding and eating disorders (51.3%) and bulimia nervosa (6.9%), respectively. In line with the findings, in the study performed by Zanarini et al. [2, 38], eating disorders not otherwise specified (i.e., diagnosis of other specified feeding and eating disorders in DSM-5) were the most common FEDs among patients with BPD. Moreover, the low rate of bulimia nervosa in patients with BPD has been contrary to much prior research [2–4, 38]. This is because FEDs frequency among patients with BPD has been investigated based on DSM-III-R and

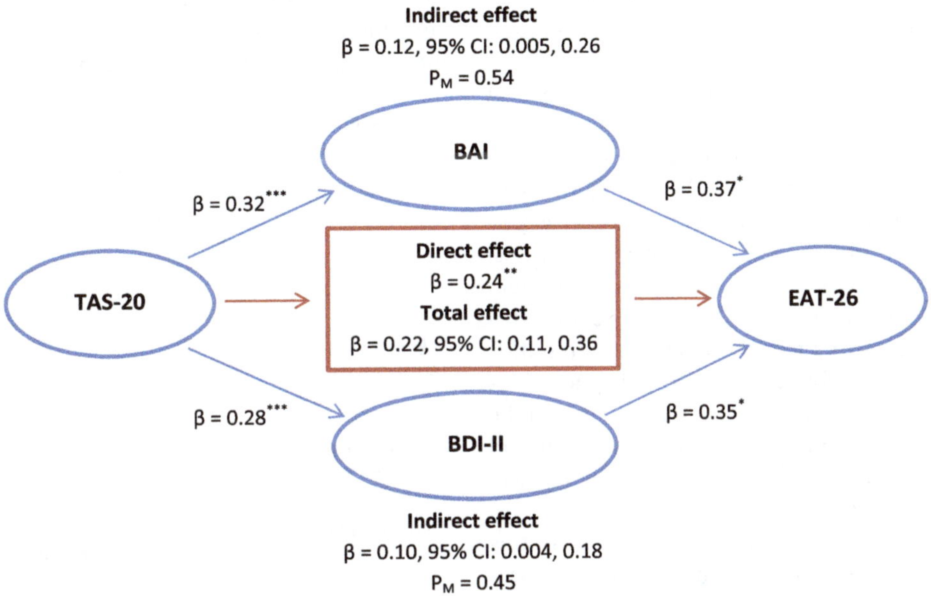

Fig. 3 Illustration of the results of the mediation analysis described in the text, which tested BAI and BDI-II total scores (the measures of anxiety and depression, respectively) as the potential mediators of the relationship between TAS-20 and EAT-26 total scores (the measures of alexithymia and disordered eating behaviors, respectively) by controlling for sociodemographic variables (included age, gender, marital status, degree level, and income) in BPD + FEDs group (n = 72). *Note.* P_M: Effect size (ratio of indirect to total effect) $^{*}p < 0.05$; $^{**}p < 0.01$; $^{***}p < 0.001$.

DSM-IV-TR criteria in previous studies, which are different from DSM-5 criteria. In addition, avoidant/restricted food intake disorder is a new diagnosis in DSM-5 that is very similar to anorexia nervosa, aside from the fact that there is no distress about body shape/size or fear of fatness in avoidant/restricted food intake disorder [28]. No subcategory of FEDs was observed in the only BPD group trough interviewing, suggesting that EAT-26 can be assumed as a useful screening instrument (with a cutoff point of above 20) [25] for diagnosing different types of FEDs in patients with BPD.

Although the highest mean score of TAS-20 in this study was related to anorexia nervosa, there was no significant difference between the scores of different types of FEDs. This finding was consistent with the results of the studies performed by Cochrane et al. [9], Troop et al. [39], and Berthoz et al. [40]. However, it was inconsistent with the studies performed by Eizaguirre et al. [16], Nowakowski et al. [12], and Gilboa-Schechtman et al. [18], who showed that mean score of TAS-20 in patients with anorexia nervosa was significantly higher than that in other types of FEDs. However, the findings may reflect insufficient power as there were not many anorexia nervosa cases in the study sample. Thus, it may represent a Type 2 error rather than a sign that anorexia nervosa does not present with high alexithymia.

Together the results demonstrated a considerable positive correlation between the scores of EAT-26 and BAI, BDI-II, and TAS-20. Moreover, there was a significant positive correlation between the scores of TAS-20 and BAI and BDI-II. These findings suggested that, in patients affected by BPD + FEDs, alexithymia was closely related to anxiety and depression. Here, this question is raised: "Is alexithymia either a state variable or a trait variable?" There is strong evidence that alexithymia is not only a by-product of FEDs symptomatology. However, there is mixed evidence of whether alexithymia is independent of general distress [12, 16, 18]. Nevertheless, several studies have indicated that elevated alexithymia scores become eliminated by controlling the effect of distress. However, some other studies have suggested that, in patients with FEDs, elevated alexithymia scores remain constant even by controlling the effect of anxiety and depression [12]. In this study, the mediation analysis showed that the role of alexithymia in the prediction of eating-disordered behaviors remained unchanged even by controlling the effect of anxiety and depression. Accordingly, alexithymia may be a trait rather than a state. In this regard, Schmidt et al. [41] stated that pharmacotherapy with antidepressants can only decrease depression level in patients with high levels of alexithymia and depression. Moreover, genetic studies have concluded that alexithymia has its own heritability component that cannot be fully explained by depression or genetic susceptibility to general distress and psychopathology [42]. As a result, although the relevant evidence is mixed, it is recommended that clinical attention should be paid to alexithymia as a distress-independent construct [12].

However, the cross-sectional design of this study prevents an understanding of relationships' exact nature, particularly with respect to causality.

The findings have many implications for nosology and interventions. First, the FEDs among patients with BPD are likely to be a subtype of emotional disorders that, in turn, should affect the prediction of the course of these afflictions. For example, if depressive episodes as a primary disorder constitute the core of these conditions, the risk of developing depressive episodes remains high, even with the recovery from the FEDs. Second, this nosological shift may also affect the type of treatment. If anxiety and depression, for instance, are diagnosed as primary or secondary disorders, the treatment will be different. Third, emotional awareness normalization and emotion regulation may be regarded as recovery markers beyond symptom reduction [18].

However, there were some limitations faced in this study. First, the cross-sectional design avoided the precise understanding of relationships' nature, especially concerning causality. It is essential to differentiate between primary and secondary alexithymia since cognitive therapies are more effective in primary alexithymia than dynamic ones [43]. However, secondary alexithymia responds to a wide range of treatments. Second, due to the small sample size (particularly among different types of FEDs in BPD + FEDs group) and participant selection from a narrow age-range and specific geographical region, the study results should be generalized to other societies with caution. Third, the adults may report different levels of alexithymia in response to certain life events based on the individual difference model. Thus, future studies should focus on some methodological constraints, including sole reliance on self-report measures of alexithymia (due to memory bias and demand characteristics), lack of longitudinal and experimental studies, lack of ethnic differences, limited age range, and negative emotions exclusively.

Conclusions

In conclusion, this study showed that BPD + FEDs patients found it difficult to identify and describe emotions. However, there was no significant difference in the level of alexithymia among different types of FEDs. The results also suggested that other specified feeding and eating disorders may be the most prevalent FEDs in patients with BPD. Besides, anxiety and depression could mediate the relationship between alexithymia and eating-disordered behaviors in patients with BPD. Accordingly, the FEDs treatment protocols among patients with BPD need to concentrate on emotions and emotion regulation to assess alexithymia, anxiety, and depression conveniently, and determine whether alexithymia precedes FEDs. Nonetheless, further longitudinal and experimental studies with a larger variety of measures to explore psychopathology could contribute to clarifying all these questions and ascertaining primary and secondary alexithymia in FEDs.

Abbreviations

ANOVA: Analysis of variance; BAI: Beck Anxiety Inventory; BDI-II: Beck Depression Inventory-II; BPD: Borderline personality disorder; BPI: Borderline Personality Inventory; EAT-26: 26-item Eating Attitudes Test; FEDs: Feeding and eating disorders; GHQ-28: 28-item General Health Questionnaire; SCID-5-RV: Structured Clinical Interviews for DSM-5: Research Version; SCID-5-PD: Structured Clinical Interview for DSM-5 Personality Disorders; TAS-20: 20-item Toronto Alexithymia Scale

Acknowledgments

The author would like to thank the patient, who contributed in conducting the present study.

Author's contributions

The author read and approved the final manuscript.

Competing interests

The author declares that he has no competing interests.

References

1. Leichsenring F, Leibing E, Kruse J, New AS, Leweke F. Borderline personality disorder. Lancet. 2011;377(9759):74–84. https://doi.org/10.1016/S0140-6736(10)61422-5.
2. Zanarini MC, Reichman CA, Frankenburg FR, Reich DB, Fitzmaurice G. The course of eating disorders in patients with borderline personality disorder: a 10-year follow-up study. Int J Eat Disord. 2010;43(3):226–32. https://doi.org/10.1002/eat.20689.
3. Rosenvinge JH, Martinussen M, Østensen E. The comorbidity of eating disorders and personality disorders: a metaanalytic review of studies published between 1983 and 1998. Eat Weight Disord. 2000;5(2):52–61. https://doi.org/10.1007/bf03327480.
4. Martinussen M, Friborg O, Schmierer P, Kaiser S, Øvergård KT, Neunhoeffer AL, et al. The comorbidity of personality disorders in eating disorders: a meta-analysis. Eat Weight Disord. 2017;22(2):201–9. https://doi.org/10.1007/s40519-016-0345-x.
5. Sansone RA, Sansone LA. Personality pathology and its influence on eating disorders. Innov Clin Neurosci. 2011;8(3):14.
6. Dolan-Sewell, Regina T., Robert F. Krueger, and M. Tracie Shea. Co-occurrence with syndrome disorders. In W. J. Livesley (Ed.), Handbook of personality disorders: Theory, research, and treatment. New York: Guilford Press; 2001.
7. Sloan E, Hall K, Moulding R, Bryce S, Mildred H, Staiger PK. Emotion regulation as a transdiagnostic treatment construct across anxiety, depression, substance, eating and borderline personality disorders: a systematic review. Clin Psychol Rev. 2017;57:141–63. https://doi.org/10.1016/j.cpr.2017.09.002.
8. Berenbaum H. Childhood abuse, alexithymia and personality disorder. J Psychosom Res. 1996;41(6):585–95. https://doi.org/10.1016/s0022-3999(96)00225-5.
9. Cochrane CE, Brewerton TD, Wilson DB, Hodges EL. Alexithymia in the eating disorders. Int J Eat Disord. 1993;14(2):219–22. https://doi.org/10.1002/1098-108x(199309)14:2<219::aid-eat2260140212>3.0.co;2-g.
10. Zlotnick C, Mattia JI, Zimmerman M. The relationship between posttraumatic stress disorder, childhood trauma and alexithymia in an outpatient sample. J Trauma Stress. 2001;14(1):177–88.
11. Wolff S, Stiglmayr C, Bretz HJ, Lammers CH, Auckenthaler A. Emotion identification and tension in female patients with borderline personality disorder. Br J Clin Psychol. 2007;46(3):347–60. https://doi.org/10.1348/014466507X173736.
12. Nowakowski ME, McFarlane T, Cassin S. Alexithymia and eating disorders: a critical review of the literature. J Eat Disord. 2013;1(1):21. https://doi.org/10.1186/2050-2974-1-21.
13. Connelly M, Denney DR. Regulation of emotions during experimental stress in alexithymia. J Psychosom Res. 2007;62(6):649–56. https://doi.org/10.1016/j.jpsychores.2006.12.008

14. Zautra A, Smith B, Affleck G, Tennen H. Examinations of chronic pain and affect relationships: applications of a dynamic model of affect. J Consult Clin Psychol. 2001;69(5):786. https://doi.org/10.1037//0022-006x.69.5.786.
15. Pandey R, Mandal MK. Eysenckian personality dimensions and alexithymia: examining the overlap in terms of perceived autonomic arousal. Personal Individ Differ. 1996;20(4):499–504. https://doi.org/10.1016/0191-8869(95)00214-6.
16. Eizaguirre AE, de Cabezón AO, de Alda IO, Olariaga LJ, Juaniz M. Alexithymia and its relationships with anxiety and depression in eating disorders. Personal Individ Differ. 2004;36(2):321–31. https://doi.org/10.1016/S0191-8869(03)00099-0.
17. Westwood H, Kerr-Gaffney J, Stahl D, Tchanturia K. Alexithymia in eating disorders: systematic review and meta-analyses of studies using the Toronto alexithymia scale. J Psychosom Res. 2017;99:66–81. https://doi.org/10.1016/j.jpsychores.2017.06.007.
18. Gilboa-Schechtman E, Avnon L, Zubery E, Jeczmien P. Emotional processing in eating disorders: specific impairment or general distress related deficiency? Depress Anxiety. 2006;23(6):331–9. https://doi.org/10.1002/da.20163.
19. Forbush KT, South SC, Krueger RF, Iacono WG, Clark LA, Keel PK, et al. Locating eating pathology within an empirical diagnostic taxonomy: evidence from a community-based sample. J Abnorm Psychol. 2010;119(2):282. https://doi.org/10.1037/a0019189.
20. Lane DM, Scott D, Hebl M, Guerra R, Osherson D, Zimmer H. An introduction to statistics. Houston: Rice University; 2017.
21. Taber KS. The use of Cronbach's alpha when developing and reporting research instruments in science education. Res Sci Educ. 2018;48(6):1273–96. https://doi.org/10.1007/s11165-016-9602-2.
22. Besharat MA. Reliability and factorial validity of a Farsi version of the 20-item Toronto alexithymia scale with a sample of Iranian students. Psychol Rep. 2007;101(1):209–20. https://doi.org/10.2466/pr0.101.1.209-220.
23. Kaviani H, Mousavi AS. Psychometric properties of the Persian version of Beck anxiety inventory (BAI). Tehran Univ Med J TUMS Publ. 2008;66(2):136–40 Persian.
24. Ghassemzadeh H, Mojtabai R, Karamghadiri N, Ebrahimkhani N. Psychometric properties of a Persian-language version of the Beck depression inventory-second edition: BDI-II-PERSIAN. Depress Anxiety. 2005;21(4):185–92. https://doi.org/10.1002/da.20070.
25. Ahmadi S, Moloodi R, Zarbaksh MR, Ghaderi A. Psychometric properties of the eating attitude Test-26 for female Iranian students. Eat Weight Disord. 2014;19(2):183–9. https://doi.org/10.1007/s40519-014-0106-7.
26. Mohammadzadeh A. Validation of the borderline personality inventory in Iran. Int J Behavioral Sci. 2011;5(3):269–77. https://doi.org/10.30491/IJBS.2011.67743.
27. First MB, Williams JB, Benjamin LS, Spitzer RL. User's guide for the SCID-5-PD (structured clinical interview for DSM-5 personality disorder). Arlington: American Psychiatric Association; 2015.
28. First MB, Williams JB, Karg RS, Spitzer RL. User's guide for the SCID-5-CV: structured clinical interview for DSM-5 disorders, clinician version. Arlington: American Psychiatric Association; 2016.
29. Taghavi S. Validity and reliability of the general health questionnaire (GHQ-28) in college students of Shiraz University. J Psychol. 2002;5(4):381–98 Persian.
30. Hayes AF. Introduction to mediation, moderation, and conditional process analysis: a regression-based approach. New York: Guilford Press; 2017.
31. Preacher KJ, Hayes AF. SPSS and SAS procedures for estimating indirect effects in simple mediation models. Behav Res Methods Instrum Comput. 2004;36(4):717–31. https://doi.org/10.3758/bf03206553.
32. Pillay AL, Sargent CA. Relationship of age and education with anxiety, depression, and hopelessness in a South African community sample. Percept Mot Skills. 1999;89(3):881–4. https://doi.org/10.2466/pms.1999.89.3.881.
33. Ta VP, Gesselman AN, Perry BL, Fisher HE, Garcia JR. Stress of singlehood: marital status, domain-specific stress, and anxiety in a national US sample. J Soc Clin Psychol. 2017;36(6):461–85. https://doi.org/10.1521/jscp.2017.36.6.461.
34. Faravelli C, Scarpato MA, Castellini G, Sauro CL. Gender differences in depression and anxiety: the role of age. Psychiatry Res. 2013;210(3):1301–3. https://doi.org/10.1016/j.psychres.2013.09.027
35. Carvalhais SM, Lima-Costa MF, Peixoto SV, Firmo JO, Castro-Costa E, Uchoa E. The influence of socio-economic conditions on the prevalence of depressive symptoms and its covariates in an elderly population with slight income differences: the Bambui health and aging study (BHAS). Int J Soc Psychiatry. 2008;54(5):447–56. https://doi.org/10.1177/0020764008090792.
36. Bussolotti D, Fernández-Aranda F, Solano R, Jiménez-Murcia S, Turón V, Vallejo J. Marital status and eating disorders: an analysis of its relevance. J Psychosom Res. 2002;53(6):1139–45. https://doi.org/10.1016/s0022-3999(02)00336-7.
37. Hay P, Girosi F, Mond J. Prevalence and sociodemographic correlates of DSM-5 eating disorders in the Australian population. J Eat Disord. 2015;3(1):19. https://doi.org/10.1186/s40337-015-0056-0.
38. Zanarini MC, Frankenburg FR, Dubo ED, Sickel AE, Trikha A, Levin A, et al. Axis I comorbidity of borderline personality disorder. Am J Psychiatry. 1998;155(12):1733–9. https://doi.org/10.1176/ajp.155.12.1733.
39. Troop NA, Schmidt UH, Treasure JL. Feelings and fantasy in eating disorders: a factor analysis of the Toronto alexithymia scale. Int J Eat Disord. 1995;18(2):151–7. https://doi.org/10.1002/1098-108x(199509)18:2<151::aid-eat2260180207>3.0.co;2-e.
40. Berthoz S, Perdereau F, Godart N, Corcos M, Haviland MG. Observer-and self-rated alexithymia in eating disorder patients: levels and correspondence among three measures. J Psychosom Res. 2007;62(3):341–7. https://doi.org/10.1016/j.jpsychores.2006.10.008.
41. Schmidt U, Jiwany A, Treasure J. A controlled study of alexithymia in eating disorders. Compr Psychiatry. 1993;34(1):54–8. https://doi.org/10.1016/0010-440x(93)90036-4.
42. Picardi A, Fagnani C, Gigantesco A, Toccaceli V, Lega I, Stazi MA. Genetic influences on alexithymia and their relationship with depressive symptoms. J Psychosom Res. 2011;71(4):256–63. https://doi.org/10.1016/j.jpsychores.2011.02.016.
43. Sexton MC, Sunday SR, Hurt S, Halmi KA. The relationship between alexithymia, depression, and axis II psychopathology in eating disorder inpatients. Int J Eat Disord. 1998;23(3):277–8. https://doi.org/10.1002/(sici)1098-108x(199804)23:3<277::aid-eat5>3.0.co;2-g.

3

Impact of COVID-19 lockdown measures on a cohort of eating disorders patients

Paulo P. P. Machado[1*], Ana Pinto-Bastos[1], Rita Ramos[1], Tânia F. Rodrigues[1], Elsa Louro[1], Sónia Gonçalves[1], Isabel Brandão[2] and Ana Vaz[1]

Abstract

Background: Lockdown implemented to prevent the COVID-19 spread resulted in marked changes in the lifestyle. The objective of the current study was to assess the impact of lockdown measures on a cohort of eating disorder (ED) patients being followed as part of an ongoing naturalistic treatment study.

Methods: Ninety-nine patients aged 18 or older, currently or previously, in treatment at a Portuguese specialized hospital unit were contacted by phone and invited to participate in the current survey. Fifty-nine agreed to be interviewed by phone, and 43 agreed to respond to a set of self-report measures of ED symptoms, emotion regulation difficulties, clinical impairment, negative urgency, and COVID-19 impact, during the week after the end of the lockdown period.

Results: Data showed that of the 26 patients currently in treatment: 8 remained unchanged (31%), 7 deteriorated (27%), and 11 reliably improved (42%). Of the 17 participants not currently in treatment: 3 deteriorated (18%), 9 remained unchanged (53%), and 5 (29%) improved after the lockdown period. The Coronavirus Impact Scale showed that most patients considered their routines moderately or extremely impacted, experienced stress related to coronavirus, and showed difficulty in maintaining physical exercise and feeding routines. Results suggest that higher impact of COVID-19 lockdown was significantly correlated with eating disorder symptoms and associated psychopathology, impulsivity, difficulties in emotion regulation and clinical impairment measured at post-lockdown. In addition, the impact of COVID-19 and lockdown measures on clinical impairment was mediated by difficulties in emotion regulation.

Conclusions: Findings suggest that some ED patients may experience worsening of their condition, especially if associated with difficulties in emotion regulation, and these difficulties might be exacerbated in the context of a stressful crisis and lockdown measures, highlighting the need for intervention strategies to mitigate its negative impact.

Keywords: COVID-19, Lockdown, Eating disorders, Clinical impairment

* Correspondence: pmachado@psi.uminho.pt
[1]Psychotherapy and Psychopathology Research Unit – Psychology Research Centre, University of Minho, School of Psychology, Braga, Portugal
Full list of author information is available at the end of the article

Plain English summary

The current study assessed the impact of the COVID-19 pandemic crisis and the government implemented lockdown measures on a group of patients diagnosed with eating disorders, attending a specialized treatment center in Portugal. We found that those struggling with eating disorders may experience worsening of their condition, especially if they tend to have difficulties in emotion regulation, and their living routines and access to care are disrupted. This can be especially the case during stressful and disrupting events like when the state of emergency was declared in Portugal to curb the spread of COVID-19.

Background

Lockdown measures implemented by the government to prevent the coronavirus disease 2019 (COVID-19) pandemic spread resulted in marked changes in the lifestyle of the general population (e.g., closure of schools, businesses, gyms, and restaurants). During the confinement period, people were instructed to stay at home, refrain from unnecessary outings, leaving home was allowed to shop for basic needs (e.g., food, and medication), short walks around home for light exercise or walk dogs.

People with eating disorders might be disproportionally affected both by the pandemic crisis and the mitigating measures implemented to contain it [1]. For example, data, from a pilot study in Spain [2], showed that 12 out of 32 patients reported impairments in their eating disorder (ED) symptomatology, and most presented worries about increased uncertainty in their lives, being it, work, treatment, or loved ones related. Another survey [3], carried in Australia, showed that in a group of participants with ED, there was an increase in restricting, binge eating, purging, and exercise behaviors.

Rodgers and colleagues [4] proposed three pathways by which the COVID-19 pandemic might cause ED symptomatic exacerbation: 1) disruptions of daily routines, and constrains in outdoors, and social activities, that are useful in terms of emotional regulation; 2) exposure to ED-specific and anxiety-provoking media content; and 3) emotional distress caused by fears of contagion and increased health concerns. The combination of these pathways to increased risk combined with a potential lack of availability of protective factors, like social support and access to care have the potential to affect in a unique way people with eating disorders. Social distancing, lack of in-person social contact, and confinement to own home may increase negative affect, that associated with difficulties in emotional regulation might pose specific challenges to people with eating disorders.

However, results regarding the impact of lockdown in eating disorders are not consistent. For instance, most recent preliminary research [5] showed that patients with a diagnosis of Anorexia Nervosa reported significant decreases on their eating symptoms, after confinement due to COVID-19. However, these results were based on retrospective self-reported evaluation of symptoms using a novel instrument.

There is currently an urgent need for research addressing the mental health impact of the COVID-19 crisis, especially amongst those already suffering from a mental disorder [6], and an assessment of potential symptomatic mitigating or aggravating factors. The objective of the current study was to assess the impact of COVID-19 and lockdown measures on a cohort of ED patients being followed as part of an ongoing naturalistic treatment study.

Methods

Participants

Participants were recruited from an ongoing naturalistic longitudinal study conducted by our research team, focusing on treatment monitoring and follow up of patients with a diagnosis of eating disorders. In the context of that study, 99 patients aged 18 or older, currently or previously, in treatment at a Portuguese specialized hospital unit were contacted by phone in order to invite them to participate in the current survey.

Four patients refused to participate in this additional survey, and 36 weren't reachable (10 had changed their contact number, 7 had their mobile phone turned off, and 19 did not answer the call). Fifty-nine participants agreed to participate and were interviewed to obtain clinical information regarding the lockdown period. In addition, they were asked to complete a set of self-report questionnaires, of which were received 43 responses.

Of these 43 participants, 26 reported to be currently in treatment.

For the purpose of this study, we used data collected in the last available evaluation prior to COVID-19 lockdown period. Data collection regarding the impact of COVID-19 lockdown started when the end of the state of emergency, in Portugal, was announced (April 30th), and finished two weeks later (May 15th). During this data collection period, the country was under a "state of calamity" where the population had the civic duty of home confinement, in spite of the reopening of some commercial establishments and public services, and a gradual deconfinement.

Measures

Clinical interview: participants were asked about clinical information regarding the COVID-19 lockdown period, namely weight change during lockdown, current medication, if they were still under ED treatment, date of the last ED appointment, and current diagnosis.

Eating Disorder Examination-Questionnaire (EDE-Q) [7, 8]: is a 28-item measure used to assess eating disorder psychopathology focusing on the last 28 days. It generates four subscales (restraint, eating concern, shape concern, and weight concern) and a global score.

Clinical Impairment Assessment (CIA) [9, 10]: is a 16-item self-report questionnaire used to evaluate psychosocial impairment secondary to eating disorders, in the personal, social and cognitive domains, over the last 28 days. A higher score represents more impairment.

Impulsive Behavior Scale-Negative Urgency Subscale (UPPS-P) [11]: this subscale is composed of 12-item and is used to assess impulsivity when accompanied by negative emotions. Higher scores represent greater negative urgency.

Difficulties in Emotion Regulation Scale - Short Form (DERS-SF) [12, 13]: is an 18-item self-report questionnaire used to assess difficulties in emotion regulation. It contains six subscales: 1) Difficulties Engaging in Goal-Directed Behavior, 2) Lack of Emotional Clarity, 3) Non-acceptance of Emotional Responses, 4) Limited Access to Emotion Regulation Strategies, 5) Lack of Emotional Awareness, and 6) Impulse Control Difficulties and also generate a total score. Higher scores represent greater emotion regulation difficulties.

Coronavirus Impact Scale (CIS) [14]: is an 11-item questionnaire that assesses the extent to which COVID-19 pandemic changed participant's lives in the following areas: routines, family income/employment, food access, mental health care access, access to social support, experience of stress related to COVID-19 pandemic, stress/family discord, personal diagnosis of coronavirus, immediate family members diagnosed with coronavirus, and extended family members and/or close friends diagnosed with COVID-19. In the current study, we also asked participants to rate how COVID-19 pandemic changed their lives in terms of two additional areas: feeding and physical exercise. Items were answered on a 4-point Likert scale, varying from 0 ("None/No change") to 3 ("Severe"). Total score was computed by the sum of the 13 items of this adapted scale.

Procedure

In order to assess the impact of COVID-19 lockdown in this population, all participants were contacted by phone. Those who accepted to participate were interviewed by a psychologist specialized in EDs assessment and were asked to complete a set of online questionnaires, using Google Forms. Telephone interviews were conducted in a semi-structured format by 2 interviewers (APB, EL). Information regarding the aims of the study and the voluntary nature of participation were provided. This study was approved by the ethical committee of the hospital involved.

Statistical analysis

Statistical analyses were conducted using the IBM SPSS Statistics software, version 26.0. For the characterization of the sample, descriptive statistics were used.

We first assessed the impact of the lockdown period by computing change scores (CS) between post and pre-lockdown on the CIA total scores. A CS was considered reliable (reliable change) if exceeded the standard error of the measure.

Pearson correlations were conducted to test the association between variables under study and COVID-19 lockdown impact, and to inform the candidate variables to include in the mediation model. In order to examine the indirect effects of difficulties in emotion regulation (DERS-SF total) on the relationship between impact of COVID-19 lockdown and clinical impairment (CIA total), a regression-based bootstrapping approach with 5000 bias-corrected resamples and 95% confidence intervals was conducted using the PROCESS macro (v3.5) for SPSS (2020). A simple mediation model was tested in which: impact of COVID-19 lockdown was included as the independent variable (X); CIA total was included as the dependent variable (Y); and DERS-SF total was introduced in the model as the mediator variable (M). The inference on mediation was based on the analysis of the indirect effects' estimates, considered significant if the interval between the lower and the upper bound of the 95% bias-corrected bootstrap confidence intervals did not contain zero [15, 16].

Results

Participant's clinical status

Forty-three ED patients with ages ranging from 18 to 55 years old (M = 27.60, SD = 8.45) completed all assessments in the post confinement period. Most were women (95.3%). Twenty had a diagnosis of anorexia nervosa, 14 of bulimia nervosa, 2 binge eating disorder, and 7 other specified feeding or eating disorder.

During the COVID-19 lockdown period, only 8 participants still went to work regularly, 6 were unemployed, 5 in layoff, 9 in prophylactic isolation, and the remaining 13 were in telework or involved in remote academic work (e.g., online classes).

Thirteen ED patients (31.0%) reported a weight increase due to COVID-19 lockdown, 8 (19.0%) decrease on weight, 4 (9.5%) do not know their current weight, and 17 (40.5%) report having maintained the weight during this period.

Participants' mean body mass index (BMI) based on self-reported weight and height during COVID-19 lockdown period was 21.58 kg/m^2 (SD = 6.85), significantly different from the BMI in the last assessment 20.53 kg/m^2 (SD = 6.60) ($t_{40} = -2.26$, $p = .030$).

Table 1 presents in detail participants' clinical and demographical data.

Table 1 Clinical and demographical characteristics

	N	%	M	SD	Min-Max
Age			27.60	8.45	18–55
Sex					
Women	41	95.3			
Men	2	4.7			
Diagnosis					
Bulimia Nervosa	14	32.6			
Anorexia Nervosa	20	46.5			
BED	2	4.7			
OSFED	7	16.3			
Currently on ED treatment					
No	17	39.5			
Yes	26	60.5			
Social Lockdown					
Yes, I'm in prophylactic isolation	9	20.9			
Yes, I'm working from home	3	7.0			
(telework)	5	11.6			
Yes, I'm in lay off	6	14.0			
Yes, I'm unemployed	10	23.3			
Yes, I'm having videoconferencing	8	18.6			
classes	0	0.0			
No, I still go to work regularly	2	4.7			
No, I still go to work sporadically					
Other					
Social Lockdown Period (weeks)			6.71	1. 64	2–9
Lockdown weight change					
Gained weight	13	31.0			
Lost weight	8	19.0			
Unchanged	17	40.5			
Doesn't know or doesn't care	4	9.5			

Note. $N = 43$, *BED* Binge Eating Disorder, *OSFED* Other Specified Feeding or Eating Disorder, *BMI* Body Mass Index, *ED* Eating Disorders, *M* Mean, *SD* Standard Deviation

Impact of COVID-19 lockdown

Table 2 presents mean and standard deviation for all self-report measures in both assessment times, last available data for each participant and post-lockdown assessment. Group differences between pre-COVID-19, and post lockdown, were not significant after Bonferroni correction for multiple comparisons. Trying to extrapolate the possible impact of the lockdown period on our participants, at the individual level, we computed change scores on our measure of clinical impairment (CIA) between the previously available time point and the end of the lockdown period. Using Jacobson and Truax [17] criteria for reliable change, 16 patients improved since previously available assessment, 17 remained unchanged, and 10 deteriorated. Data showed that of the 26 patients currently in treatment: 8 remained unchanged (31%), 7 deteriorated (27%), and 11 reliably improved (42%). Of the 17 participants not currently in treatment: 3 deteriorated (18%), 9 remained unchanged (53%), and 5 (29%) improved after the lockdown period.

Table 2 Pre and post lockdown self-reported measures of eating disorder, clinical impairment, impulsivity, and difficulties in emotion regulation

	Previous Assessment M (SD)	COVID-19 Assessment M (SD)
EDE-Q Total	2.92 (1.57)	2.93 (1.58)
CIA Total	23.33 (12.94)	19.93 (13.16)
UPPS-P	2.59 (0.66)	2.65 (0.75)
DERS-SF Total	43.35 (15.94)	47.56 (14.85)

Note. $N = 43$, *EDE-Q* Eating Disorder Examination-Questionnaire, *UPPS-P* Impulsive Behavior Scale, *DERS-SF* Difficulties in Emotion Regulation Scale-Short Form, *CIA* Clinical Impairment Assessment

Results suggest that most participants, whether currently in treatment or not, considered that COVID-19 changed moderately to extremely their life in terms of routines, experiences of stress related to coronavirus pandemic, physical exercise and eating habits. The data are summarized in Table 3.

Associations between the impact of COVID-19 lockdown, eating psychopathology and psychological distress during lockdown

Table 4 shows the correlations between impact of COVID-19 lockdown, eating psychopathology and psychological distress during lockdown. Results suggest that higher impact of COVID-19 lockdown was significantly correlated with eating disorder symptoms and associated psychopathology, impulsivity, difficulties in emotion regulation and clinical impairment measured at post-lockdown. Considering the significant correlations, we tested a model including impact of COVID-19 lockdown, clinical impairment and difficulties in emotion regulation.

The mediational role of emotion regulation difficulties in the relationship between the coronavirus impact and clinical impairment secondary to ED

The total effect of the impact of COVID-19 lockdown (CIS total) on clinical impairment (CIA total) was significant, $c = 1.24$, $t = 4.43$, $p < .001$. Also, the CIS total was positively associated to difficulties in emotion regulation (DERS-SF total), $a = 0.97$, CI [.26, 1.69], which was, in turn, positively associated with CIA total, $b = 0.42$, CI [.21, .64]. After introducing the mediator in the model, the association between the CIS total on CIA total remained significant, $c' = 0.83$, $t = 3.18$, $p = .003$. Finally, the indirect effect of CIS total on CIA total via DERS-SF total was positive and statistically significant,

Table 3 Impact of COVID-19 lockdown in ED patients

	Currently in treatment				Total	
	Yes		No			
	N	%	N	%	N	%
Routines						
No change/Mild	6	23.1	4	23.5	10	23.3
Moderate/ Severe	20	76.9	13	76.5	33	76.7
Family Income/Employment						
No change/Mild	16	61.5	16	94.1	32	74.4
Moderate/ Severe	10	38.5	1	5.9	11	25.6
Food Access						
No change/Mild	26	100.0	16	94.1	42	97.7
Moderate/ Severe	0	0.0	1	5.9	1	2.3
Medical health care access						
No change/Mild	15	57.7	10	58.8	25	58.1
Moderate/ Severe	11	42.3	7	41.2	18	41.9
Mental health treatment access						
No change/Mild	14	53.8	13	76.5	27	62.8
Moderate/ Severe	12	46.2	4	23.5	16	37.2
Access to extended family and non-family social supports						
No change/Mild	21	80.8	15	88.2	36	83.7
Moderate/ Severe	5	19.2	2	11.8	7	16.3
Experiences of stress related to coronavirus pandemic						
None/Mild	11	42.3	7	41.2	18	41.9
Moderate/ Severe	15	57.7	10	58.8	25	58.1
Stress and discord in the family						
No change/Mild	21	80.8	15	88.2	36	83.7
Moderate/ Severe	5	19.2	2	11.8	7	16.3
Physical Exercise						
No change/Mild	10	38.5	8	47.1	18	41.9
Moderate/ Severe	16	61.5	9	52.9	25	58.1
Feeding						
No change/Mild	9	34.6	8	47.1	17	39.5
Moderate/ Severe	17	65.4	9	52.9	26	60.5

Note. N = 43

ab = 0.41, CI [.11, .81]. The final model (Fig. 1), accounted for a total of 51% of the final variance of CIA total (Table 5).

Discussion

To our knowledge, this was one of the first studies to examine the impact of COVID-19 pandemic and the associated confinement measures on a cohort of patients diagnosed with eating disorders. Because these patients were participating on a naturalistic study and there was previously available data on several aspects of their psychosocial functioning, it was possible to prospectively measure the potential impact of the COVID-19 pandemic and the lockdown confinement measures.

The COVID-19 pandemic and the lockdown-imposed measures had a significant impact on patients with eating disorders. The vast majority of patients reported that the lockdown measures had impacted, moderately to severely, their life routines. Around half of the patients reported to have significant difficulties assessing medical health care and even more so accessing mental health care. Other significant changes noted were related to exercise and eating routines. This change in life routines and the increased time spent at home, in a potentially

Table 4 Correlations between impact of COVID-19 during lockdown, eating psychopathology and psychological distress variables

Variable		CIS	CIA	EDE-Q	UPPS-P	DERS-SF
1. CIS	Pearson's r	–				
	Upper 95% CI	–				
	Lower 95% CI	–				
2. CIA Total	Pearson's r	0.569***	–			
	Upper 95% CI	0.742	–			
	Lower 95% CI	0.323	–			
3. EDE-Q Total	Pearson's r	0.451**	0.819***	–		
	Upper 95% CI	0.662	0.898	–		
	Lower 95% CI	0.175	0.687	–		
4. UPPS-P	Pearson's r	0.380*	0.384*	0.392**	–	
	Upper 95% CI	0.611	0.614	0.620	–	
	Lower 95% CI	0.090	0.095	0.104	–	
5. DERS-SF Total	Pearson's r	0.393**	0.626***	0.505***	0.682***	–
	Upper 95% CI	0.620	0.780	0.699	0.816	–
	Lower 95% CI	0.106	0.401	0.241	0.480	–

* $p < .05$, ** $p < .01$, *** $p < .001$

CIS Coronavirus Impact Scale, *CIA* Clinical Impairment Assessment, *EDE-Q* Eating Disorder Examination-Questionnaire, *UPPS-P* Impulsive Behavior Scale, *DERS-SF* Difficulties in Emotion Regulation Scale-Short Form

triggering environment, might have created additional challenges to ED patients.

Curiously only a minority of patients reported moderate to severe difficulty in access to extended family and non-family social support. The fact that this was a relatively young cohort of patients with easy access to social media and internet-based communication tools, and the advertised benefit of keeping in touch with social support groups (i.e., social distancing does not mean social isolation) might have contributed to this fact.

Our data suggest that patients that experience significant changes in their living routines and report highest impact of COVID-19 crisis and lockdown measures, also experience increased psychological distress, which, in turn, may result in more disordered eating and clinical impairment. The changes imposed by the COVID-19 lockdown were significantly associated with clinical impairment. Most importantly, this impact was mediated by emotion regulation difficulties.

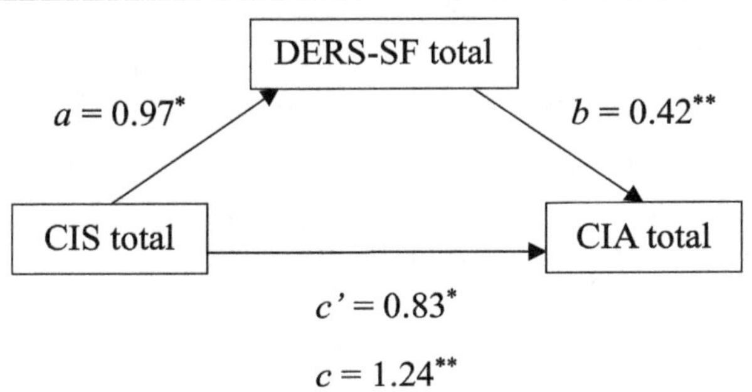

Fig. 1 Statistical diagram of the simple mediation model of the relationship between the coronavirus impact and clinical impairment, mediated by emotion regulation difficulties. CIS - Coronavirus Impact Scale; DERS-SF - Difficulties in Emotion Regulation Scale-Short Form; CIA - Clinical Impairment Assessment. * $p < .05$, ** $p < .01$

Although the COVID-19 crisis had impacted the general population as well, there are reasons to believe that those struggling with a mental health problem, and transient difficulties in accessing regular mental health care services, might be disproportionally affected by the pandemic crisis and associated measures [18]. However, further research that includes control group comparisons are needed to understand whether ED patients are significantly more affected than the general population.

To the best of our knowledge, this is one of the first studies to assess the impact of COVID-19 and lockdown measures in a cohort of ED patients that is not completely retrospective. The timing of the data collection, and the availability of data from pre-COVID-19 provided a unique opportunity to assess the impact of the pandemic crisis and associated lockdown measures. However, the current study has limitations, namely: 1) the use of a convenient, relatively small, sample based on an ongoing naturalistic study, 2) the use of phone interviews in the second wave of data collection as opposed to face-to-face in the first one; 3) the use of self-report measures and self-report height and weight that might have introduced some bias; 4) most patients that we approached, for various reasons, did not take part of the study; and, 5) findings reflect the experience of a sample of patients in Portugal.

Table 5 Model coefficients for the mediation model

Antecedent	Consequent	M (DERS-SF total)				Y (CIA total)		
		Coeff.	SE	p		Coeff.	SE	p
X (CIS total)	a	0.97	0.35	.009	c′	0.83	0.26	.003
M (DERS-SF total)		–	–	–	b	0.42	0.11	< .001
Constant	i_M	35.07	5.02	< .001	i_Y	−10.85	5.05	.038
		$R^2 = 0.15$				$R^2 = 0.51$		
		$F(1, 41) = 7.51$, $p = .009$				$F(2, 40) = 21.20$, $p = < .001$		

Note. N = 43, *CIS* Coronavirus Impact Scale, *DERS-SF* Difficulties in Emotion Regulation Scale - Short Form, *CIA* Clinical Impairment Assessment

Conclusions

Those struggling with eating disorders may experience worsening of their condition, especially if associated with difficulties in emotion regulation, and these difficulties might be exacerbated in the context of a stressful crisis and lockdown measures. Given the need to plan for future adjustments to deal with COVID-19 is important to take these findings into consideration. Future interventions need to include self-help strategies that provide structure when usual routines are disrupted and adaptive emotion regulation strategies to deal with stressful events.

Abbreviations

ED: Eating Disorders; COVID-19: Coronavirus disease 2019;; EDE-Q: Eating Disorder Examination-Questionnaire; CIA: Clinical Impairment Assessment; UPPS-P: Impulsive Behavior Scale-Negative Urgency Subscale; DERS-SF: Difficulties in Emotion Regulation Scale - Short Form; CIS: Coronavirus Impact Scale; CS: Change scores; SPSS: Statistical package for the social sciences

Acknowledgements

The authors wish to acknowledge, Sertório Timóteo, MD and Patrícia Nunes, MD, at the University Hospital Center of São João, for their collaboration in collecting data for this study. Also, we would like to thank the participants for their willingness to contribute to this study.

Authors' contributions

All authors contributed to the planning and design of the study. PPM took primary responsibility for the manuscript, including reviewing relevant literature and drafting the paper for publication. APB was responsible for recruitment of participants and data collection, contributed to its analysis and interpretation. RR managed the database, contributed to its analysis, and interpretation. TFR contributed to its analysis and interpretation. EL collaborated in data collection and participants recruiting. IB conducted diagnostic interviews. All authors assisted with literature review and editing of the manuscript. All authors read and approved the final manuscript.

Competing interests

The authors declare that they have no competing interests.

Author details

[1]Psychotherapy and Psychopathology Research Unit – Psychology Research Centre, University of Minho, School of Psychology, Braga, Portugal. [2]Faculty of Medicine, Psychiatry Department, University Hospital Center of São João, 4200-319 Porto, Portugal.

References

1. Touyz S, Lacey H, Hay P. Eating disorders in the time of COVID-19. J Eat Disord. 2020;8:8–10. https://doi.org/10.1186/s40337-020-00295-3..
2. Fernández-Aranda F, Casas M, Claes L, Bryan DC, Favaro A, Granero R, et al. COVID-19 and implications for eating disorders. Eur Eat Disord Rev. 2020;28: 239–45. https://doi.org/10.1002/erv.2738.
3. Phillipou A, Meyer D, Neill E, Tan EJ, Toh WL, Van Rheenen TE, et al. Eating and exercise behaviors in eating disorders and the general population during the COVID-19 pandemic in Australia: initial results from the COLLATE project. Int. J. Eat. Disord. 2020;53:1158–65. https://doi.org/10.1002/eat.23317.
4. Rodgers RF, Lombardo C, Cerolini S, Franko DL, Omori M, Fuller-Tyszkiewicz M, et al. The impact of the COVID-19 pandemic on eating disorder risk and symptoms. Int J Eat Disord. 2020;53:1166–70. https://doi.org/10.1002/eat.23318.
5. Fernández-Aranda F, Munguía L, Mestre-Bach G, et al. COVID Isolation Eating Scale (CIES): Analysis of the impact of confinement in eating disorders and obesity—A collaborative international study. Eur Eat Disord Rev. n/a(n/a). https://doi.org/10.1002/erv.2784.
6. Holmes EA, O'Connor RC, Perry VH, Tracey I, Wessely S, Arseneault L, et al. Multidisciplinary research priorities for the COVID-19 pandemic: a call for action for mental health science. Lancet Psychiatry. 2020;7:547–60. https://doi.org/10.1016/S2215-0366(20)30168-11.
7. Fairburn CG, Beglin SJ. Eating Disorder Examination Questionnaire (6.0). In: Fairburn CG, editor. Cogn. Behav. Ther. Eat. Disord. New York: Guilford Press; 2008. p. 309–13.
8. Machado P, Martins C, Vaz A, Conceição E, Pinto-Bastos A, Gonçalves S. Eating disorder examination questionnaire (EDE-Q): psychometric properties and norms for the Portuguese population. Eur Eat Disord Rev. 2014;22:448–53. https://doi.org/10.1002/erv.2318.
9. Bohn K, Fairburn CG. The Clinical Impairment Assessment Questionnaire (CIA 3.0). In: Fairburn CG, editor. Cogn. Behav. Ther. Eat. Disord. New York, NY: Guilford Press; 2008. p. 315–8.
10. Vaz AR, Conceição E, Pinto-Bastos A, Silva D, Machado PPP. Validation of the Portuguese version of the clinical impairment assessment (CIA) in eating disorders' patients. Eat Weight Disord. 2020;25:627–35. https://doi.org/10.1007/s40519-019-00661-4.
11. Whiteside SP, Lynam DR, Miller JD, Reynolds SK. Validation of the UPPS impulsive behavior scale: a four factor model of impulsivity. Eur J Personal. 2005;574:559–74. https://doi.org/10.1002/per.556.
12. Kaufman EA, Xia M, Fosco G, Yaptangco M, Skidmore CR, Crowell SE. The difficulties in emotion regulation scale short form (DERS-SF): validation and replication in adolescent and adult samples. J Psychopathol Behav Assess. 2016;38:443–55. https://doi.org/10.1007/s10862-015-9529-3.
13. Moreira H, Gouveia MJ, Canavarro MC. A bifactor analysis of the difficulties in emotion regulation scale - short form (DERS-SF) in a sample of adolescents and adults. Curr Psychol Current Psychol. 2020. https://doi.org/10.1007/s12144-019-00602-5.
14. Kaufman J, Stoddard J. Coronavirus impact scale. 2020; https://disasterinfo.nlm.nih.gov/search/?source=2587. Accessed 28 April 2020.
15. Hayes AF, Rockwood NJ. Regression-based statistical mediation and moderation analysis in clinical research: observations, recommendations, and implementation. Behav Res Ther. 2017;98:39–57. https://doi.org/10.1016/j.brat.2016.11.001.

16. Hayes AF. Introduction to mediation, moderation, and conditional process analysis: A regression-based approach. 2nd ed: New York: Guilford Press; 2018.
17. Jacobson NS, Truax P. Clinical significance: a statistical approach to defining meaningful change in psychotherapy research. J Consult Clin Psychol. 1991; 59:12–9. https://doi.org/10.1037/10109-042.
18. Moreno C, Wykes T, Galderisi S, et al. How mental health care should change as a consequence of the COVID-19 pandemic. Lancet Psychiatry. 2020;7(9):813–24. https://doi.org/10.1016/S2215-0366(20)30307-2.

4

Exploring the impact of the COVID-19 pandemic and UK lockdown on individuals with experience of eating disorders

Dawn Branley-Bell* and Catherine V. Talbot

Abstract

Background: The coronavirus disease 2019 (COVID-19) pandemic may raise unique challenges for individuals with experience of eating disorders. Many factors have potential for detrimental impacts on psychological wellbeing and eating disorder recovery, including: Disruption to living situations, 'social distancing' restrictions, difficult access to healthcare, and societal changes to food behaviours and technology usage. To date, little is known on the impact of the pandemic on this population, particularly within the UK.

Method: A mixed-methods online survey was developed for the purpose of this study. Data was collected from 129 individuals currently experiencing, or in recovery from, an eating disorder during the early stages of the UK pandemic lockdown. Participants were aged between 16 and 65 years, with 121 participants identifying as female, 7 male and 1 participant preferring not to disclose their gender.

Results: Findings suggest that the pandemic is having a profound, negative impact upon individuals with experience of eating disorders. Eight key themes were generated: Disruption to living situation, increased social isolation and reduced access to usual support networks, changes to physical activity rates, reduced access to healthcare services, disruption to routine and perceived control, changes to relationship with food, increased exposure to triggering messages, and positive outcomes. The results suggest detrimental impacts on psychological wellbeing including decreased feelings of control, increased feelings of social isolation, increased rumination about disordered eating, and low feelings of social support.

Conclusions: Individuals with eating disorders are at significant risk of negative impacts of the pandemic. There is a vital need for interventions to support this population. Inequalities in healthcare provision were identified, emphasising a need for a more cohesive approach to remote treatment across UK healthcare services. Positive aspects of technology use were identified but the results suggest a need to address and/or limit the potential for negative impacts of public messages around food and exercise behaviours, and to co-design technologies with end-users to facilitate effective treatment.

Keywords: Pandemics, Coronavirus, COVID-19, Eating disorders, anorexia nervosa, Bulimia nervosa, Vulnerable populations, Healthcare

* Correspondence: dawn.branley-bell@northumbria.ac.uk
Department of Psychology, Northumbria University, Newcastle upon Tyne, England, UK

Plain English summary

This research uses an online survey to gather data from individuals in the UK with experience of eating disorders during the coronavirus disease 2019 (COVID-19) pandemic. The results suggest that disruptions to daily life as a result of lockdown and 'social distancing' may have a negative impact on individuals' wellbeing. Negative effects may be due to changes to individuals': regular routine, living situation, time spent with friends and family, access to treatment, engagement in physical activity, relationship with food and use of technology. The research discusses how these issues can be addressed via further developments within healthcare, research, governance and policy. This could benefit those experiencing eating disorders and also mental health issues more broadly.

Introduction

Individuals with, or in recovery from, eating disorders (EDs) are likely to be negatively impacted by the COVID-19 pandemic. ED symptoms may be exacerbated by media exposure, disruption to daily activities, social isolation, modified physical activity and sleep, and negative affect and fear of contagion [1]. The pandemic may also lower protective capacity and access to care, by restricting access to social support, treatment, and adaptive coping strategies [1]. Psychological factors linked to ED symptoms will likely be exacerbated by the pandemic and associated lockdown. For example, stress [2, 3], health anxieties and contamination fears [2, 4, 5], perceived lack of control and problems with emotional regulation [5, 6], reliance upon routine, structure [4, 5], and social isolation [3, 5].

Technology may play an important role at this pivotal time when physical socialisation is limited and virtual interaction comes into its own. Internet use has been linked to both negative and positive consequences for this population [7]. Thus, it is important to investigate the role that technology is playing at the current time. As a result of the pandemic, healthcare organisations also find themselves suddenly relying more heavily on virtual methods to deliver treatment and support. Research is already underway to identify how therapy for EDs can be translated to online delivery [8, 9]. Despite these efforts, healthcare organisations - and those receiving treatment – may face significant challenges with the move to remote healthcare [4]. For a population that can require regular in-person appointments [5], this reduction in service provision could be catastrophic.

Researchers from across the globe have started to investigate the impact of the pandemic upon individuals experiencing EDs. Early studies from Singapore and Barcelona highlight how increased anxiety is having a negative impact [2, 10]. In Australia, Phillipou et al. [11] found evidence of increased restricting, binge eating, purging, and exercise among this population. Many reports focus upon countries with greater experience of infectious disease outbreaks (e.g., [4, 5, 12]). These countries are generally more prepared for dealing with the pandemic than others [5] due to previous experience of contact tracing and disease surveillance, provision of emergency healthcare resources needed for isolation, and co-ordinated public health messaging. There are other global studies in progress, e.g., in Australia [11], the United States [13] and the Netherlands [13]. However, research within the United Kingdom (UK) is limited. Fernández-Aranda et al. [10] conducted a small, qualitative UK study ($N = 8$) describing some of the challenges faced by those with EDs during COVID-19. However, no quantitative data was reported, and the sample was specific to those with Anorexia. To the best of our knowledge, there has been no empirical work conducted with people with EDs in the UK during the pandemic. The current research addresses this, with the aim of investigating the impact of the pandemic and UK lockdown on the lives of people with experience of EDs. In addition to raising awareness, the results could influence future health service provisions, guidance and policies.

Methods

Sample

One hundred fifty-three participants were recruited via social media (Twitter and Facebook) using opportunistic and snowball sampling. Inclusion criteria was: Over 16 years of age, current UK resident, experience of an ED (including those in recovery). Recruitment was limited to the UK to allow the researchers to accurately identify the stage of the pandemic and the lockdown, and to ensure that data was comparable in this regard. Twenty-four participants were excluded due to not proceeding past the first page of the survey or not meeting the inclusion criteria. The final sample consisted of 129 participants, aged between 16 and 65 years ($M = 29.27$ yrs., $SD = 8.99$ yrs). One hundred twenty-one participants identified as female (93.8%), 7 male (5.4%) and 1 (0.8%) participant preferring not to disclose their gender. The majority ($N = 80$, 62%) of the sample described themselves as currently experiencing an ED (including those in a period of relapse), 8 (6.2%) described themselves as "in recovery <3 months", 8 (6.2%) "in recovery between 3-12 months", and 33 (25.6%) "in recovery >12 months".

Procedure and measures

Recruitment took place in early April 2020, 2 weeks after UK lockdown restrictions were first enforced. Participants completed an anonymous online survey containing questions around their experience of EDs and the pandemic. This included closed and open-ended questions about: the social impact of the lockdown; internet usage;

food and exercise behaviours; and the overall impact of the pandemic on their EDs. Established scales were used to measure: Mental wellbeing, perceived stress, social support, perceived control and rumination (see Supplementary Material 1).

Short Warwick-Edinburgh mental wellbeing scale

The 7-item Short Warwick-Edinburgh Mental Wellbeing Scale (SWEMWBS: [14, 15]) was used to measure emotional and functioning aspects of mental wellbeing. Scores range from 7 to 35, with higher scores indicative of greater mental wellbeing. Cronbach's alpha for the scale in the current study = .81.

Perceived stress scale

The Perceived Stress Scale (PSS: [16]) is one of the most widely applied measures of perceived stress, i.e., the degree to which an individual perceives situations within their life as stressful. The shortened 4-item version was used in the current study as it has been shown to maintain good validity and reliability [17]. The PSS-4 gives a score out of 16, with higher scores indicating greater perceived stress. Cronbach's alpha = .72.

ENRICHD social support instrument

The ENRIHD Social Support Instrument (ESSI: [22, 23]) is a 7-item measure of social support, i.e., the existence or availability of people on who an individual can rely. Scores range between 8 to 34, with higher scores indicating greater social support. Cronbach's alpha = .86.

Shapiro control inventory

To measure perceived control we used the Shapiro Control Inventory (SCI, [24]) general domain sense of control scale. This 16-item scale encompasses positive and negative sense of control. Scores range between 16 and 112 with higher scores indicating greater perceptions of control. Cronbach's alpha = .86.

Rumination response scale for ED

The Rumination Response Scale for Eating Disorders (RRS-ED, [25]) is a 9-item measure of preoccupation with ruminative themes of eating, weight and shape. It is the first self-report measure to specifically capture ED rumination. The measure gives a total score between 9 and 36, with higher scores indicative of greater rumination. Cronbach's alpha = .86.

Analytical approach

A mixed methods approach was applied. Descriptive statistics, and between group comparisons (current ED group vs. recovery group) were complemented with thematic analysis of the qualitative data (using NVivo12). The second author coded the dataset independently using both an inductive and deductive approach, whereby some categories were developed prior to the analysis and others were generated from the data. Codes were collated to identify initial themes. To increase rigor, a team approach was taken with the first author providing critical feedback on themes and coding. Amendments were made where appropriate. The finalised themes were then generated and agreed upon by both authors.

Results

Quantitative measures

Mean scores for the five scales are provided for participants categorised into two groups: those currently experiencing an ED, and those who report being in recovery (Table 1).

Significant differences were found between the two groups for all measures except the rumination scale which just failed to reach significance ($p = .052$). The group differences are in the direction that would be expected with the recovery group showing higher mental wellbeing, lower perceived stress [2, 3], higher social support [3, 5] and higher perceived control [5, 6]. The borderline significant result was also in the expected direction with those in recovery scoring lower for ED rumination [26].

Overall impact of the pandemic

When asked about the overall impact of the pandemic on their ED symptoms, an overwhelming majority (86.7%) reported that their symptoms had worsened as a result of the pandemic, with over 30% reporting that their symptoms were *much* worse. In contrast, only 2 participants reported a slight improvement in their symptoms (Table 2).

We explore potential factors for this detrimental impact further in the following section.

Themes

The analysis generated eight themes relating specifically to the effects of the pandemic and associated lockdown: (1) Disruption to living situation; (2) Increased social isolation and reduced access to usual support networks;

Table 1 Participant scores for mental wellbeing, perceived stress, social support, perceived control and ED rumination

	Current ED			In Recovery		
	N	*M*	*SD*	*N*	*M*	*SD*
Mental Wellbeing (WEMWBS)	80	16.35*	3.24	49	17.66*	2.48
Perceived Stress (PSS)	80	14.66**	2.61	49	13.10**	2.71
Social Support (ESSI)	80	19.76*	5.71	49	21.94*	6.47
Control (SCI-general)	77	54.52**	13.15	48	62.71**	12.74
Rumination (RRS-ED)	76	22.67†	6.96	47	20.04†	7.59

Significant differences between the groups are indicated. ** $p = .001$ * $p < .05$
†p = borderline (.052)

Table 2 Participants' reported overall impact of the pandemic on their ED symptoms ($N = 129$)

	N	%
Symptoms much worse	38	30.9
Moderately worse	48	37.2
Slightly worse	24	18.6
No change	11	8.5
Slightly better	2	1.6
Moderately better	0	0
Symptoms much better	0	0
Missing	6	4.7

(3) Changes to physical activity rates; (4) Reduced access to healthcare services; (5) Disruption to routine and perceived control; (6) Increased exposure to triggering messages; (7) Changes to the individual's relationship with food; (8) Positive outcomes.

Disruption to living situation

Over a fifth of participants reported a change to their normal living situation due to the pandemic (Table 3). When asked whether they felt this change had affected their ED symptoms, 85.2% reported that the change had worsened their symptoms. Reasons included: Increased interpersonal stresses, hiding their ED from others, increased scrutiny and/or pressure from others to eat more, and a loss of control over diet. For example, one participant describes how their relationship is impacting upon their ED:

> My relationship with my partner significantly impacts my eating behaviours and this has been worse since the pandemic.

Whilst hiding their ED from others left some participants reporting feelings of being "trapped", "incredibly low" and "unhappy":

> I'm trapped at home with people who don't know I have anorexia. I am hiding and lying constantly.

When describing the challenges associated with being in lockdown with partners or family members, participants tended to refer to mealtimes. Specifically, participants felt that the people they lived with were often critical of their eating behaviours:

> I have much less choice of what I eat and I have to eat most of my meals in front (and in scrutiny) of others and that is causing enormous stress.

This pressure to eat appears to be worsened by others worrying that the individual will be unable to recover if they contract COVID-19, due to not correctly fuelling their body:

> My mother is particularly concerned about me because I "do not give my body enough energy to overcome the virus" if I contracted it, and she wants me to eat more because of this. This is weighing on my mind because I absolutely do not want to do this.

Suddenly living with others resulted in many participants losing control over the meals they were able to eat, for example due to others taking responsibility for cooking:

> My partner is making more of our meals so I'm less certain about the ingredients and amounts, so less able to track this using MyFitnessPal. I'm also less in control of what I eat for breakfast and lunch, when usually I would have full control over this in the office.

In the likely event of the pandemic continuing for some time, the prolonged stress of living in challenging environments could be particularly detrimental for those experiencing EDs.

Social isolation and reduced access to usual social support networks

The vast majority (86.4%) of our sample reported greater feelings of social isolation as a result of the pandemic (Table 3). For many individuals, spending time with friends and family represents a vital factor in their ED recovery. Lockdown has resulted in many participants being unable to access and/or physically engage with these support networks. Impacts of this include worsened ED symptoms and reduced motivation for recovery:

> Unable to see friends, who are supportive and boost my mood (which affects my eating).

The social aspect of eating can be particularly important for helping some individuals manage their symptoms. Going 'out' for food can provide an important coping mechanism to encourage them to eat. The lockdown clearly impedes this:

> The MAJORITY of my "safe" eating takes place outside of the house. E.g. getting coffees, going to Pret for food I am familiar and comfortable with. There is something less shameful and "holding" for me about eating out, and that isn't the case at home. Now I have to eat more at home, on my own, and the isolation around eating and exercise is not a good place for me to be.

Unfortunately, isolation can also impact recovery through reduced feelings of accountability. Whilst individuals who find themselves suddenly living with others may experience increased feelings of scrutiny and pressure to recover (refer to Disruption to living situation section), the opposite can occur for those who find themselves isolated from others. Over 20% of our sample reported feeling less social pressure to recover due to the pandemic:

> Not seeing those close to me who would recognise my losing weight and deterioration has put me under less pressure to challenge my ED as I can unwitnessed lose weight without challenge from others which is less pressure for me.

Some participants felt that they were becoming more restrictive with their diet and expressed concerns around the impacts that this could have, not only now, but to their future recovery:

> I am concerned that I am becoming more rigid about what I eat when I had moved on from this. I worry it will be harder to go back to social eating.

Here, we are provided with a crucial reminder that the impacts of the pandemic are likely to be felt for a prolonged period of time; continuing after cessation of the lockdown and the return to 'normality'. It is also important to recognise that ED behaviour that occurred during the pandemic may have been reinforced by repetition during a lengthy lockdown period. These reinforced or 'habitual' behaviours can be resistant to change.

Changes to physical activity rates

Participant responses to the impact of the pandemic upon physical activity were varied. The researchers initially assumed that physical activity rates may drop as a result of lockdown, and indeed almost half of our sample reported a reduction in physical activity. However, 36.5% reported an *increase* in physical activity (Table 3). Qualitative responses indicate that activity increases were primarily driven by anxieties about weight gain and a desire to counteract the effects of inactivity during lockdown:

> I was doing lots before but even more now partly because I actually like it, partly to fill the time, partly from an unhealthy driven mentality. Rest days now feel unnecessary because I'm resting every day if I'm not working.

Not being able to freely engage in ED behaviours such as bingeing and purging provided another driver:

> Now people are home with me my binge purge has reduced to every other day. However, my exercise has increased to compensate for this.

It can be easier for others to monitor or 'police' eating behaviours than it is to identify when an individual has crossed the line between healthy exercise and excessive, detrimental activity levels. It can also be easier for individuals to defend and rationalise physical activity, especially during lockdown when daily exercise was so widely discussed in government daily COVID-19 updates. Participants were aware of this tension between healthy activity and over-exercise, and reported finding it difficult to manage their relationship with exercise during lockdown:

> There is part of me that wants to do all of the exercise, to 'get thin' and to listen to the disorder. But there is also part of me that knows I need to moderate my exercise because it's so triggering for me.

For those who did report a *decrease* in activity, the same anxieties around weight gain provided a driver for engaging in restrictive eating behaviours:

> Can't exercise as much / the way I was, and not getting as many steps, so being more restrictive with foods eaten, calories, and timing of eating (doing intermittent fasting again).

This demonstrates that the pandemic can increase symptoms both in relation to eating behaviours and/or excessive exercise, depending upon the individual and the context they find themselves in during lockdown (Table 3).

Reduced access to healthcare services

One of the major challenges faced by participants was a reduction in healthcare service provision and/or discrepancies in access to healthcare services. Participants reported being prematurely discharged from inpatient units, having treatment suspended or remaining on a waiting list for treatment, and receiving limited post-diagnostic support:

> The pandemic meant that I was discharged suddenly and prematurely from inpatient treatment, and has also meant that my post-discharge support is limited.

It was clearly a distressing time for participants, and a reduction in service provision caused some participants to feel like a *"burden"*, an *"inconvenience"*, and *"forgotten"* by the government and NHS. The consequences of not being able to access professional treatment during

Table 3 Reported changes due to COVID-19 pandemic and effect on ED symptoms

Factor	Changed due to pandemic	*N*	%	Effect of change on symptoms (of those who indicated change)	*N*	%
Living situation	Yes	27	20.9	Symptoms much worse	1	3.7
	No	98	76	Moderately worse	11	40.7
	Other	4	3.1	Slightly worse	11	40.7
	Total	129	–	No change	2	7.4
				Slightly better	1	3.7
				Moderately better	1	3.7
				Symptoms Much better	0	0
				Missing	0	0
				Total	27	–
Social isolation	Much more isolated	56	43.4	Symptoms much worse	33	28.2
	Moderately more isolated	35	27.1	Moderately worse	45	38.5
	Slightly more isolated	17	13.2	Slightly worse	24	20.5
	No change	8	6.2	No change	12	10.3
	Slightly less isolated	5	3.9	Slightly better	2	1.7
	Moderately less isolated	4	3.1	Moderately better	0	0
	Much less isolated	0	0	Symptoms Much better	0	0
	Missing	4	3.1	Missing	1	0.9
	Total	129	–	Total	117	–
Usual support network(s)	Yes	93	72.1	Symptoms much worse	14	15.1
	No	31	24	Moderately worse	26	28
	Missing	5	3.9	Slightly worse	27	29
	Total	129	–	No change	23	24.7
				Slightly better	3	3.2
				Moderately better	0	0
				Symptoms Much better	0	0
				Missing	0	0
				Total	93	–
Physical activity	Much less physical activity	36	27.9	Symptoms much worse	41	36.9
	Moderately less	15	11.6	Moderately worse	32	28.8
	Slightly less	13	10.1	Slightly worse	28	25.2
	No change	13	10.1	No change	8	7.2
	Slightly more	16	12.4	Slightly better	1	0.9
	Moderately more	13	10.1	Moderately better	0	0
	Much more	18	14	Much better	1	0.9
	Missing	5	3.9	Missing	0	0
	Total	129	–	Total	111	–

the pandemic could be severe, and in some cases even fatal. These concerns were echoed by one participant:

> People are going to die during this from their ED because they are unable to be physically monitored.

Unfortunately, this reduced physical monitoring links back to the aforementioned lack of accountability (refer to Social isolation and reduced access to usual social support networks section) with participants reporting feeling greater 'opportunity' to engage in undetected ED behaviours:

> Because I no longer can go to the day service, my anorexia makes me believe it's a chance to 'get away' with me e.g. losing a ton of weight.

Despite the reduction in service provision, some participants stated that they were still able to access professional healthcare services via technology, such as video-calling software. However, whilst online support was described as a positive factor, participants described this as falling short of treatment and support received in-person. They did not view online treatment as a direct replacement for face-to-face support, but rather the 'next best thing' or the 'only alternative' when traditional support mechanisms were unavailable:

> I wouldn't usually access phone support or video chat. I dislike doing these, but felt I had to having lost my face to face support.

Unfortunately, participants reported discrepancies in access to services. Not all services are using technology to support individuals during the pandemic – or they have been delayed in their provision of such services. One participant described the inequality in service provision across the UK as a *"postcode lottery"*:

> There is a postcode lottery in terms of what services are now providing, some patients in some areas were offered video chat straight away, my service still haven't got this up and running.

Remote services also raised their own, perhaps unexpected, issues. For example, some participants felt that video calling was having a detrimental effect on their ED. Seeing their own video during the call, made some participants more aware and more critical of their appearance:

> Have seen myself more and made me question if I good enough or look good. Also, things have changed to online video conferencing. It's just the amount of time seeing yourself.

It is vital that researchers and service providers accurately assess the appropriateness of technologies for remote service provision.

Some participants were also concerned about being asked to self-monitor by healthcare professionals, whilst relying on remote treatment. Many individuals experiencing EDs choose not to keep weighing scales in their homes as this can lead to an unhealthy fixation on their weight. This is in direct conflict with being asked to self-monitor to enable remote treatment:

> Many of us trying to recover have gotten rid of our scales as for some they fuel the compulsive nature of the ED - I wonder how many will worsen due to being told to buy scales from ED services.

> The challenges of physical monitoring - the ED service that I am under would prefer for me to have own scales and self-report weight whereas GP sees this as a big risk in itself (I would become dangerously fixated on the number).

Our findings highlight discrepancies in service provision, a lack of consistency in advice between services, concerns around the suitability of some remote treatment methods, and the need to develop clear evidence-based guidelines for best practice.

Disruption to routine and perceived control

For many, keeping to a regular routine is vital for ED recovery and relapse prevention. Unfortunately, many routines have been significantly impacted as a result of lockdown:

> Feeling frustrated because I've been learning how to control the bulimic symptoms and normally able to manage them. Yet the change in routine (or lack of) and general stress/anxiety is unsettling it and noticed my thoughts and behaviours changing.

The majority of participants (65.9%) reported some change to their usual coping mechanisms as a result of the pandemic. A lack of routine and/or distractions created more time for rumination about weight, exercise habits, and meals. Routine can also contribute to an individual's perceived sense of control; another significant factor in recovery and general psychological wellbeing. When perceived control is low (such as during the pandemic), disordered eating can represent one thing that the individual *can* control:

> Normally when I am in control over everything I am able to do better. I currently have less control of being able to go out, my studying, work etc and I feel subconsciously I am controlling this with food.

Due to the pandemic's overwhelming impact on routines, we may see an increase in ED behaviours as a coping mechanism.

Increased exposure to triggering messages

Unsurprisingly, given the current lockdown, the majority (81.4%) of participants reported spending more time online. This is a trend seen in the population more generally, with digital spaces switching from an amenity to a necessity . When asked whether this had an effect upon their ED symptoms, over half (55%) of our sample reported that this increase in time online had worsened their symptoms (Table 4).

Table 4 Changes to time spent online due to the COVID-19 pandemic

Time spent online	*N*	%	Effect on ED symptoms[a]	*N*	%
Much more time	47	36.4	Symptoms much worse	11	9.9
Moderately more time	34	26.4	Moderately worse	24	21.6
Slightly more time	24	18.6	Slightly worse	27	24.3
No change	13	10.1	No change	44	39.6
Slightly less time	3	2.3	Slightly better	4	3.6
Moderately less time	3	2.3	Moderately better	0	0
Much less time	0	0	Much better	0	0
Missing	5	3.9	Missing	1	0.9
Total	129	–	Total	111	–

[a]excludes those participants who reported 'no change' for time spent online

There are numerous reasons why time online could have a negative impact for those experiencing an ED. For example, it is possible that without their usual social support networks and professional healthcare services, individuals may find support from less helpful sources, encounter extreme content (such as pro-anorexia content) or come across misinformation online [7]. This was supported by some participants mentioning that they accessed pro-ana websites and/or searched for "thinspo" content. However, for many participants, the main contributing factors appeared to be the increase in food and exercise-related messages dominating public discourse. For example, many social media posts refer to the general public's *"fear of gaining weight"* during lockdown. These messages can be particularly triggering for individuals living with EDs:

> There is a lot going around social media such as putting on weight during COVID-19 due to not doing as much and that is really triggering for people like myself as straight away my head thinks, that can't happen to me! I must change the way I am towards food etc.

There has also been an increase in posts about physical activity, for example, people sharing information on their 'daily exercise' or sharing content to encourage others to stay active at home (including increased availability of workout content, e.g., the free daily YouTube workouts delivered by 'body coach' Joe Wicks). Excessive exercise is a major factor in many EDs and participants reported finding it difficult to cope with this increased emphasis around physical activity:

> There is a heavier push on ALL social platforms to 'stay for' and 'stay in shape'. Any coping mechanisms I did have before have changed. I struggle with exercise mainly, and with everything being in the spotlight it's harder to look away from it and ignore it.

Content promoting exercise, also caused participants to engage in social comparisons (e.g., comparing their body to others, or comparing their level of exercise):

> Watching work out videos judging myself for my lack of motivation to do anything and just how disgusting my body is compared to everyone else's out there. Everyone is doing self-improvement and I'm not.

These messages not only dominated social media, but also mass media stories:

> I think the messages we are given through the media right now are that by eating "healthy" and "keeping active" we are somehow protecting ourselves from the virus. Actually, I don't think there is sufficient, scientifically valid evidence that this is the case. I can be rational about this, but nonetheless, I find these constant reminders quite triggering.

Whilst public health initiatives that promote healthy eating and exercise might be beneficial for some members of the general public, it is clear from participants' statements that a focus on exercise and food can be triggering for people with EDs. This is particularly important when screen time is likely to be increased due to lockdown.

Changes to relationship with food

The lockdown has resulted in a change in food behaviours across the population, for example we have seen evidence of food hoarding leading to supply shortages. Of the participants in our study, 66.7% reported that their relationship with food has changed due to the pandemic. Lockdown can result in individuals having a shortage of food in the house (or provide them with a reason to justify a lack of supplies), or excess amounts if they are in a household that has stocked up. Any changes to food behaviours have the potential to have a significant impact upon individuals with experience of EDs. We can see some of the range of impacts in our data. Some participants raised concerns about being more likely to binge during the pandemic due to increased access to food in the household:

> Being at home makes me more likely to binge as there is more food in the house.

Participants also reported increased levels of rumination over their food intake, which they attributed to its *"scarcity"* and being unable to purchase *"safe foods"*, referring to food that is often low in calories that a person feels is safe to eat:

> I feel like I am thinking more and more about food. Part of it is scarcity and the inability to eat healthy food - this has made me feel a bit trapped and like it's all I can focus on.

A perceived scarcity of food during the pandemic caused some participants to feel guilty for eating food. These participants said they felt *"less deserving"* of food than other people:

> Restriction can become a 'reasonable' thing to do because you're saving food for later or someone else.

For these participants, the pandemic reinforced their ED behaviours by providing them with a way of rationalising food restriction. In addition to experiencing increased feelings of guilt, many participants also expressed that their relationship with food had become more negative and purely functional as a result of the pandemic:

> Totally unenjoyable; purely functional, seeing as a 'prescription medication', a means to an end, almost resentful of food.

Interestingly, some participants used the pandemic to rationalise their food restrictions for other reasons stating that they felt they were *"less likely to get sick with anything if I don't eat"*. This is a stark contrast from the attitudes they reported from friends and family who encourage them to eat to prevent getting sick (see Disruption to living situation section).

Positive outcomes

It was uplifting to also see positive signs of adaptive coping mechanisms within our data, primarily in response to the use of technology to access support. Due to reduced physical access to usual support networks, some participants reported using the internet and social media (e.g., Facebook groups, WhatsApp, and YouTube) to speak to friends, access support from ED communities, and to follow others' journeys to/of recovery. These platforms can represent an important resource during periods of isolation. Social media appears to facilitate social connection and support, thus combatting some of the challenges of the pandemic:

> Looking at support networks for bulimia and talking to friends who know I'm fearing a relapse due to this pandemic.

Some participants identified unexpected, positive impacts of the pandemic. For example, for some individuals the restrictions on ED behaviour attributed with changes in their living situation were identified as a positive:

> Binging [sic] and purging has reduced. I was doing this 5 times a day. Now people are home with me my binge purge has reduced to every other day.

This stands in stark contrast with many participants' experiences, who found changes in living situation to be incredibly stressful (see Disruption to living situation section).

Others found positives in the social distancing imposed by lockdown. For example, explaining that reduced social interaction also reduced social comparisons, thereby reducing anxiety:

> Fewer social interactions with others maybe mean fewer self-comparisons with others & also not experiencing same level of anxieties about being 'at fault' in some way

Others reflected on their choice of clothing during the lockdown period, reporting that they wore more comfortable clothing that was less triggering of their symptoms:

> I have been less critical of and aware of my body and its day to day changes. This is because I have been wearing only leggings or tracksuits and yoga bras and haven't been 'triggered' by uncomfortable clothing -previously my Jeans would dig in after lunch and I would fall into a spiral of thinking I'd gained weight/body checking etc.

However, it should be noted that these individuals are not representative of the vast majority of participants, with many experiencing increased pressures and stress as a result of the pandemic. Also some positives, such as those associated with a lack of social interaction, may not represent a healthy long-term solution.

Discussion

Our findings highlight eight key themes describing how the COVID-19 pandemic is affecting individuals with experience of EDs: (1) Disruption to living situation; (2) Increased social isolation and reduced access to usual support networks; (3) Changes to physical activity rates; (4) Reduced access to healthcare services; (5) Disruption to routine and perceived control; (6) Changes to relationship with food; (7) Increased exposure to triggering messages; and (8) Positive outcomes.

In keeping with previous research, our findings suggest that patients (and their loved ones) may be grateful of opportunities for remote treatment and support when in-person alternatives are not available [5, 10] – something also suggested in the recent COVID-19 call to action [3]. Preliminary findings suggest that health treatment delivered remotely via technology may be effective for those experiencing EDs, however it is noted that there is still limited evidence in this regard and more research is necessary [5]. It is also noted that serious consideration must be given beyond digital interventions due to potential inequalities in access to technology [3].

Alarmingly, our data shows inequalities in UK health service provision during the pandemic, this must be addressed to ensure consistency in service provision across the UK. In addition to ensuring equality of access, our findings highlight other barriers to effective remote treatment, such as how to monitor health and recovery progress without having a detrimental impact on mental wellbeing. This includes not requiring weighing scales within the individual's household, and providing alternatives to technologies, such as video-calling software, which may inadvertently make users critical of their appearance (this supports previous findings (e.g., [8, 10]). In other instances, software may have the required functions available - such as an option to 'hide self-view' - but users may not be aware of this; increasing awareness or setting this option as a default should be considered. Clear guidelines are required for the design and implementation of appropriate remote/digital health services.

Our findings demonstrate the importance of social support from friends and family. Social relationships can have a protective buffering effect from stressful events [3]. This protective effect can be diminished during lockdown periods. Future research should look to identify ways to minimise the detrimental effects of physical distancing, and develope and/or encourage alternative positive coping mechanisms.

Media coverage and social media posts were a source of anxiety for our participants, due to a public preoccupation with food, weight gain and exercise. Although positive messages about diet and exercise can be beneficial for the majority of the population, it is important for healthcare and government to acknowledge that these can be triggering or upsetting for vulnerable populations, and work to establish guidelines to help address this. Risk-elevating messages designed to nudge individuals towards social distancing and safe behaviour can also lead to increased anxiety and reduced feelings of control over the situation; again, factors linked to negative impacts on psychological wellbeing and ED symptoms. As described by Holmes et al. [3] 'research is needed to inform future approaches, including strategies to help individuals to stay informed by authoritative sources, prevent over-exposure to media, and mitigate and help manage the effect of viewing [...] traumatic content' (p. 552). Our findings suggest a need for clear guidelines - driven by the insight of those with lived experience - around media reporting, social media policies and positive strategies to manage emotional and psychological consequences.

Crucially, our findings illustrate why we must not underestimate the longevity of the impact of the pandemic. Individuals with experience of EDs will likely experience a long-term effect on their symptoms and/or recovery. It is important that this is recognised by healthcare services, and beyond, in order to offer the necessary resources to support this vulnerable population now and on an on-going basis.

The lessons learned as a consequence of the COVID-19 pandemic have the potential to be relevant to other public health emergencies, other ED populations, and to future circumstances which involve periods of lockdown, food shortages, and/or social isolation. As there are international studies in progress (e.g., [11]), cross-cultural comparisons could be an interesting area for future research – particularly in relation to how different countries have addressed ED treatment and healthcare during, and after, the pandemic.

Limitations

While this study provides an in-depth examination of the impact of the pandemic on the lives of people with EDs, it does have some limitations. Firstly, all participants were recruited via social media, resulting in the sample being biased toward those who have access to and are familiar with technology. This opportunistic approach may also have resulted in the sample being biased towards people who are currently experiencing difficulties, rather than those who are not facing challenges related to their EDs. Secondly, information about specific diagnoses was not collected. This information could be collected in future research to enable comparisons between different groups of people experiencing EDs.

Finally, data were only collected at a single time point during the early stages of the UK lockdown. The pandemic will likely continue for some time, potentially having long-lasting impacts upon the lives of individuals experiencing EDs. Thus, longitudinal research is required to investigate the long-term effects of the pandemic on this population.

Due to not having a baseline measure (i.e., pre-pandemic) it is not possible to make assumptions about the impact of the pandemic on the quantitative scale scores within our sample. Again, longitudinal research could be beneficial in this regard - allowing the comparison of data from the start of lockdown with data from later time points. This would help identify the ongoing, and potentially evolving, impact of the pandemic as it progresses. The researchers are planning a follow-up study to address this. Future research may also wish to include further quantitative analysis of the relationships between the facilitators (e.g., low perceived control) and barriers to ED (high social support) behaviour during periods of lockdown.

Conclusions

In summary, this research suggests that the ED population is at significant risk of negative impacts of the pandemic; the consequences of which may be felt long after a societal return to 'normality'. There is a vital need for interventions to support this population during the current pandemic and beyond. Interventions should be co-designed with end-users to facilitate effective treatment. Our findings also highlight inequalities in healthcare provision that must be addressed; a more cohesive approach to remote treatment is required across all UK healthcare services. Positive aspects of technology use were identified but it is also necessary to consider potential negative impacts of public messages around food and exercise behaviours.

Abbreviations

COVID-19: Coronavirus Disease 2019; ED: Eating Disorder; ESSI: ENRICHD Social Support Instrument; NHS: National Health Service; PSS: Perceived Stress Scale; RRS-ED: Rumination Response Scale for Eating Disorders; SCI: Shapiro Control Inventory; WEMWBS: Warwick-Edinburgh Mental Wellbeing Scale

Acknowledgements

Not applicable.

Authors' contributions

DB led initial idea formation and project management. Both authors were involved in designing the survey and data collection. DB led on quantitative analysis; CT led on thematic coding of qualitative data. Both authors played a major role in the write up of the results. DB led on initial preparation of the manuscript. The author(s) read and approved the final manuscript.

Competing interests

The authors declare that they have no competing interests.

References

1. Rodgers RF, Lombardo C, Cerolini S, Franko DL, Omori M, Fuller-Tyszkiewicz M, et al. The impact of the COVID-19 pandemic on eating disorder risk and symptoms. Int J Eat Disord. 2020;53:1166–70. https://doi.org/10.1002/eat.23318.
2. Yao H, Chen JH, Xu YF. Patients with mental health disorders in the COVID-19 epidemic. Lancet Psychiatry. 2020;7:e21. https://doi.org/10.1016/S2215-0366(20)30090-0.
3. Holmes EA, O'Connor RC, Perry VH, Tracey I, Wessely S, Arseneault L, et al. Multidisciplinary research priorities for the COVID-19 pandemic: a call for action for mental health science. Lancet Psychiatry. 2020;7:547–60. https://doi.org/10.1016/S2215-0366(20)30168-1.
4. Davis C, Chong NK, Oh JY, Baeg A, Rajasegaran K, Elaine Chew CS. Caring for children and adolescents with eating disorders in the current COVID-19 pandemic: a Singapore perspective. J Adolesc Health. 2020. https://doi.org/10.1016/j.jadohealth.2020.03.037.
5. Gordon CM, Katzman DK. Lessons learned in caring for adolescents with eating disorders: the Singapore experience. J Adolesc Health. 2020. https://doi.org/10.1016/j.jadohealth.2020.03.041.
6. Manasse SM, Schumacher LM, Goldstein SP, Martin GJ, Crosby RD, Juarascio AS, et al. Are individuals with loss-of-control eating more prone to dietary lapse in behavioural weight loss treatment? An ecological momentary assessment study. Eur Eat Disord Rev. 2018;26:259–64. https://doi.org/10.1002/erv.2583.
7. Branley DB, Covey J. Pro-ana versus pro-recovery: a content analytic comparison of social media users' communication about eating disorders on twitter and Tumblr. Front Psychol. 2017;8:1356. https://doi.org/10.3389/fpsyg.2017.01356.
8. Murphy R, Calugi S, Cooper Z, Dalle GR. Challenges and opportunities for enhanced cognitive behaviour therapy (CBT-E) in light of COVID-19. Cogn Behav Ther. 2020;13. https://doi.org/10.1017/S1754470X20000161.
9. Waller G, Pugh M, Mulkens S, Moore E, Mountford VA, Carter J, et al. Cognitive-behavioral therapy in the time of coronavirus: clinician tips for working with eating disorders via telehealth when face-to-face meetings are not possible. Int J Eat Disord. 2020;53:1132–41. https://doi.org/10.1002/eat.23289.
10. Fernández-Aranda F, Casas M, Claes L, Bryan DC, Favaro A, Granero R, et al. COVID-19 and implications for eating disorders. Eur Eat Disord Rev. 2020;28:239–45. https://doi.org/10.1002/erv.2738.
11. Phillipou A, Meyer D, Neill E, Tan EJ, Toh WL, Van Rheenen TE, et al. Eating and exercise behaviors in eating disorders and the general population during the COVID-19 pandemic in Australia: initial results from the COLLATE project. Int J Eat Disord. 2020;53:1158–65. https://doi.org/10.1002/eat.23317.
12. Wong JEL, Leo YS, Tan CC. COVID-19 in Singapore - current experience: critical global issues that require attention and action. J Am Med Assoc. 2020;323:1243–4. https://doi.org/10.1001/jama.2020.2467.
13. Temorshuizen JD, Watson HJ, Thornton LM, Borg S, Flatt RE, MacDermod CM, et al. Early Impact of COVID-19 on Individuals with Eating Disorders: A survey of ~1000 Individuals in the United States and the Netherlands. MedRxiv Prepr Serv Heal Sci. 2020;2020(05):28.20116301. https://doi.org/10.1101/2020.05.28.20116301.
14. Tennant R, Hiller L, Fishwick R, Platt S, Joseph S, Weich S, et al. The Warwick-Edinburgh mental well-being scale (WEMWBS): development and UK validation. Health Qual Life Outcomes. 2007;5:1–13. https://doi.org/10.1186/1477-7525-5-63.
15. NHS Health Scotland. Warwick-Edinburgh Mental Well-being Scale (WEMWBS) user guide. 2016.
16. Cohen S, Kamarck T, Mermelstein R. A global measure of perceived stress. J Health Soc Behav. 1983;24:386–96. https://doi.org/10.2307/2136404.
17. Karam F, Bérard A, Sheehy O, Huneau M-C, Briggs G, Chambers C, et al. Reliability and validity of the 4-item perceived stress scale among pregnant women: results from the OTIS antidepressants study. Res Nurs Health. 2012;35:363–75. https://doi.org/10.1002/nur.21482.
18. Vaglio J, Conard M, Poston WS, O'Keefe J, Haddock CK, House J, et al. Testing the performance of the ENRI CHD social support instrument in cardiac patients. Health Qual Life Outcomes. 2004. https://doi.org/10.1186/1477-7525-2-2.
19. Blumenthal J, Babyak M. Al. E. Enhancing recovery in coronary heart disease patients (ENRI CHD): study design and methods. Am Heart J. 2000;139:1–9. https://doi.org/10.1016/S0002-8703(00)90301-6.
20. Shapiro Jr. DH. Shapiro control inventory (SCI) manual 1994. http://controlresearch.net/shapiro-control-inventory-manual.html Accessed 4 May 2020.
21. Cowdrey FA, Park RJ. Assessing rumination in eating disorders: principal component analysis of a minimally modified ruminative response scale. Eat Behav. 2011;12:321–4. https://doi.org/10.1016/j.eatbeh.2011.08.001.
22. Smith KE, Mason TB, Lavender JM. Rumination and eating disorder psychopathology: a meta-analysis. Clin Psychol Rev. 2018;61:9–23. https://doi.org/10.1016/j.cpr.2018.03.004.
23. Gardner B, Rebar AL, Gardner B, Rebar AL. Habit formation and behavior change. Oxford Res Encycl Psychol. 2019. https://doi.org/10.1093/acrefore/9780190236557.013.129.

24. Beaunoyer E, Dupéré S, Guitton MJ. COVID-19 and digital inequalities: reciprocal impacts and mitigation strategies. Comput Human Behav. 2020; 106424. https://doi.org/10.1016/j.chb.2020.106424.
25. Southey F. Panic buying amid coronavirus fears. [Online] Available at: https://www.foodnavigator.com/Article/2020/03/27/Panic-buyingamidcoronavirus-fears-How-much-are-we-spending-and-why-is-it-a-problem. Accessed 22 Apr 2020.
26. Anderson KE, Byrne CE, Crosby RD, Le Grange D. Utilizing Telehealth to deliver family-based treatment for adolescent anorexia nervosa. Int J Eat Disord. 2017;50:1235–8. https://doi.org/10.1002/eat.22759.

5

Eating disorders amongst Aboriginal and Torres Strait Islander Australians: A scoping review

Adam Burt[1], Deborah Mitchison[2,3*], Kerrie Doyle[1] and Phillipa Hay[2,4]

Abstract

Background: Aboriginal and Torres Strait Islander Australians (Indigenous Australians) have poorer mental health compared to other Australians. Yet, there is a lack of research into mental disorders among this population, especially for eating disorders (ED), which are amongst the most lethal and debilitating mental disorders.

Aim: We aimed to answer 2 questions: 1. What is the volume and content of literature on ED among Indigenous Australians? 2. Has a screening or diagnostic tool/instrument been developed for the assessment of ED amongst Indigenous Australians?

Method: We conducted a scoping review of electronic databases (Pubmeb, Embase, PsychInfo, Proquest, Cochrane Library, Indigenous HealtInfoNet and Scopus), for studies addressing ED, body image, muscle dysmorphia, weight and shape concern among Indigenous Australians, as well as diagnostic and screening tools. All relevant studies were reviewed in full by 2 researchers. Narrative synthesis of the data was performed.

Results: There is limited evidence for ED among Indigenous Australians, however, the evidence available strongly suggests that ED are more common among Indigenous Australians compared to other Australians. Eating disorders among Indigenous Australians are also associated with high levels of overvaluation of weight and shape. The increased risk of ED among Indigenous Australians was largely explained by factors such as poorer psychosocial wellbeing. No evidence was found for the existence of validated diagnostic or screening tools for ED in Indigenous Australians.

Conclusion: The evidence suggests ED are common among Indigenous Australians, and there are no diagnostic or screening tools available to assist clinicians in assessing them. More research is required in this field, especially towards the development of a validated and culturally specific screening or diagnostic tool for ED among Indigenous Australians.

Keywords: Feeding and eating disorders, Oceanic ancestry group, Aboriginal and Torres Strait islander, Diagnosis, Screening

* Correspondence: deborah.mitchison@westernsydney.edu.au
[2]Translational Health Research Institute, School of Medicine, Western Sydney University, Campbelltown, Australia
[3]Centre for Emotional Health, Department of Psychology, Macquarie University, North Ryde, New South Wales, Australia
Full list of author information is available at the end of the article

Plain English summary

Indigenous-Australians are known to have poorer mental health compared to other Australians, yet there is a lack of research into mental disorders for Indigenous-Australians, especially for eating disorders. It is important to conduct research into eating disorders because they are among the most debilitating and lethal of all mental disorders.

We reviewed all the available research evidence addressing eating disorders amongst Indigenous-Australians, including for any tools used to assist in the screening and diagnosis of eating disorders among Indigenous-Australians. We included 7 research papers in the study. We found that there is limited evidence for eating disorders amongst Indigenous-Australians and the evidence available suggests that eating disorders are common amongst Indigenous-Australians, more common than amongst other-Australians. The most common eating disorders among Indigenous-Australians are those with overeating symptoms, including night eating syndrome amongst adolescents, and unspecified feeding and eating disorder with binge eating among Indigenous adults. Evidence from the studies we reviewed suggested that the increased risk of eating disorders among Indigenous-Australians was explained poorer social and psychological wellbeing. We found that there needs to be more research in this area as well as increased awareness of eating disorders amongst those caring for Indigenous-Australian patients.

Introduction

Mental health of Aboriginal and Torres Strait Islander Australians

Aboriginal and Torres Strait Islander Australians (Indigenous Australians) have poorer health, especially mental health, compared to other Australians. The Australian Burden of Disease Study is a large report produced by the Australian Government and provides data on the burden of fatal and non-fatal disease in the Australian population, including Indigenous Australians. According to the study, mental illness makes up the greatest burden of non-fatal disease amongst Indigenous Australians; the top 3 conditions being anxiety disorders, depressive disorders and alcohol use disorders [1]. Indigenous Australian adolescents also have a greater burden of conduct disorder, intentional self-harm and suicide, and 3-fold more hospital separations for psychosis and substance use disorders [1–3]. Indigenous Australians are also burdened with significant risk factors for physical and mental illness such as psychological distress. Numerous large studies have suggested up to a third of Indigenous Australians suffer high to very high levels of psychological distress, which is 3-fold higher than the rest of the Australian population [2, 4, 5]. The evidence suggests factors such as social and civic distrust, negative perception of neighborhoods, low socioeconomic status and an inability to access help from family have been found to explain the higher levels of psychological distress among Indigenous Australians [4]. Indigenous Australians are also a younger population than other Australians (21.8 years vs. 37.6 years) [1, 2, 6, 7]. Thus, many young Indigenous Australians are suffering debilitating mental illnesses in the prime of their lives and will likely live for many years with chronic mental illness and its associated medical and social complications. Aside from the significant psychosocial burden, these rates of psychological distress and mental disorders significantly increase the risk of medical conditions. Conditions such as eating disorders are also known to arise in young people [8] and are associated with physical comorbidities [9]. However, there is little consideration of these conditions in young Indigenous people.

Eating disorders and rationale for a scoping review

Eating disorders are a group of mental disorders characterised by persistent disturbances in eating or eating related behaviour resulting in altered consumption or absorption of food, with accompanying psychopathology such as excessive body image concern and significant psychosocial impairment and distress [10]. Unique amongst mental health problems they are associated with significant physical morbidity involving many organ systems as a result of starvation, obesity or eating disorder related behaviours such as purging [9]. Eating disorders are also amongst the most life-threatening mental disorders, with a 6-fold increase in attempted suicide in those affected, and a persistently elevated risk of suicide after recovery [11–13]. Eating disorders are also very common, being prevalent in up to 22% of young Australians [14] and in 2011 accounting for 1.4% of the burden of non-fatal disease in Australia [15].

Despite the severity of eating disorders as mental illnesses and their prevalence in Australia, very little has been published on eating disorders in Indigenous Australians, and to date no review articles have been published specifically addressing eating disorders in this group. A systematic review aimed to identify the prevalence of psychiatric disorders among Indigenous Australians. The study included 17 articles, yet the authors found no prevalence data for several psychiatric disorders, including eating disorders [3]. It is unclear why there has been a lack of research into this area to date. A lack of identification of eating disorders and Indigenous Australians in epidemiological studies, and a lack of treatment seeking or identification of eating disorders, especially in primary care, may be reflected in the lack of data. There are similar issues in New Zealand where low rates of ethnicity reporting data and low inclusion rates of Māori in eating disorder research have left a gap in the evidence base, despite the equal prevalence of eating disorders between Māori and non- Māori New Zealanders [16, 17].

Identification of eating disorders relies on appropriate means of assessment, such as validated screening or diagnostic tools and interviews. This is especially important when they are used to screen or diagnose conditions in Indigenous Australians, as they differ from other Australians both in terms of culture, general health and wellbeing [18–20]. The adapted patient health questionnaire version 9 (aPHQ-9) is a recently developed, rigorously validated and culturally specific screening tool for depression in Indigenous Australians and is an exemplar in this regard. This tool was designed and validated with multiple Indigenous communities across Australia and is free to use [21]. However, a systematic review of diagnostic methods for psychiatric disorders in Indigenous Australians did not identify any culturally specific or validated diagnostic or screening tools for eating disorders among Indigenous Australians [22].

Methods

We chose to conduct a scoping review of the literature in this emerging field to guide future research on this group of disorders for Indigenous Australians. Thus, our specific aim was to answer two questions: 1. What is the volume and content of literature on eating disorders among Indigenous Australians? 2. Has a screening or diagnostic tool/instrument been developed for the assessment of eating disorders amongst Indigenous Australians?

We developed a scoping review protocol (registered with The Open Science Framework (OSF), registration: osf.io/ptmdg. We utilised the framework for scoping reviews described by Arskey and O'Malley (2005): identify the research question, identify relevant studies, select studies, chart the data, collate and summarise the results, report, and consult with others in the field, in our case with Indigenous Australian academics and members of the Indigenous community [23]. We reported all items suggested by the Preferred Reporting Items for Systematic reviews and Meta-Analyses extension for Scoping Reviews (PRISMA-ScR) checklist [24]. The actual protocol used in the study was closely followed as registered on OSF.

Search procedure

Given the aim, we opted to search widely, using multiple databases. We performed a systematic search of the electronic databases: Pubmeb, Embase, PsychInfo, Proquest, Cochrane Library, Indigenous HealtInfoNet and Scopus (for grey literature) using the search terms: [Indigenous Australian OR Aboriginal and Torres Strait Islander OR First Australians] AND [Eating Disorder OR Anorexia Nervosa OR Bulimia nervosa OR Binge eating OR body image OR body dysmorphia OR muscle dysmorphia OR weight/shape overvaluation]. Search terms such as body image, body dysmorphia and weight/shape overvaluation were included because they cover important areas of psychopathology in eating disorders and are areas of interest in research with Indigenous Australians. Manual searches of reference lists of articles used in this review were also conducted.

Selection criteria

Studies included were: 1) prevalence surveys, review articles, clinical trials, case reports and observational studies published in English with no date limits, addressing Indigenous Australians with eating disorders or disordered eating, of all ages; 2) studies addressing eating disorder screening or diagnostic tools for Indigenous Australians; 3) inclusive of rural, remote, urban and metropolitan communities of Australia. The last search was conducted on 19th September 2020. Articles were screened by 1 reviewer, and if they met the selection criteria they were fully reviewed by 2 reviewers. Any disagreements were resolved by consultation with a 3rd reviewer.

Data extraction and synthesis

Figure 1 displays the article selection process. A table was developed for each research question extracting and summarising study characteristics:

1 *What is the volume and content of literature on eating disorders and disordered eating amongst indigenous Australians?*

Study details and characteristics: citation, country, context, participants, ethical considerations for Indigenous Australians. Results extracted from the study: type or quality of assessment of eating disorders/disordered eating (self-report, diagnostic or symptomatic, representative or convenience sample), what was assessed, what was reported in regard to epidemiology.

2. *Has a screening or diagnostic tool/instrument been developed for the assessment of eating disorders amongst indigenous Australians?*

Study details and characteristics: citation, country and context. Numbers, gender, response rate and ethnicity of participants. As well as ethical considerations for Indigenous Australians. Results extracted from the study (in relation to question 2: an assessment tool) such as quality of life domains assessed, number of items in the tool, details of psychometric validation of the tool.

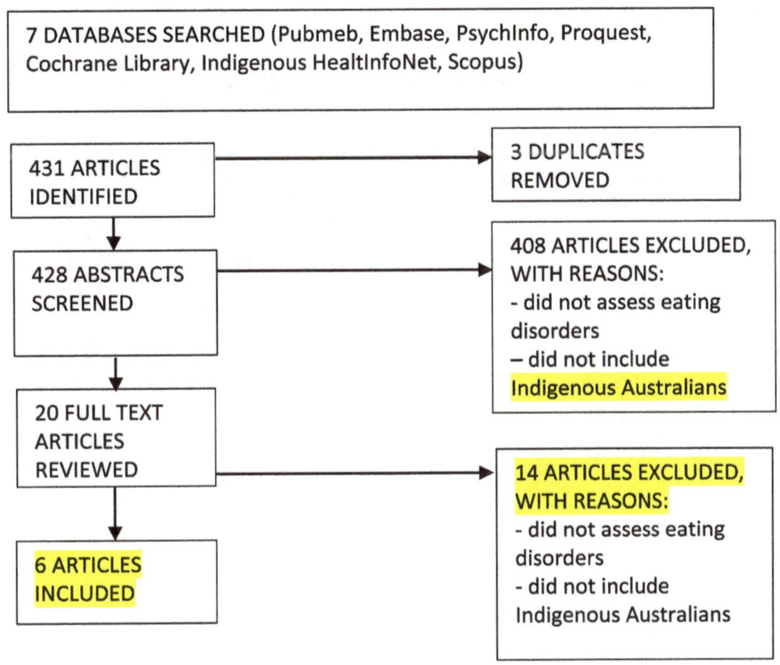

Fig. 1 Flow diagram of study selection process

A narrative synthesis of the data was performed, this type of synthesis is appropriate for studies scoping research such as this and is frequently used in scoping and systematic reviews [25, 26].

Results

Of the 6 studies included, 5 were cross sectional, 1 was a systematic synthesis of population data. Two of the studies estimated eating disorders in Indigenous Australians to the diagnostic threshold level, and 2 estimated disordered eating features in Indigenous Australians. One study measured the impact of media messaging on body dissatisfaction in Indigenous compared other Australian adolescents. No studies were identified that directly assessed a screening or diagnostic tool for eating disorders in Indigenous Australians.

The 2 reviewers assessed all included articles for the reporting items in the protocol. The timeframe of the studies was from 2005 to 2020. All studies included both male and female participants. Details of the studies are found in Table 1 and attached online file.

Prevalence and correlates of eating disorders in the general population

A systematic synthesis of population data by Azzopardi et al., (2018) [2] aimed to report the health and wellbeing of Indigenous Australian adolescents based on 3 domains: health outcomes (mortality, avoidable mortality, disease and injuries), health risks (health behaviours and states) and sociocultural determinants (culture, family, physical wellbeing, education, employment etc). Data were included from 4 national surveys and 4 administrative data sets from national databases which were mapped to the 3 domains. No sample size estimate was provided. The authors suggested eating disorders were more common amongst other Australian adolescents compared to Indigenous Australian adolescents. The paper did not comment on community consultation, however, it did involve an Indigenous author.

The findings of the former study were contrasted by two more recent representative general population studies by Burt et al., (2020) [29, 30]. The authors estimated the diagnostic prevalence of eating disorders to be higher in adult (27%) and adolescent (29%) Indigenous Australians compared to non-Indigenous Australians. Indigenous Australian status did not explain the greater prevalence of eating disorders among the adult or adolescent groups. In the adult group the greater prevalence of eating disorders was associated with the higher body mass index (BMI), poorer mental health related quality of life (MHRQoL) and younger age of Indigenous Australians, Indigenous adults also experienced higher levels of overvaluation of weight and shape compared to other Australians. Similarly, in the adolescent group the higher eating disorder prevalence was largely explained by poorer psychosocial quality of life (Psychosocial QoL) experienced by the Indigenous Australian group, they did not however differ significantly in weight and shape concern compared to the other Australian adolescents. The most common eating disorder among Indigenous Australian adults was unspecified feeding or eating disorder with recurrent binge eating (UFED), among

Table 1 Articles included addressing eating disorders and eating disorder screening or diagnostic tools for Indigenous Australians

Study Details and Characteristics						
Study citation details	Mulders-Jones 2017 [27]	Hay 2012 [28]	Azzopardi 2018 [2]	Burt 2020 [29]	Burt 2020 [30]	McCabe 2005 [31]
Country	Australia	Australia	Australia	Australia	Australia	Australia
Context	Rural, urban and metropolitan	Rural, urban and metropolitan	Rural, urban and metropolitan	Rural, urban and metropolitan	Rural, urban and metropolitan	Urban (Melbourne)
1.Participants 2.Survey response rate	1.Male 2960 - Female 3081 - Total 6041, - Indigenous 118 2. Data from 2 surveys, 62.8% & 59.3%	1.Total 5926 -Female 3017 -Male 2909 Indigenous 155 -Female 91 -Male 64 2.Not given	360 papers sampling 10-24yo Indigenous adolescents.	1. Total 5068 -Male 3003 -Female 2065 Indigenous 402 -Female 143 -Male 259 -Did not disclose 80 2.Not given	1.Total 6041 Indigenous 92 -Female 53 -Male 42 2. Data from 2 surveys, 53.7% & 58.4%.	1.Total 100 Indigenous 50 -Female 25 -Male 25 12-16yo 2.Not given
Ethical considerations in regards to Indigenous Australian research.	Nil	Nil	Nil	Nil	Nil	Consultation from Aboriginal cooperatives and elders in the community where data gathered.
Details						
Quality or type of assessment: 1. self-report or interview 2. Diagnostic or symptoms. 3.Representative or convenience sample	1. Interview. 2. Symptoms. 3.Representative sample.	1.Interview. 2.Symptoms. 3.Representative sample.	N/A	1.Interview. 2.Diagnostic. 3.Representative sample.	1.Interview. 2.Diagnostic. 3.Representative sample.	1.Self report. 2. Symptomatic. 3. Convenience sample.
What was assessed?	Socioeconomic status and DE features.	Prevalence of DE features.	Population health data.	Prevalence of ED in Indigenous adolescents, and moderating effects of independent variables.	Prevalence of ED in Indigenous adults, and moderating effects of Independent variables.	BD using 5 subscales of body image and body image inventory.
What was reported in regards to epidemiology of DE/ED	There was an equal likelihood to report DE/ED features, regardless of identification as Indigenous. Those who did not report their Indigenous status reported higher levels of overvaluation of weight and shape.	Higher prevalence of DE/ED features amongst Indigenous.	Reported ED less common in Indigenous adolescents v. other Australians, more common in urban v. rural Indigenous adolescents (they did not identify a non-urban case). Population health data. Also reported more mood disorders, psychosis and psychological distress in Indigenous.	Indigenous Australians had higher prevalence of ED, mostly due to higher OSFED-NES in Indigenous Australians. OSFED-NES 7.14% (95%CI 4.81–10.49) of IA vs. 3.72% (95%CI 3.17–4.36) in other Australians. The greater NES was due to poorer Psychosocial QoL in Indigenous.	Indigenous Australians had a higher prevalence of ED, 27%. Most prevalent was UFED with binge eating. On logistic regression analysis independent variables: higher BMI, younger age and poorer MHRQoL were retained in model were the dependent variable was having an ED. ED were associated with high levels of overvaluation.	Indigenous Australians more BD than other Australians and undertook more strategies to decrease weight and increase weight and increase muscles. Indigenous girls had lower levels of BD than other Australian girls. Indigenous adolescents received less media messages although they had more impact.

ED Eating Disorder, *DE* Disordered Eating behaviour, *BD* Body Dissatisfaction

Indigenous adolescents the most common eating disorder was other specified feeding or eating disorder – night eating syndrome (OSFED-NES). Whilst neither study consulted the Indigenous community in the design of their research, both were written and informed by an Indigenous lead author. A limitation of the adult study by Burt et al. [30], was the small number of Indigenous participants (n = 92), and missing data due to a number of participants not disclosing their Indigenous status, albeit this was adjusted for in the analyses. Moreover, it is suggested the estimates may be conservative.

The contrasting findings between Burt et al. [29, 30], and Azzopardi et al. [2], may be because the latter was based on data from the national hospital morbidity and other databases for mental disorders. These data miss those who have not been admitted to hospital, which is almost certainly the majority of cases of eating disorders [32].

The former are further supported by two general population studies by Hay and Carriage (2012) and Mulders-Jones, Mitchison, Girosi and Hay (2017) who reported on prevalence of eating disorder behaviours. The authors found eating disorder behaviours to be of similar or increased frequency in Indigenous compared to non-Indigenous Australians. Neither reported on consultation with the Indigenous community, although the former included an Indigenous Australian author [27, 28].

When considered together, the findings from the adult and adolescent studies by Burt et al. [29, 30], and the former study by Hay and Carriage [28], suggest that eating disorders are more common among Indigenous Australians compared to other Australians, particularly eating disorders with overeating features such as UFED with recurrent binge eating and OSFED-NES.

Body image concern

One study by McCabe et al., (2005) [31] measured the effect of media influences on the body dissatisfaction amongst 50 Indigenous Australian adolescents compared to a matched cohort of other Australian adolescents. The authors' aims were to examine the extent of differences in body image and body change strategies and awareness of media messages to change weight and shape for Indigenous and non-Indigenous adolescents from urban areas, and to examine the extent to which these media messages predicted body image and body change strategies in these groups. Overall, Indigenous adolescents engaged in more activities to lose weight, increase weight and increase muscles than non-Indigenous adolescents; however in sex-stratified analyses, Indigenous girls reported less body image dissatisfaction compared to non-Indigenous girls. The authors suggest the Indigenous adolescents may have been less aware of the media messages' impact on their behaviour or were more reluctant to report that media messaging impacted their behaviour. The high levels of weight and shape concern among Indigenous adolescents found in this study accords with the findings of research by Burt et al. [29, 30].

The authors of this study consulted local Indigenous elders in preparation for the research.

Screening or diagnostic tools

No studies were identified that directly assessed a diagnostic or screening tool for eating disorders.

Discussion

There is limited evidence addressing mental disorders amongst among Indigenous Australians, especially for eating disorders, which is both a major finding and a limitation of the research literature. The majority of evidence available on eating disorders amongst Indigenous Australians comes from 3 cross sectional papers by members of this research team: the adult and adolescent studies by Burt et al., (2020) [29, 30], the study by Hay and Carriage, (2012) [28], supported by the body image study by McCabe et al., (2005) [31]. When these studies are considered together with well demonstrated significant burden of mental illness [1] and mental illness risk factors [4] in the Indigenous population, they strongly suggest that eating disorders are more common among Indigenous Australians compared to other Australians. This suggestion is supported by the consistency in the types of disorders (those with overeating features) prevalent in the Indigenous community, the explanatory variables (poorer psychosocial wellbeing) for those disorders and the prominent psychopathology (overvaluation of weight and shape), supported across multiple studies and in different age groups. We suggest that within the Indigenous population there exists a relatively larger pool of younger people with poorer mental health, high levels body image concern that ostensibly does not diminish with adulthood, and severe socioeconomic disadvantage, leaving that population more vulnerable to developing an eating disorder. These findings of elevated general psychosocial impairment also accord with other studies that have found an increased risk for a range of mental disorders among Indigenous Australians, that is, this risk is not specific to eating disorders [33, 34].

No studies were identified in this review that directly assessed a diagnostic or screening tool for eating disorders among Indigenous Australians. One systematic review aimed to examine the cultural validity of the methods used to diagnose psychiatric disorders among Indigenous Australians, however, it not include any articles directly assessing eating disorders, thus it was not included in this review [22].

The implications of these findings are the need for greater awareness of eating disorders among those who work in Indigenous health, among parents of Indigenous children, as well as schoolteachers who may be among the first to notice eating disorder behaviours in young people. Further research is needed to assess the uptake of treatment for eating disorders among Indigenous Australians to guide future research into effective treatments as well as identification of eating disorders in this population. Indigenous Australians are culturally and linguistically different to other Australians, even in areas where the Indigenous Australian population speak English almost exclusively. There are very few Indigenous

Australian healthcare workers, especially those likely to come into contact with undifferentiated patients with eating disorder symptoms such as Nurses, Psychologists, General Practitioners and Psychiatrists. The assessment and treatment of eating disorders is a specialised field, and not always easily accessible for patients in Australia. Moreover, the majority of clinicians who treat Indigenous Australian patients are not eating disorder experts, therefore, the absence of a culturally specific, validated screening tool is of directly clinical relevance and importance and should be a priority for researchers in order to assist those who see Indigenous Australian patients. This field of research, including qualitative research conducted within an Indigenous paradigm and within the Indigenous community should aim to understand the nature of eating disorders so that effective treatments may also be developed, such as psychotherapies.

Conclusions

The evidence available strongly suggests that eating disorders are more common amongst Indigenous Australians compared to other Australians and are associated with high levels of overvaluation of weight and shape. To the best of our knowledge no research has been published addressing diagnostic or screening instruments to help detect eating disorders amongst Indigenous Australians. More research is required in this field, especially towards the development of a validated and culturally specific screening or diagnostic tool/instrument for eating disorders amongst Indigenous Australians, ideally conducted in collaboration with Indigenous communities and Indigenous researchers.

Abbreviations

ABS: Australian Bureau of Statistics; AMS: Aboriginal Medical Service; aPHQ-9: Adapted Patient Health Questionnaire; BED: Binge Eating Disorder; BMI: Body Mass Index; BN: Bulimia Nervosa; CI: Confidence Interval; df: Degrees of freedom; DSM-5: Diagnostic and Statistical Manual of Mental Disorders 5th edition; ED: Eating Disorder; IA: Indigenous Australian; HOS: Health Omnibus Survey; n: Number of participants; NES: Night Eating Syndrome; OR: Odds Ratio; OSFED: Other Specified Feeding or Eating Disorder; UFED: Unspecified Feeding or Eating Disorder; YLD: Years Lived with Disability.

Acknowledgements

We acknowledge and respect the Darug, Gundungurra, D'harawal, Wiradjuri and Bundjalung Peoples, upon which Western Sydney University campuses now stand, and all Traditional Owners of the Lands across Australia, and their contribution to the generation of knowledge herein this manuscript.

Authors' contributions

Adam Burt conceived the study, conducted the data search and data extraction, appraisal, and interpretation, and lead the manuscript preparation; Deborah Mitchison contributed to data appraisal and writing of the manuscript; Kerrie Doyle, contributed to data interpretation and writing of the manuscript; Phillipa Hay, contributed to data appraisal, interpretation and writing of the manuscript. The author (s) read and approved the final manuscript.

Competing interests

Professor Hay receives/has received sessional fees and lecture fees from the Australian Medical Council, Therapeutic Guidelines publication, and New South Wales Institute of Psychiatry and royalties/honoraria from Hogrefe and Huber, McGraw Hill Education, and Blackwell Scientific Publications, Biomed Central and PlosMedicine and she has received research grants from the NHMRC and ARC. She is Chair of the National Eating Disorders Collaboration Steering Committee in Australia (2012-), was Member of the ICD-11 Working Group for Eating Disorders (2012–2018), and was Chair Clinical Practice Guidelines Project Working Group (Eating Disorders) of RANZCP (2012–2015). In the past 5 years she has prepared a report under contract for Shire Pharmaceuticals and received honoraria for education of psychiatrists from Shire Pharmaceuticals (Takeda group). All views in this paper are her own. She is an Editor of this Journal.

Author details

[1]School of Medicine, Western Sydney University, Campbelltown, Australia. [2]Translational Health Research Institute, School of Medicine, Western Sydney University, Campbelltown, Australia. [3]Centre for Emotional Health, Department of Psychology, Macquarie University, North Ryde, New South Wales, Australia. [4]Campbelltown Hospital, SWSLHD, Campbelltown, Australia.

References

1. Al-Yaman F. Australian Burden of Disease Study: impact and causes of illness and death in Aboriginal and Torres Strait Islander people, 2011. Public Health Res Pract. 2017;27(4):2741732.
2. Azzopardi PS, Sawyer SM, Carlin JB, Degenhardt L, Brown N, Brown AD, et al. Health and wellbeing of indigenous adolescents in Australia: a systematic synthesis of population data. Lancet. 2018;391(10122):766–82.
3. Black EB, Ranmuthugala G, Kondalsamy-Chennakesavan S, Toombs MR, Nicholson GC, Kisely S. A systematic review: identifying the prevalence rates of psychiatric disorder in Australia's indigenous populations. Aust N Z J Psychiatry. 2015;49(5):412–29.
4. Markwick A, Ansari Z, Sullivan M, McNeil J. Social determinants and psychological distress among Aboriginal and Torres Strait islander adults in the Australian state of Victoria: a cross-sectional population based study. Soc Sci Med. 2015;128:178–87.
5. McNamara BJ, Banks E, Gubhaju L, Joshy G, Williamson A, Raphael B, et al. Factors relating to high psychological distress in indigenous Australians and their contribution to indigenous-non-indigenous disparities. Aust N Z J Public Health. 2018;42(2):145–52.
6. 2016 Census: Aboriginal and/or Torres Strait Islander Peoples QuickStats: Australian Bureau of Statistics 2016 [Available from: https://quickstats.censusdata.abs.gov.au/census_services/getproduct/census/2016/quickstat/IQS036.
7. 2016 Census QuickStats: Australian Bureau of Statistics 2016 [Available from: https://quickstats.censusdata.abs.gov.au/census_services/getproduct/census/2016/quickstat/036?opendocument.
8. Volpe U, Tortorella A, Manchia M, Monteleone AM, Albert U, Monteleone P. Eating disorders: what age at onset? Psychiatry Res. 2016;238:225–7.
9. Mehler PS, Brown C. Anorexia nervosa – medical complications. J Eat Disord. 2015;3(1):11.
10. Diagnostic and Statistical Manual of Mental Disorders (DSM-5): American Psychiatric Association 2013.
11. Arcelus J, Mitchell AJ, Wales J, Nielsen S. Mortality rates in patients with anorexia nervosa and other eating disorders. A meta-analysis of 36 studies. Arch Gen Psychiatry. 2011;68(7):724–31.
12. Papadopoulos FC, Ekbom A, Brandt L, Ekselius L. Excess mortality, causes of death and prognostic factors in anorexia nervosa. Br J Psychiatry. 2009;194(1):10–7.
13. Udo T, Bitley S, Grilo CM. Suicide attempts in US adults with lifetime DSM-5 eating disorders. BMC Med. 2019;17(1):120.
14. Mitchison D, Mond J, Bussey K, Griffiths S, Trompeter N, Lonergan A, et al. DSM-5 full syndrome, other specified, and unspecified eating disorders in Australian adolescents: prevalence and clinical significance. Psychol Med. 2020;50(6):981–90.

15. Australian Burden of Disease Study Impact and causes of illness and death in Australia 2011. Canberra Australian Institute of Health and Welfare; 2016.
16. Lacey C, Clark M, Manuel J, Pitama S, Cunningham R, Keelan K, et al. Is there systemic bias for Māori with eating disorders? A need for greater awareness in the healthcare system. N Z Med J (Online). 2020;133(1514):71.
17. Lacey C, Cunningham R, Rijnberg V, Manuel J, Clark MTR, Keelan K, et al. Eating disorders in New Zealand: Implications for Maori and health service delivery. Int J Eat Disord. 2020;1-9.
18. Australian Standard Classification of Languages. Australian Bureau of Statistics. 1997.
19. Shahid S, Finn L, Bessarab D, Thompson SC. Understanding, beliefs and perspectives of Aboriginal people in Western Australia about cancer and its impact on access to cancer services. BMC Health Serv Res. 2009;9:132.
20. Crowe R, Stanley R, Probst Y, McMahon A. Culture and healthy lifestyles: a qualitative exploration of the role of food and physical activity in three urban Australian indigenous communities. Aust N Z J Public Health. 2017; 41(4):411–6.
21. Getting it Right Collaborative G. Getting it right: validating a culturally specific screening tool for depression (aPHQ-9) in Aboriginal and Torres Strait islander Australians. Med J Aust. 2019;211(1):24–30.
22. Black EB, Toombs MR, Kisely S. The cultural validity of diagnostic psychiatric measures for indigenous Australians. Aust Psychol. 2018;53(5):383–93.
23. Arksey H, O'Malley L. Scoping studies: towards a methodological framework. Int JSoc Res Methodol. 2005;8(1):19–32.
24. Tricco AC, Lillie E, Zarin W, O'Brien KK, Colquhoun H, Levac D, et al. PRISMA extension for scoping reviews (PRISMA-ScR): checklist and explanation. Ann Intern Med. 2018;169(7):467–73.
25. Fuglset TS, Landro NI, Reas DL, Ro O. Functional brain alterations in anorexia nervosa: a scoping review. J Eat Disord. 2016;4:32.
26. Piat M, Pearson A, Sabetti J, Steiger H, Israel M, Lal S. International training programs on eating disorders for professionals, caregivers, and the general public: A scoping review. J Eat Disord. 2015;3:28.
27. Mulders-Jones B, Mitchison D, Girosi F, Hay P. Socioeconomic correlates of eating disorder symptoms in an Australian population-based sample. PLoS One. 2017;12(1):e0170603.
28. Hay PJ, Carriage C. Eating disorder features in indigenous Aboriginal and Torres Strait islander Australian peoples. BMC Public Health. 2012;12:233.
29. Burt A, Mitchison D, Dale E, Bussey K, Trompeter N, Lonergan A, et al. Prevalence, features and health impacts of eating disorders amongst first-Australian Yiramarang (adolescents) and in comparison with other Australian adolescents. J Eat Disord. 2020;8:10.
30. Burt A, Mannan H, Touyz S, Hay P. Prevalence of DSM-5 diagnostic threshold eating disorders and features amongst Aboriginal and Torres Strait islander peoples (first Australians). BMC Psychiatry. 2020;20(1):449.
31. McCabe MP, Ricciardelli L, Mellor D, Ball K. Media influences on body image and disordered eating among indigenous adolescent Australians. Adolescence. 2005;40(157):115–27.
32. Hart LM, Granillo MT, Jorm AF, Paxton SJ. Unmet need for treatment in the eating disorders: a systematic review of eating disorder specific treatment seeking among community cases. Clin Psychol Rev. 2011;31(5):727–35.
33. Twizeyemariya A, Guy S, Furber G, Segal L. Risks for mental illness in indigenous Australian children: a descriptive study demonstrating high levels of vulnerability. Milbank Q. 2017;95(2):319–57.
34. Shepherd CC, Li J, Mitrou F, Zubrick SR. Socioeconomic disparities in the mental health of indigenous children in Western Australia. BMC Public Health. 2012;12:756.

6

An open trial of app-assisted acceptance and commitment therapy (iACT) for eating disorders in type 1 diabetes

Rhonda M. Merwin[1*], Ashley A. Moskovich[1], Michael Babyak[1], Mark Feinglos[2], Lisa K. Honeycutt[1], Jan Mooney[1], Sara P. Freeman[1], Heather Batchelder[1] and Devdutta Sangvai[3]

Abstract

Background: Eating disorders (EDs) among individuals with type 1 diabetes (T1D) increase the risk of early and severe diabetes-related medical complications and premature death. Conventional eating disorder (ED) treatments have been largely ineffective for T1D patients, indicating the need to tailor treatments to this patient population and the unique conditions under which ED symptoms emerge (in the context of a chronic illness with unrelenting demands to control blood glucose, diet and exercise). The current study was a pilot open trial of *iACT*, a novel intervention for EDs in T1D grounded in Acceptance and Commitment Therapy (ACT). *iACT* was based on the premise that ED symptoms emerge as individuals attempt to cope with T1D and related emotional distress. *iACT* taught acceptance and mindfulness as an alternative to maladaptive avoidance and control, and leveraged personal values to increase willingness to engage in T1D management, even when it was upsetting (e.g., after overeating). A tailored mobile application ("app") was used in between sessions to facilitate the application of ACT skills in the moment that individuals are making decisions about their diabetes management.

Methods: Adults with T1D who met criteria for an ED completed 12 sessions of *iACT* (with three optional tapering sessions). In addition to examining whether treatment was acceptable and feasible (the primary aim of the study), the study also examined whether *iACT* was associated with increased psychological flexibility (i.e., the ability to have distressing thoughts/feelings about diabetes while pursuing personally meaningful values), and improvements in ED symptoms, diabetes management and diabetes distress.

Results: Treatment was acceptable to T1D patients with EDs and feasible to implement. Participants reported increased psychological flexibility with diabetes-related thoughts/feelings, and less obstruction and greater progress in pursuing personal values. There were large effects for change in ED symptoms, diabetes self-management and diabetes distress from baseline to end-of-treatment (Cohen's $d = .90–1.79$). Hemoglobin A_{1c} also improved, but the p-value did not reach statistical significance, $p = .08$.

Conclusions: Findings provide preliminary evidence for *iACT* to improve outcomes for T1D patients with EDs and support further evaluation of this approach in a controlled trial.

(Continued on next page)

* Correspondence: rhonda.merwin@duke.edu
[1]Department of Psychiatry and Behavioral Sciences, Duke University Medical Center, DUMC Box 3842, Durham, NC 27712, USA
Full list of author information is available at the end of the article

(Continued from previous page)
Keywords: Eating disorders, Type 1 diabetes, Acceptance and commitment therapy, Experiential avoidance, Psychological flexibility, Diabetes distress, Mobile health

Plain English summary

Eating disorders (EDs) are fairly common among individuals with type 1 diabetes (T1D) and can be deadly. Treatments for anorexia and bulimia nervosa that are currently available are not as effective for individuals with T1D. This preliminary study examined whether a new treatment, *i*ACT, was acceptable to T1D patients with EDs and feasible to implement, and whether it reduced eating disorder (ED) symptoms and improved diabetes management. *i*ACT was based on Acceptance and Commitment Therapy (ACT) and focused on helping individuals with T1D cope effectively with emotional distress and choose actions based on personal values. A mobile application ("app") was also used in between sessions to help patients practice new behaviors at home. The treatment was acceptable and feasible, with good participation and few unwanted side effects. Participants reported improvements in their ED symptoms and emotional distress. They also reported improvements in their responses to diabetes-related thoughts and feelings and greater ability to pursue their personal values over the course of treatment, suggesting that treatment worked the way it was intended. The current study suggests that a larger study is needed comparing this treatment to a waitlist (to determine whether improvements are greater than what would happen with time alone) or to other, currently available interventions.

Background

Type 1 diabetes (T1D) is an endocrine disorder in which the immune system attacks the beta cells of the pancreas, eliminating the body's ability to produce insulin. Individuals with T1D survive by self-monitoring blood glucose and administering insulin multiple times a day to attempt to achieve near-normal glycemia. It is a complex and burdensome regimen that requires careful planning of diet, exercise and insulin dosing to prevent immediately life-threatening circumstances and slow the progression of macro- and microvascular complications and premature death [1, 2].

Eating disorder (ED) symptomatology is fairly common among adolescents and young women with T1D and has severe negative consequences for diabetes management [3–6]. In a longitudinal study of 126 adolescent girls interviewed 7 times over 14 years, 32.4% (23/71) met the criteria for a current ED at Time 7, and an additional 8.5% (6/71) had a subthreshold ED [4]. The cumulative probability of ED onset was 60% by age 25 [4]. This is consistent with other studies that have found elevated rates of eating disorders (EDs) and disordered eating behavior among young women with T1D (e.g., [5, 6]).

ED symptoms are associated with elevated hemoglobin A_{1c} (HbA_{1c}) [6], a key metric of glycemic control that reflects the percentage of hemoglobin in red blood cells that is glycated, i.e. attached to a glucose molecule. HbA_{1c} provides an estimate of average blood glucose over the past 2 to 3 months. Target HbA_{1c} for individuals with T1D is typically between 7.0–7.5% [7]. In previous studies of EDs in T1D mean HbA_{1c} is typically 9% or higher [8]. Higher HbA_{1c} predicts microvascular (e.g., retinopathy, neuropathy, nephropathy) and macrovascular complications (e.g., cardiovascular disease) [2].

ED behaviors in T1D include the dangerous practice of administering less insulin than is needed to maintain or lose weight. While insulin restriction may be effective at producing weight loss (particularly when prolonged), it is extremely dangerous. When insulin is restricted, excess glucose remains in the blood stream, causing hyperglycemia that damages the blood vessels, advancing vascular disease [2]. Glucose is eventually excreted via urination, effectively "purging" calories, but damaging the kidneys. Further, when the body has insufficient insulin, it is unable to use glucose for energy and begins to break down fat for fuel. The breakdown products include ketones that, when released into the bloodstream at high levels, are toxic and can be immediately life-threatening. Food restriction can have a similar, although less severe, effect (with too little glucose available for energy and the body drawing from fat stores, ketones are subsequently released into the bloodstream). When these two behaviors are combined, mortality is particularly high [9]. T1D patients with EDs have an increased incidence of life-threatening diabetic ketoacidosis and hospitalizations [10]. Insulin restriction is the single best predictor of early mortality among individuals with T1D and triples the risk of premature death [11, 12].

Existing treatments for anorexia and bulimia nervosa are largely ineffective for individuals with T1D [13–15]. Even when eating and weight-related attitudes improve, T1D management and glycemic control may not [14]. This suggests the need to tailor interventions to T1D, and the unique needs and experiences of this patient population and the conditions under which ED symptoms emerge.

ED symptomatology is more prevalent among individuals with T1D than the general population [4–6]. Factors that contribute to the increased prevalence of EDs in T1D are unknown, however it is hypothesized that it is directly related to the T1D treatment regimen which encourages perfectionism in blood glucose control achieved via careful carbohydrate counting and intensive insulin therapy [16]. Among vulnerable individuals, attempting to achieve near normal glycemia may lead to maladaptive attention to food choices and attempts to control eating and weight gain associated with insulin therapy [16]. There is empirical evidence that emotional distress specific to diabetes (diabetes distress; e.g., feeling overwhelmed by diabetes or like a failure in diabetes management) could have an important role in EDs in T1D, as both a precipitant and a consequence of disordered eating [12, 17]; however, pathways from this emotional distress to ED symptoms have not been fully specified.

Hypothesized functional pathways to EDs in T1D

Perfectionism is a trait feature that is highly correlated with EDs in nondiabetic populations [18]. Research differentiates negative perfectionism (i.e., perfectionistic concerns, including fear of failure and making mistakes) and positive perfectionism (i.e., perfectionistic strivings), with a stronger correlation between negative perfectionism and EDs [19]. In the context of T1D, negative perfectionism might lead to extreme responses to the T1D treatment regimen and associated distress that inadvertently contribute to an ED. For example, T1D patients with elevated perfectionism may be more prone to "clamp down" on eating, attempting to follow extremely strict dietary rules (which paradoxically increases risk for bouts of disinhibited eating [20]). Alternatively, they may "give up," eating or overeating highly palatable foods, and avoid giving insulin to reduce the impact of eating on weight. While these responses may help individuals feel better in the short-term, they would perpetuate poor glycemic control, increasing feelings of failure and further disrupting mood. See Fig. 1.

A novel treatment approach

Acceptance and Commitment Therapy (ACT) is a contemporary cognitive behavioral therapy that may be well-suited for chronic illnesses such as T1D [21]. While traditional cognitive behavioral therapy focuses on challenging and changing beliefs [22], ACT emphasizes changing how individuals respond to their distressing thoughts/feelings [21]. Thus, ACT may be well-matched to T1D, in which distressing cognitions (e.g., the possibility of medical complications) are often not irrational or illogical and thus not easily disputed, and may be cued multiple times a day as individuals engage in T1D management.

ACT uses acceptance and mindfulness strategies to decouple the typical relationship between distressing thoughts/feelings and behavior, such that behavior may be more flexible and aligned with personal values (i.e., who the person wants to be or how they want to live

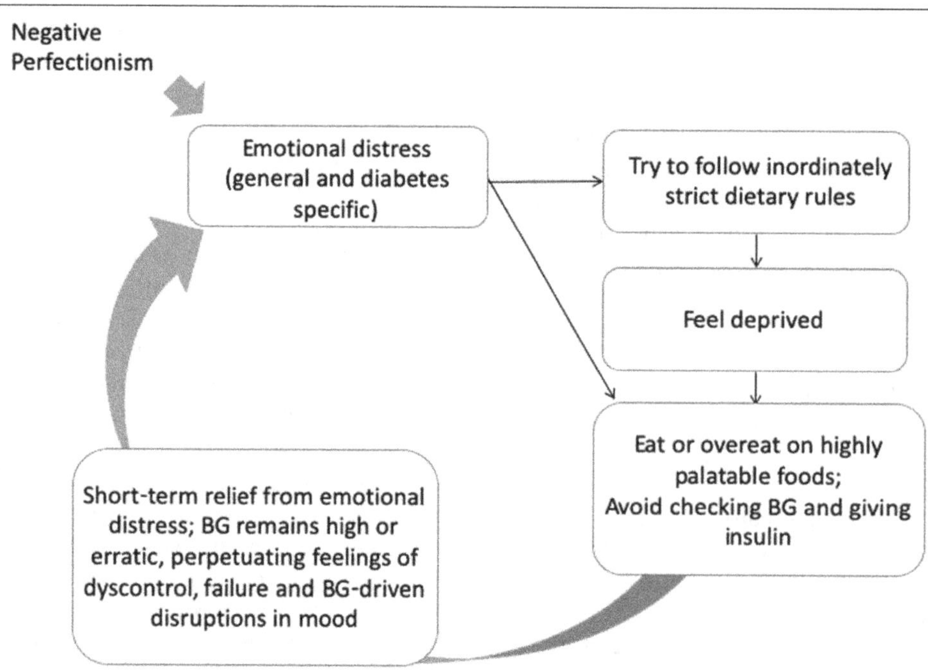

Fig. 1 Hypothesized functional pathways of eating disorder behavior in type 1 diabetes

their lives) [21, 23]. ACT's values orientation might help T1D patients persist in diabetes management tasks, even when doing so is not immediately reinforcing or is even punishing (e.g., patients may experience edema as they begin to administer more insulin which creates physical and emotional discomfort). The ability to be fully in the present moment with one's internal experience and choose behavior based on personal values is described as psychological flexibility, and the primary process of change in ACT interventions [21, 23].

Preliminary evidence suggests ACT may improve diabetes management in individuals with type 2 diabetes and that it may be useful for EDs (e.g., [24, 25]), including more intractable conditions such as anorexia nervosa [26, 27]. However, ACT has not been adapted for use with T1D patients with EDs.

iACT protocol

*i*ACT is a novel treatment protocol based on ACT that was designed to target functional pathways to ED development and maintenance among individuals with T1D. *i*ACT combined individual in-person sessions with a mobile application ("app") (denoted with the "*i*" in *i*ACT), used in between sessions to facilitate ACT skills practice and behavior change. *i*ACT focused on the unique emotional antecedents and consequences of ED behaviors among individuals with T1D (e.g., feelings of failure in diabetes). Individuals were taught to recognize ED antecedents in the moment and cope more effectively using acceptance and mindfulness skills. The individual's personal values were also clarified and used to encourage individuals to engage in T1D management tasks, even when it was upsetting (e.g., testing BG or giving insulin after overeating). Acceptance interventions extended to the individual, and encouraged a more compassionate and less punitive approach to managing oneself and T1D (e.g., viewing blood glucose as data rather than a marker of personal success/failure).

The *i*ACT app was a modified version of Recovery Record, an existing mobile app designed to help individuals with EDs recover [28]. The decision to include an app was based on previous research that has found individuals with T1D and ED do not fare well in outpatient treatment, but may do better in inpatient or residential settings (e.g., [29, 30]). These settings have the advantage of providing therapeutic support in the moment that individuals are making decisions about their T1D management. A mobile app can similarly provide additional therapeutic support anytime, including in the late afternoon or overnight when individuals may be more prone to skip insulin [31]. The app was also included to expedite skill acquisition and generalization to daily life (a common obstacle in cognitive behavioral therapy) [32] and it allowed T1D patients to track daily behavior change goals, rather than relying on distal outcomes, such as HbA_{1c}. As individuals with T1D engage in new behaviors more regularly, and glycemic control improves, changes may be maintained without app support.

The original Recovery Record app has interactive features such as logs to track thoughts, feelings and behaviors (particularly at mealtimes), the ability to set personal goals, coping skills and affirmations, among other features [28]. This app was modified for our model of ED maintenance in T1D and our strategy for intervention [33]. This included adding T1D-specific feelings (e.g., feeling overwhelmed or like a failure in T1D) to the logs and T1D-specific management behaviors and goals (e.g., taking insulin at each meal). It also included: 1) creating ACT specific coping skills presented at times of heightened emotional distress (e.g., mindfulness exercises, such as watching thoughts like "Leaves on a Stream" [21, 34] or observing emotions as waves) [34], 2) adapting general affirmations to recontextualize T1D with messages of strength, humor or compassion ("*You don't know how strong you are until strong is the only option you have: TYPE ONE*" [33], and 3) building a new values feature that presented participants' personalized values images to encourage skill use at times of heightened emotional distress. Before conducting the open trial, the app modifications were vetted with adults with T1D in two focus groups (total $N = 10$) and online questionnaires ($N = 33$). The fully functioning app was then beta tested with 9 T1D patients with eating and weight concerns. Participants used the fully functioning app for 14 days. On average, participants accessed the app 47.56 times over 14 days (or an average of 3.40 times per day) and reported no functionality errors or concerns with the app, indicating it was appropriate to continue to the open trial examining the acceptability and feasibility of the full intervention.

Study aims

The primary aim of the current study was to examine the acceptability and feasibility of *i*ACT, an app-assisted, tailored ACT intervention for EDs in T1D. Secondary aims of the study were to 1) assess whether the intervention functioned as intended, increasing psychological flexibility with distressing thoughts and feelings about diabetes and decreasing the extent to which these experiences interfered with taking effective action or pursuing values, and 2) the potential of *i*ACT to decrease ED symptoms and improve diabetes management, which has not been shown with previous outpatient treatments. This is the first study of a tailored intervention for EDs in individuals with T1D, which might be more effective in reducing symptoms and improving glycemic control than more generic ED treatments.

Method

Participants

Participants were older adolescents and adults with T1D with clinically significant ED symptomatology. To be eligible for the study, T1D patients had to be at least 17 years old, meet diagnostic criteria for an ED, and have a physician managing their diabetes whom they agreed to follow up with throughout the study. They also had to consent to the study team contacting their physician as needed for the study or to maintain safety. Original study criteria also included baseline $HbA_{1c} \geq 7.5\%$ (indicating that average blood glucose over the past 2–3 months was elevated above recommended levels); however, this requirement was dropped because some individuals who presented for the study met full criteria for an ED but did not have $HbA_{1c} \geq 7.5\%$ (due to maladaptive compensatory behaviors, such as severe food restriction between binge episodes that resulted in an overall lower average blood sugar). These individuals were part of the target population and thus included in the study. Individuals with T1D were excluded if they reported an inability to manage their diabetes independently (e.g., due to cognitive impairments) or a thought disorder (e.g., psychosis), or hypoglycemic unawareness (assessed via the Gold Method [35]) which would pose additional safety concerns or suggest another treatment may be more appropriate (e.g., blood glucose awareness training).

The recruitment target was $N = 25$, for a final sample of $N = 21$ with attrition. Assuming two-tailed $\alpha = .05$, a pre-post mean of average 3-day blood glucose correlation of 0.7, and $SD = 58.08$ mg/dL (calculated from prior data [17, 31], a sample size of 21 provided 80% power to detect a reduction of at least 32 mg/dL in average daily blood glucose, equivalent to a .5% reduction in HbA_{1c}, which is considered clinically significant [36].

Participants were recruited from endocrinology clinics at two major medical centers in the Southeast, directly by their treatment providers or by flyers placed in the clinic, or via an email announcement sent to a T1D participant research registry. The study was described as a treatment study for patients with T1D who sometimes take less insulin than they need and/or have concerns about their eating, weight and diabetes management. Interested individuals contacted the Clinical Research Coordinator for eligibility screening. Individuals with Diabetes Eating Problems Survey – Revised (DEPS-R [37];) scores ≥20 were invited onsite for a diagnostic interview to confirm ED diagnosis. Participants provided informed consent for screening and again for study participation. All study procedures were approved by the Institutional Review Board (IRB).

Eating disorder diagnosis

The Eating Disorder Examination (EDE [38];) is a gold standard semi-structured diagnostic interview that was used to confirm ED diagnosis. The EDE was administered by a Masters or PhD level assessor who was trained in the EDE, and specifically how to administer and score the EDE with T1D patients (e.g., how to discriminate when the individual's attitudes or behavior are beyond that expected or necessary for diabetes management). Intentionally transdiagnostic, clinical presentation could vary and eligible individuals could present with one or several ED behaviors (e.g., severe caloric restriction, binge eating, self-induced vomiting or insulin restriction for weight control) in any combination if these behaviors were associated with significant distress or impairment.

Procedure

Individuals who enrolled in the study had height/weight measurements taken and blood drawn to determine HbA_{1c}. They also completed questionnaires via Qualtrics® (See Measurements). Participants were then assigned to a therapist (RM, AM). They completed a clinical intake and 12 weekly therapy sessions (50–60 min in duration) with 3 optional tapering sessions (occurring every 2–3 weeks), and used a tailored mobile app between sessions. During the study, participants maintained care with the physician currently managing their diabetes. Medical oversight for study tasks was provided by the study's endocrinologist (MF) and safety was monitored by an independent safety officer (DS).

Baseline assessments (i.e., EDE, height/weight measurements, questionnaires and HbA_{1c}) were repeated after Session 12 (3 months). This was considered end-of-treatment and the primary assessment point. Assessments (with the exception of the EDE) were repeated at two additional time points, administered 3 months after the previous assessment (approximately 6 and 9 months after treatment initiation). In some cases, HbA_{1c} and height/weight measurements for these assessments were obtained from proximal medical visits (rather than asking participants to repeat these measures within a short time frame).

Participants also completed a questionnaire at each therapy session. The questionnaire asked about frequency and severity of hypoglycemia, edema, and other physical and emotional symptoms and medical utilization (routine and emergency visits). This questionnaire was expanded to include the Valuing Questionnaire (VQ [39];) after participants completed session material reviewing core content (typically Session 2).

Process of change measures

Acceptance and action diabetes questionnaire (AADQ; [23])

The AADQ is a diabetes-specific version of the Acceptance and Action Questionnaire [40], a measure widely used in ACT clinical trials to capture change in psychological flexibility. The AADQ consists of 11 items that measure willingness to experience diabetes-related thoughts and feelings, or the inverse, the extent to which experiential *unwillingness* (rejection or suppression of diabetes-related thoughts and feelings) interferes with diabetes management using a Likert-type scale. Sample items include "When I have an upsetting feeling or thought about my diabetes, I try to get rid of that feeling or thought" and "I do not take care of my diabetes because it reminds me that I have diabetes." Gregg et al. [24] reported a Cronbach's $\alpha = .94$ for the AADQ.

Valuing questionnaire (VQ; [38])

The VQ is a 10-item measure that was designed to be administered weekly in clinical and research contexts to capture ongoing change. The VQ measures the extent to which personal values were obstructed by unwanted thoughts and feelings and progress in valued life domains. Unlike the AADQ, the VQ does not require individuals to have explicit awareness of the avoidant function of their behavior, and items extend beyond chronic illness management. Sample items include "I had unpleasant thoughts and emotions that stopped me from achieving my goals." (Obstruction) and "I made progress in areas of life that I care most about." (Progress).

Outcome measures

Eating disorder examination (EDE; [37])-global score

In addition to diagnostic information, the EDE quantifies ED symptom severity with 62 items that assess the frequency and severity of disordered eating behaviors and attitudes within the preceding 4 weeks. The EDE has demonstrated high inter-rater reliability and test-retest reliability as well as convergent validity with daily food records and measures of similar constructs [41, 42].

Diabetes eating problems survey – revised (DEPS-R; [36])

The DEPS-R is a 16-item self-report measure specifically designed to assess disordered eating in individuals with T1D. Respondents rate the frequency with which they have experienced relevant attitudes and behaviors over the past 4 weeks on a 6-point Likert scale ranging from 'never' to 'always.' Sample items include: "I feel fat when I take all my insulin," "I would rather be thin than have good control of my diabetes," "After I overeat, I don't take enough insulin to cover my food," and "I avoid checking my blood sugar when I feel like it is out of range." Scores range between 0 and 80, with higher total scores indicating more ED symptoms. Scores ≥ 20 are considered clinically significant and have been associated with higher HbA_{1c} [37]. Although originally validated with adolescent patients, the DEPS-R has been used with adults with T1D and has demonstrated satisfactory internal consistency and construct validity among adult samples (e.g., [43]).

Diabetes self-management questionnaire (DSMQ; [43])

The DSMQ is a measure of engagement in self-care activities associated with glycemic control. The self-report questionnaire includes 16 items describing self-care behaviors. Respondents rate the extent to which each item applies to them over the past 8 weeks using a four-point Likert scale (3 – 'applies to me very much' to 0 'does not apply to me'). The DSMQ yields a global score estimate of self-care and five subscale scores (Physical Activity, Dietary Control, Medication Adherence, Physician Contact, and Glucose Management). Schmitt et al. [44] reported good internal consistency ($\alpha = 0.84$) for the DSMQ.

Hemoglobin A1c (HbA_{1c})

Blood for HbA_{1c} assessment was drawn by a trained phlebotomist in the Behavioral Diabetes Research Laboratory and analyzed by LabCorp using the Roche Tina Quant assay.

Diabetes distress scale (DDS; [44])

The DDS is a 17-item questionnaire that assesses diabetes-related emotional distress. Sample items include "Feeling angry, scared, and/or depressed when I think about living with diabetes," and "Feeling that I am often failing with my diabetes regimen." Respondents rate the degree to which each item was problematic during the last month on a scale ranging from 1 ('no problem') to 6 ('serious problem'). Item scores are averaged resulting in an estimate of total diabetes distress ranging between 1 and 6. Scores of 3 or higher are considered to reflect clinically meaningful levels of distress [45]. Polonsky et al. [46] report good internal reliability and validity ($\alpha = 0.93$).

Patient-reported outcomes measurement information system (PROMIS; [46]) anxiety and depression scales

The PROMIS research tools were developed by the National Institutes of Health (NIH) to allow for comparison of physical, mental, and social health related outcomes across studies. The PROMIS Short Form-Anxiety 8a (PROMIS Anxiety) and PROMIS Short Form-Depression 8a (PROMIS Depression) are self-report instruments, each containing 8 items, which are rated on a 5-point response scale. The Anxiety 8a measures symptoms of anxiety, including fear, nervousness, and tension, whereas the Depression 8a measures symptoms of depression, including worthlessness, helplessness, and unhappiness. Measures assess frequency of symptoms during the past 7 days with response options ranging from 1 ('never') to 5 ('always'). Raw scores of these instruments are converted into standardized *T*-scores, based on a normative sample with a mean of 50 and standard deviation of 10 (higher scores reflect more severe symptomatology). These measures demonstrate robust psychometric properties established by the PROMIS instrument development and validation standards [47].

Data analysis

Continuous data were examined for normality assumptions and were acceptable with the exception of HbA_{1c}, which was transformed (natural log transformation). Paired sample *t*-tests were used to compare participants' AAQ-D, EDE, DEPS-R, DSMQ, HbA_{1c}, DDS, and PROMIS scores at baseline and end-of-treatment (Session 12, 3 months) and Cohen's *d* effect sizes were calculated. In the case of an outlier, analyses were run with and without the outlier (which did not change the results). Data from the VQ were first analyzed using a flexible curve fitting procedure (3 knot restricted cubic spline) to determine whether a linear model was adequate. Data from the VQ were then analyzed using mixed models. Session number was treated as a continuous variable, with the intercept and session specified as random effects. An unstructured covariance matrix was used based on a comparison of fit indices.

Data from one participant who completed treatment was excluded from all analyses due to late reveal of psychosis which made her ineligible for the study. This individual had paranoid delusions directly related to her insulin pump which interfered with her diabetes management.

Results

Sample characteristics

Complete demographics are provided for the full recruited sample ($n = 28$) as well as treatment completers ($n = 20$) for comparison purposes (Table 1). The recruited sample was 79% White and 100% female. Average age of onset of T1D was 16.2 ($SD = 11.6$). Thirty-nine percent of the sample ($n = 11$) reported using an insulin pump as their mode of insulin delivery, rather than multiple daily injections, which has been associated with lower $HbA1_c$ [48]. Seventy-five percent ($n = 21$) reported that they had major or minor complications associated with diabetes; 7.1% ($n = 2$) indicated they did not have any diabetes-related complication; 17.9 ($n = 5$) did not complete this part of the assessment. The most common complications were diabetes ketoacidosis after initiation of insulin therapy (diabetic ketoacidosis prior to diagnosis is not included here) (50%), bladder, yeast or other urinary tract infection (46%), stomach or intestinal problems (39%) and retinopathy (36%). Skin problems or infections, slow healing cuts or other wounds and decreased vision were also common, with 25% of the sample reporting each of these complications. A few participants also reported neuropathy (11%) and nephropathy (7%).

Participants reported clinically significant ED symptomatology with DEPS-R scores ranging from 25 to 76 ($M = 41.25$; $SD = 12.84$). Of the 24 participants who completed the diagnostic interview, the majority (75%) met criteria for threshold ($n = 13$) or subthreshold ($n = 5$) bulimia nervosa. Subthreshold bulimia was defined as meeting all criteria for bulimia but with binge-purge frequency less than what is required for full diagnosis. Thirteen percent ($n = 3$) met criteria for purging disorder, 8% ($n = 2$) met criteria for binge eating disorder, and 4% ($n = 1$) did not meet threshold criteria for an ED (this participant was withdrawn from the study by the PI and referred to more appropriate treatment). Twenty-five percent of the full sample ($n = 28$) reported receiving treatment for an ED in the past (18%, $n = 5$ did not provide this information).

HbA_{1c} for the sample ranged from 6.1–15.5% ($M = 9.93$, $SD = 2.81$). As previously reported, five participants had HbA_{1c} below 7.5%. These individuals were either restrictive in their eating, or vacillated between binge eating and maladaptive compensatory strategies of self-induced vomiting, overexercise or fasting, which resulted in significant daily BG variability, but produced an average BG in an acceptable range. ED symptoms in the absence of elevated HbA_{1c} is perhaps the most challenging clinical presentation because problems may go undetected by physicians if patients are not regularly screened for ED symptoms.

The sample was highly distressed about their diabetes, with baseline scores on the DDS ranging between 2.12 and 4.88, with the average falling above 3, the clinically recommended cut-off for "high diabetes distress" ($M = 3.79$, $SD = .74$) [45]. Baseline descriptives for all measures at major assessment points are provided in Table 2.

Recruitment and retention

Five of the 28 individuals recruited for the study withdrew after completing some or all of the baseline assessment but before starting treatment, for personal reasons unrelated to the intervention (e.g., distance to travel). Of the 23 individuals who started treatment, 87% ($n = 20$) completed treatment. As previously noted, one participant (4%) was withdrawn by the PI at mid-treatment and referred for more appropriate treatment (this participant had attention-deficit disorder as the primary issue impacting T1D management and was determined to not meet criteria for an ED), and two participants (9%) withdrew after beginning treatment (one withdrew

Table 1 *Participant Demographics*

	All Recruited Participants (*n* = 28)*	*Treatment Completers* (*n* = 20)	*Analyzed* (*n* = 19)
Characteristic	*M* (*SD*) or %	*M* (*SD*) or %	*M* (*SD*) or %
Age (yrs.)	34.8 (12.4)	35.0 (11.8)	35.4 (12.0)
Sex (% female)	100	100	100
Race/Ethnicity (%)			
Caucasian/White	78.6	80	78.9
African-American/Black	14.3	10	10.5
More than one race	7.1	10	10.5
Marital Status (%)			
Never Married	46.4	50	47.4
Married	25.0	35	36.8
Separated/Divorced	14.3	15	15.8
Unknown	14.3	0	0
Highest Level of Education (%)			
Some high school	3.6	5	5.3
Some college/technical school	25.0	20	21.1
Bachelor's degree	28.6	35	31.6
Graduate degree	28.6	40	42.1
Unknown	14.3	0	0
Body Mass Index (BMI) (*M*)	27.8 (5.5)	28.2 (5.8)	28.5 (5.7)
Normal Weight (%)	29	35	32
Overweight (%)	25	25	26
Obese (%)	29	40	42
Unknown (%)	18	0	0
Insulin Administration (%)			
Insulin Pump	39	45	47
Multiple Daily Injections	46	55	53
Unknown	14	0	0
Age at Type 1 Diabetes Diagnosis (Years)	16.2 (11.6)	17.2 (12.2)	17.3 (12.5)
Diabetes Complications (%)			
History of Retinopathy	36	40	42
History of Neuropathy	11	10	11
History of Nephropathy	7	5	5
History of Diabetes Ketoacidosis Post Initiation of Insulin Therapy	50	55	58
Eating Disorder Diagnosis (%)			
Bulimia Nervosa	46	60	63
Subthreshold Bulimia Nervosa	18	15	11
Purging Disorder	11	15	16
Binge Eating Disorder	7	10	11
Unknown	14	0	0

Note: Data analyses were conducted on 19 of the 20 treatment completers; $n = 1$ was excluded from analyses due to late reveal of psychosis directly impacting her management behavior

Table 2 Mean (SD) for Outcome Variables for the Recruited and Analyzed Sample at all Assessment Points

	Baseline (*n* = 28)*	Baseline (*n* = 19)	End-of-Treatment (3 Months) (*n* = 19)	Second Assessment (6 Months) (*n* = 16)	Third Assessment (9 Months) (*n* = 15)
EDE	3.5 (1.0)	3.5 (1.1)	2.5 (1.0)	-	-
DEPS-R	41.3 (12.8)	42.7 (13.9)	25.3 (10.8)	26.3 (11.8)	28.3 (14.9)
DSMQ	4.7 (1.6)	4.7 (1.5)	6.3 (1.5)	6.1 (1.8)	6.4 (1.0)
HbA_{1c} (%)	9.9 (2.8)	9.8 (2.7)	8.9 (2.4)	8.5 (1.9)	9.3 (2.4)
DDS	3.8 (.7)	3.8 (.6)	2.8 (.7)	2.7 (.7)	2.7 (.93)
PROMIS-D	60.2 (6.7)	61.0 (6.9)	57.0 (7.7)	56.5 (8.2)	55.8 (11.3)
PROMIS-A	61.2 (7.3)	60.84 (7.7)	58.5 (10.2)	56.1 (8.5)	58.5 (10.4)
AADQ	49.9 (7.7)	49.2 (6.9)	56.1 (4.9)	56.1 (6.1)	56.2 (7.5)

Note: *Includes all recruited participants who completed some or all of the baseline assessment
EDE Eating Disorder Examination Global Score (administered only at baseline and EOT), *DEPS-R* Diabetes Eating Problems Survey-Revised, *DSMQ* Diabetes Self-Management Questionnaire (higher scores indicate improvement), *HbA_{1c}* Hemoglobin A_{1c}, *DDS* Diabetes Distress Scale, *PROMIS-D* PROMIS Short Form-Depression 8a, *PROMIS-A* PROMIS Short Form-Anxiety 8a, *AADQ* Acceptance and Action Diabetes Questionnaire (higher scores indicate improvement)

after completing the first session and the other was lost to contact after completing two sessions).

The majority of treatment completers ($n = 18$) completed optional tapering sessions, and over half of these individuals ($n = 12$; 60%) requested to continue treatment beyond this point. Given the lack of information about appropriate treatment duration for T1D patients with EDs, the risk of continued ED symptoms (e.g., insulin restriction), and the lack of other treatment options for this high-risk patient population, participants who requested to continue to receive treatment were provided with additional therapy sessions. The total number of sessions among treatment completers ($n = 20$) ranged from 12 to 21, with the exception of two participants who continued in weekly treatment after their end-of-treatment (Session 12, 3 month) assessment. Both of these individuals presented with additional comorbid diagnoses (e.g., major depressive disorder) and complex trauma.

App engagement

All participants who initiated treatment ($n = 23$) downloaded and accessed the app at least once, with the exception of the one participant who discontinued treatment after two sessions. There was considerable variability in app use as indexed by completion of logs providing information about meals, ED and diabetes management behaviors or emotional distress. Treatment completers ($n = 20$) completed 156.2 ($SD = 109.35$; Median = 161.50) logs on average between Session 1 and Session 12, and averaged 189.9 ($SD = 152.86$; Median = 196.5) logs between Session 1 and the last study assessment (occurring approximately 9 months after treatment initiation).

Treatment tolerance

Overall, treatment was well tolerated. Therapy session questionnaires indicated mild to moderate (but not severe) bloating and edema were common, particularly mid-treatment. Hypoglycemia was also not a major problem. Six participants reported hypoglycemia was a regular occurrence (occurring multiple times a week). About half the sample ($n = 10$) reported hypoglycemic events were absent or infrequent throughout treatment. Four participants reported a mixed pattern (i.e., hypoglycemic events were absent or infrequent about 40–60% of the time, and occurred multiple times a week the remainder of the time). Participants did not require emergency intervention for hypoglycemia during the study, but one participant did have a severe episode that required this type of intervention during the follow-up period.

No participants were hospitalized during the intervention. One participant (a 17-year old with bulimia nervosa) sought residential treatment after Session 12. This participant improved her HbA_{1c} during the 12 weeks, and entering residential treatment was viewed as a positive next step to continue her progress.

BMI did not significantly change from baseline to end-of-treatment, t [19] = − 1.3, 95% CI [−.96, .25], p = .23, which is important given weight gain is often a concern for ED patients that may interfere with treatment engagement.

Completion of assessments

Of the participants who completed treatment ($n = 20$), 100% completed the first assessment (Session 12, 3 months). Ninety percent ($n = 18$) completed some or all of the second assessment (a few participants provided a blood sample for HbA_{1c} but did not complete the questionnaires or vice versa), scheduled 3 months after the individual's previous assessment. Eighty percent ($n = 16$) completed some or all of the third assessment battery, scheduled 3 months after the individual's previous assessment. Participants who did not complete all study assessments were unable to do so for the following reasons: family member illness and associated time restrictions ($n = 1$), relocation for residential treatment ($n = 1$) and unknown reasons (i.e., lost to contact) ($n = 2$).

Changes in psychological flexibility

Participants reported increased psychological flexibility with diabetes-related thoughts and feelings from baseline to end-of-treatment, as indexed by the AADQ, t [19] = − 4.1, 95% CI [− 10.53, − 3.37], $p = .001$, Cohen's $d = 0.94$.

Preliminary analyses of the VQ suggested a linear fit was probably adequate (i.e., the trajectory of change for either VQ subscale did not appear to be nonlinear, Obstruction $p = 0.89$ and Progress, $p = 0.28$). The linear slope coefficient for Obstruction was − 0.51 (95% CI = − 0.79, − 0.24, $p = 0.001$), indicating that Obstruction of Values was reduced by about a half point per session. For Progress, the linear slope coefficient was 0.30 (95% CI = 0.09, 0.51, $p = 0.006$), indicating that Progress in Values increased by about a third of a point every session.

Eating disorder symptoms

Participants reported significant improvements in ED symptoms from baseline to end-of-treatment, as indexed by the EDE Global Scores, t [19] = 4.13, 95% CI [.51, 1.57], $p = .001$, Cohen's $d = 0.90$, and the DEPS-R, t [19] = 7.8, 95% CI [12.73, 22.11], $p < .001$, Cohen's $d = 1.79$.

Diabetes management

Diabetes self-management (DSMQ scores) significantly improved, t [19] = − 4.1, 95% CI [− 2.36, −.76], $p = .001$, Cohen's $d = 0.92$. Change in HbA_{1c} did not reach statistical significance, t [19] = 1.9, $p = .08$, Cohen's $d = 0.44$. Mean decrease in HbA_{1c} was .9% (95% CI = -.07–1.77). Fifty-three percent of the participants with $HbA_{1c} \geq 7.5\%$ at baseline evidenced at least a .5% decrease from baseline to end-of-treatment, which is considered clinically significant [25].

Emotional distress

Diabetes distress (DDS scores) decreased from baseline to end-of-treatment, t [19] = 6.0, 95% CI [.69, 1.45], $p < .001$, Cohen's $d = 1.38$. There were mixed findings for change in depression and anxiety, which were not explicitly targeted by the intervention. Depression (PROMIS Depression scores) significantly improved, t [19] = 2.4, 95% CI [.51, 7.32], $p = .03$, Cohen's $d = 0.55$, but anxiety (PROMIS Anxiety scores) did not, t [18] = 1.0, 95% CI [− 2.4, 7.08], $p = .32$, Cohen's $d = 0.24$).

Discussion

The problem of EDs in T1D is significant and relatively intractable to change [4–6]. Treatments for this high-risk patient population are underdeveloped and understudied, and thus patients are without empirically-based outpatient treatment options. The current study piloted a novel intervention tailored to the unique experience of living with diabetes and the related emotional distress that may contribute to the development of maladaptive eating and weight control behaviors. This is the first study to assess the acceptability and feasibility of an outpatient intervention specifically tailored to this unique patient population. The key finding was that treatment was acceptable to T1D patients with ED symptoms and feasible to implement with minimal complications.

Changes in target processes of psychological flexibility and value-guided action were also observed, and individuals who participated in the intervention experienced significant improvements in ED symptomatology, diabetes management and diabetes distress. However, given the open trial design, we cannot infer that changes were the result of intervention, rather than nonspecific treatment effects, natural course, or regression to the mean; although it should be noted that previous studies have found that without intervention, ED behaviors in T1D tend to persist and worsen over time [4].

Many participants requested additional treatment. This suggests that the treatment was acceptable, but also indicates that participants believed that they needed more or continued support. Previous reviews have indicated typical treatment duration of 8 to 20 sessions for EDs, depending on clinical presentation [49–52]. Thus, in comparison, *i*ACT might be considered brief. Longer treatment duration could be helpful for some patients.

The current treatment paired individual therapy sessions with the use of a mobile app between sessions to evoke and reinforce behavior change in the natural environment. It did not test the individual components of the intervention, and thus it is unclear whether particular components are necessary or sufficient. This would be an important next step for potentiating treatment effects and maximizing treatment efficiency. Future studies might examine whether the app is necessary, whether engagement with particular app features predicts outcomes, or explore strategies to increase app use among some participants. Future studies might also explore whether some individuals respond to the app alone, or whether the app can be paired with a single in-person contact or with video/telehealth sessions to enhance portability. Future studies could examine the effect of the different treatment components, as well as treatment dose, using adaptive (e.g., Sequential Multiple Assignment Randomized Trial; SMART) designs.

The primary aim of the current study was to assess acceptability and feasibility of this treatment approach. However, the outcomes for HbA_{1c} are still of interest. Many participants evidenced change of .5% in HbA_{1c} from baseline to end-of-treatment, which is considered clinically significant. However, mean change in HbA_{1c} did not achieve statistical significance. The more modest effect size for HbA_{1c} (relative to the large effects observed for other outcomes) may be attributable to the amount of time necessary for behavior change to be reflected in HbA_{1c} (with the average lifespan of a red blood cell 100–120 days). Longer follow up in controlled studies is needed.

Change in HbA_{1c} might have also been attenuated due to the inclusion of patients with $HbA_{1c} \leq 7.5\%$. These patients were part of the population of interest (i.e., they met criteria for an ED) and their clinical presentation put them at risk for complications associated with both hyper- and hypoglycemia due to significant BG variability associated binge eating, purging or other ED behaviors. Future studies of EDs in T1D should adequately account for these patients in power calculations and use continuous glucose monitoring, in addition to HbA_{1c}, to index treatment related improvements in glycemic control. For example, continuous glucose monitoring might reveal decreased time spent below 70 or above 180 mg/dL, or reductions in daily BG variability as a result of intervention. This is increasingly possible with technological advancements that allow glucose sensors to be worn for longer periods of time and data loss to be minimized.

The current study allowed participants to continue in treatment if they requested to do so. This decision was made prioritizing the needs of this high-risk population, and with the understanding that necessary and appropriate treatment duration for T1D patients with EDs is unknown and may vary by individual. As with any pilot study, findings should be interpreted with caution.

The current study may have limited generalizability as the majority of participants were white females. While this is expected given that T1D is more prevalent in white individuals, and EDs are more prevalent among women and girls [53, 54], larger studies with more diverse samples are needed. The current study also recruited participants from endocrinology clinics. Individuals recruited from endocrinology may be less severe than those who would be recruited from a general psychiatry or ED practice, or have other differences that limit the generalizability of the findings.

As first noted, the most significant limitation to the current study is the single-arm trial design. However, the primary aim of the investigation was to determine whether this type of treatment is acceptable and feasible, and gather preliminary evidence that the targeted processes of change were engaged and that treatment might improve ED symptoms and T1D management. Findings from the current study suggest that a randomized controlled trial of *i*ACT is warranted.

Conclusion

In summary, *i*ACT holds promise for the treatment of ED symptoms among T1D patients. This treatment approach, which is tailored to this unique patient population and grounded in theory regarding how these behavior problems may develop or be maintained, is acceptable to T1D patients and feasible to implement. Additional research is needed to test whether improvements in ED symptoms and glycemic control exceed what would be expected with time alone or with another treatment. Future research might also investigate which treatment components are necessary and sufficient, explore options for maximizing treatment effects or portability of the intervention, and examine patient matching to treatment and treatment dose. More broadly, this study adds to a growing body of research on ACT for a variety of clinical problems [23], including EDs and diabetes management. It also provides an example of the use of mobile technology in ACT-based treatment delivery, which may inform innovative, highly scalable interventions.

Abbreviations

T1D: Type 1 diabetes; EDs: Eating disorders; ED: Eating disorder; BG: Blood glucose; HbA_{1c} : Hemoglobin $A1_c$; App : Mobile application

Acknowledgements

The authors wish to thank Jenna Tregarthen, PGDip and Stuart Argue for the use of the Recovery Record (RR) mobile application and their assistance in programming the unique features and extracting the RR data for this trial.

Authors' contributions

RM formulated the idea (conceptualization and methodology), obtained funding and directed the investigation, developed and administered the intervention and drafted the majority of the manuscript; AM managed the data (data validation), administered the intervention to subsequent participants, and drafted portions of the manuscript; MB summarized and analyzed the data; MF provided medical oversight for study participants and assisted in data interpretation; LH managed daily study operations, administered diagnostic assessments and acquired biometrics and contributed to methodology and data summarization; JM assisted with data acquisition and validation, and formulation of the idea; SF assisted with data validation, tables and figures; HB assisted with data acquisition, tables and figures; DS served as an independent safety officer and assisted with methodology. All authors reviewed, edited and approved the submitted manuscript.

Competing interests

The authors declare that they have no competing interests.

Author details
[1]Department of Psychiatry and Behavioral Sciences, Duke University Medical Center, DUMC Box 3842, Durham, NC 27712, USA. [2]Department of Medicine, Division of Endocrinology, Metabolism and Nutrition, Duke University Medical Center, Durham, NC, USA. [3]Department of Family Medicine and Community Health, Duke University Medical Center, Durham, NC, USA.

References

1. American Diabetes Association (2019). Standards of Medical Care in Diabetes—2019 Diabetes Care, 42 (Supplement 1).
2. Nathan DM, Group DER. The diabetes control and complications trial/ epidemiology of diabetes interventions and complications study at 30 years: overview. Diabetes Care. 2014;37(1):9–16.
3. Araia E, Hendrieckx C, Skinner T, Pouwer F, Speight J, King RM. Gender differences in disordered eating behaviors and body dissatisfaction among adolescents with type 1 diabetes: results from diabetes MILES youth—Australia. Int J Eat Disord. 2017;50(10):1183–93.
4. Colton PA, Olmsted MP, Daneman D, Farquhar JC, Wong H, Muskat S, et al. Eating disorders in girls and women with type 1 diabetes: a longitudinal study of prevalence, onset, remission, and recurrence. Diabetes Care. 2015; 38(7):1212–7.
5. Toni G, Berioli M, Cerquiglini L, Ceccarini G, Grohmann U, Principi N, et al. Eating disorders and disordered eating symptoms in adolescents with type 1 diabetes. Nutrients. 2017;9(8):906.
6. Young V, Eiser C, Johnson B, Brierley S, Elliott J, Heller S. Eating problems in adolescents with type 1 diabetes: a systematic review with meta-analysis. Diabet Med. 2013;30:189–98.
7. American Diabetes Association (2019). 6. Glycemic targets: standards of medical care in diabetes—2019. Diabetes Care, 41(Supplement 1), S61-S70.
8. Rydall AC, Rodin GM, Olmsted MP, Devenyi RG, Daneman D. Disordered eating behavior and microvascular complications in young women with insulin-dependent diabetes mellitus. N Engl J Med. 1997;336(26):1849–54.
9. Nielsen S, Emborg C, Molbak A. Mortality in concurrent type I diabetes and anorexia nervosa. Diabetes Care. 2002;25:309–12.
10. Scheuing N, Bartus B, Berger G, Haberland H, Icks A, Knauth B, et al. Clinical characteristics and outcome of 467 patients with a clinically recognized eating disorder identified among 52,215 patients with type 1 diabetes: a multicenter german/austrian study. Diabetes Care. 2014;37(6):1581–9.
11. Takii M, Uchigata Y, Tokunaga S, Amemiya N, Kinukawa N, Nozaki T, et al. The duration of severe insulin omission is the factor Most closely associated with the microvascular complications of type 1 diabetic females with clinical eating disorders. Int J Eat Disord. 2008;41(3):259–64.
12. Goebel-Fabbri AE, Fikkan J, Franko DL, Pearson K, Anderson BJ, Weinger K. Insulin restriction and associated morbidity and mortality in women with type 1 diabetes. Diabetes Care. 2008;31(3):415–9.
13. Custal N, Arcelus J, Agüera Z, Bove FI, Wales J, Granero R, et al. Treatment outcome of patients with comorbid type 1 diabetes and eating disorders. BMC Psychiatry. 2014;14(1):140.
14. Olmsted MP, Daneman D, Rydall AC, Lawson ML, Rodin G. The effects of psychoeducation on disturbed eating attitudes and behavior in young women with type 1 diabetes mellitus. Int J Eat Disord. 2002;32(2):230–9.
15. Peveler RC, Fairburn CG. The treatment of bulimia nervosa in patients with diabetes mellitus. Int J Eat Disord. 1992;11(1):45–53.
16. Goebel-Fabbri AE. Disturbed eating behaviors and eating disorders in type 1 diabetes: clinical significance and treatment recommendations. Current Diabetes Reports. 2009;9:133–9.
17. Merwin RM, Dmitrieva NO, Honeycutt LK, Moskovich AA, Lane JD, Zucker NL, et al. Momentary predictors of insulin restriction among adults with type 1 diabetes and eating disorder symptomatology. Diabetes Care. 2015; 38(11):2025–32.
18. Farstad SM, McGeown LM, von Ranson KM. Eating disorders and personality, 2004–2016: a systematic review and meta-analysis. Clin Psychol Rev. 2016; 46:91–105.
19. Vacca M, Ballesio A, Lombardo C. The relationship between perfectionism and eating-related symptoms in adolescents: a systematic review. Eur Eat Disord Rev. 2020.
20. Polivy J, Herman C. Dieting and bingeing: a causal analysis. Am Psychol. 1985;40:193–201.
21. Hayes SC, Strosahl KD, Wilson KG. Acceptance and commitment therapy: the process and practice of mindful change: Guilford press; 2011.
22. Beck JS. Cognitive behavior therapy: basics and beyond: Guilford press; 2011.
23. Levin ME, Luoma JB, Haeger JA. Decoupling as a mechanism of change in mindfulness and acceptance: a literature review. Behav Modif. 2015;39(6): 870–911.
24. Gregg JA, Callaghan GM, Hayes SC, Glenn-Lawson JL. Improving diabetes self-management through acceptance, mindfulness, and values: a randomized controlled trial. J Consult Clin Psychol. 2007;75(2):336–43.
25. Juarascio A, Shaw J, Forman E, Timko CA, Herbert J, Butryn M, et al. Acceptance and commitment therapy as a novel treatment for eating disorders: an initial test of efficacy and mediation. Behav Modif. 2013;37(4): 459–89.
26. Timko CA, Zucker NL, Herbert JD, Rodriguez D, Merwin RM. An open trial of acceptance-based separated family treatment (ASFT) for adolescents with anorexia nervosa. Behav Res Ther 2015;69(0):63–74.
27. Wildes JE, Marcus MD, Cheng Y, McCabe EB, Gaskill JA. Emotion acceptance behavior therapy for anorexia nervosa: a pilot study. Int J Eat Disord. 2014; 47(8):870–3.
28. Tregarthen JP, Lock J, Darcy AM. Development of a smartphone application for eating disorder self-monitoring. Int J Eat Disord. 2015;48(7):972–82.
29. Takii M, Uchigata Y, Komaki G, Nozaki T, Kawai H, Iwamoto Y, et al. An integrated inpatient therapy for type 1 diabetic females with bulimia nervosa: a 3-year follow-up study. J Psychosom Res. 2003;55(4):349–56.
30. Dickens YL, Haynos AF, Nunnemaker S, Platka-Bird L, Dolores J. Multidisciplinary residential treatment of type 1 diabetes mellitus and co-occurring eating disorders. Eat Disord. 2015;23(2):134–43.
31. Merwin RM, Moskovich AA, Honeycutt LK, Lane JD, Feinglos M, Surwit RS, et al. Time of day when type 1 diabetes patients with eating disorder symptoms most commonly restrict insulin. Psychosom Med. 2018;80(2):222–9.
32. Stokes TF, Osnes PG. An operant pursuit of generalization. Behav Ther. 1989; 20(3):337–55.
33. Merwin RM. ACT innovations for dangerous weight control: anorexia nervosa and ED-DMT1. In: Levin M, Twohig M, Krafft J, editors. Acceptance and commitment therapy: clinical advances and applications in ACT: New Harbinger Publications; 2020. –Oakland.
34. Stoddard JA, Afari N. The big book of ACT metaphors: a practitioner's guide to experiential exercises and metaphors in acceptance and commitment therapy: new harbinger publications; 2014.
35. Gold AE, Macleod KM, Frier BM. Frequency of severe hypoglycemia in patients with type 1 diabetes with impaired awareness of hypoglycemia. Diabetes Care. 1994;17(7):697–703.
36. Little RR, Rohlfing CL, Sacks DB. Status of hemoglobin A1c measurement and goals for improvement: from chaos to order for improving diabetes care. Clin Chem. 2011;57(2):205–14.
37. Markowitz J, Butler D, Volkening L, Antisdel J, Anderson B, Laffel L. Brief screening tool for disordered eating in diabetes. Internal consistency and external validity in a contemporary sample of pediatric patients with type 1 diabetes. Diabetes Care. 2010;33:495–500.
38. Fairburn C, Cooper, Z., & O'Connor, M. . Eating Disorder Examination (Edition 17.0D). 2014.
39. Smout M, Davies M, Burns N, Christie A. Development of the valuing questionnaire (VQ). J Contextual Behav Sci. 2014;3(3):164–72.
40. Bond FW, Hayes SC, Baer RA, Carpenter KM, Guenole N, Orcutt HK, et al. Preliminary psychometric properties of the acceptance and action questionnaire–II: a revised measure of psychological inflexibility and experiential avoidance. Behav Ther. 2011;42(4):676–88.
41. Berg KC, Peterson CB, Frazier P, Crow SJ. Convergence of scores on the interview and questionnaire versions of the eating disorder examination: a meta-analytic review. Psychol Assess. 2011;23(3):714.
42. Rizvi SL, Peterson CB, Crow SJ, Agras WS. Test-retest reliability of the eating disorder examination. Int J Eat Disord. 2000;28(3):311–6.
43. Wisting L, Wonderlich J, Skrivarhaug T, Dahl-Jørgensen K, Rø Ø. Psychometric properties and factor structure of the diabetes eating problem survey–revised (DEPS-R) among adult males and females with type 1 diabetes. J Eat Disord. 2019;7(1):2.
44. Schmitt A, Gahr A, Hermanns N, Kulzer B, Huber J, Haak T. The diabetes self-management questionnaire (DSMQ): development and evaluation of an instrument to assess diabetes self-care activities associated with glycaemic control. Health Qual Life Outcomes. 2013;11(1):138.

45. Fisher L, Hessler DM, Polonsky WH, Mullan J. When is diabetes distress clinically meaningful?: establishing cut points for the Diabetes Distress Scale. Diabetes Care. 2012:DC_111572.
46. Polonsky W, Fischer L, Earles J, Dudl R, Lees J, Mullan J, et al. Assessing psychosocial stress in diabetes: Development of the Diabetes Distress Scale. Diabetes Care. 2005;28:626–31.
47. Cella D, Riley W, Stone A, Rothrock N, Reeve B, Yount S, et al. The patient-reported outcomes measurement information system (PROMIS) developed and tested its first wave of adult self-reported health outcome item banks: 2005–2008. J Clin Epidemiol. 2010;63(11):1179–94.
48. Alzahrani NN, Mashrah HT, Alzahrani SM, Asiri AS, Faydh AA, Aljuaid NW, et al. Comparison of haemoglobin A1c level in insulin pump versus multi daily injections users for type one diabetes mellitus. Middle East J Family Med. 2019;7(10):22.
49. Brockmeyer T, Friederich H-C, Schmidt U. Advances in the treatment of anorexia nervosa: a review of established and emerging interventions. Psychol Med. 2018;48(8):1228–56.
50. Fairburn CG, Bailey-Straebler S, Basden S, Doll HA, Jones R, Murphy R, et al. A transdiagnostic comparison of enhanced cognitive behaviour therapy (CBT-E) and interpersonal psychotherapy in the treatment of eating disorders. Behav Res Ther. 2015;70:64–71.
51. Ghaderi A, Odeberg J, Gustafsson S, Råstam M, Brolund A, Pettersson A, et al. Psychological, pharmacological, and combined treatments for binge eating disorder: a systematic review and meta-analysis. PeerJ. 2018;6:e5113.
52. Wonderlich SA, Peterson CB, Crosby RD, Smith TL, Klein MH, Mitchell JE, et al. A randomized controlled comparison of integrative cognitive-affective therapy (ICAT) and enhanced cognitive-behavioral therapy (CBT-E) for bulimia nervosa. Psychol Med. 2014;44(3):543–53.
53. Pettitt DJ, Talton J, Dabelea D, Divers J, Imperatore G, Lawrence JM, et al. Prevalence of diabetes in US youth in 2009: the SEARCH for diabetes in youth study. Diabetes Care. 2014;37(2):402–8.
54. Hudson JI, Hiripi E, Pope HG Jr, Kessler RC. The prevalence and correlates of eating disorders in the National Comorbidity Survey Replication. Biol Psychiatry. 2007;61(3):348–58.

7

Associations between autism spectrum disorder and eating disorders with and without self-induced vomiting

Noriko Numata[1*], Akiko Nakagawa[1], Kazuko Yoshioka[2], Kayoko Isomura[3], Daisuke Matsuzawa[1], Rikukage Setsu[4,5], Michiko Nakazato[6,7] and Eiji Shimizu[1,4]

Abstract

Background: Although approximately 23% of anorexia nervosa (AN) patients have concomitant autism spectrum disorder (ASD), it is clinically difficult to determine ASD coexistence in patients with eating disorders. Restrictive AN is more common in younger patients and self-induced vomiting usually appears during adolescence/young adulthood, in order to prevent gaining weight caused by overeating. However, some patients are tolerant of weight gain even if they start overeating. It is important to understand the essential difference between those who vomit and those who do not vomit. In this study, we hypothesised that the absence of self-induced vomiting may be associated with the presence of ASD and aimed to assess the presence of ASD traits in each eating disorder (EDs). Clarifying this association helps to consider the coexistence of ASD in the clinical setting and can lead to the next detailed ASD evaluation, and as a result, helps to determine the appropriate treatment and support individually.

Methods: We retrospectively evaluated 43 females aged 15–45 years who attended Chiba University Hospital between 2012 and 2016 using the Eating Disorder Examination Questionnaire (EDE-Q) and Autism-Spectrum Quotient (AQ) to quantify the severity of the EDs and to identify whether ASD traits were present.

Results: There was no difference in the AQ score between bingeing-purging type AN and restricting type AN. However, there was significant difference in the AQ score between bulimia nervosa and binge EDs (BED). Of the 4 ED subtypes, BED had the highest ASD traits. The non-vomiting group with illness duration < 4 years had a significantly higher AQ communication score than the vomiting group with illness duration ≥4 years.

Conclusions: There was a difference in the AQ score by the presence or absence of self-induced vomiting. The results of this study suggest an association between high scores on AQ and non-vomiting. Thus, evaluation of patients for the absence of self-induced vomiting while assessing them for EDs may help us to understand the association with ASD traits.

Keywords: Eating disorder, Subtype, Autism spectrum disorder, Self-induced vomiting, Autism-Spectrum quotient

* Correspondence: n_numata@chiba-u.jp
[1]Research Center for Child Mental Development, Chiba University, 1-8-1 Inohana, Chuo-ku, Chiba 260-8670, Japan
Full list of author information is available at the end of the article

Plain English summary

Although about 23% of anorexia nervosa (AN) patients have concomitant autism spectrum disorder (ASD), it is clinically difficult to determine ASD coexistence in patients with eating disorders (EDs). Restrictive AN is more common in younger patients and self-induced vomiting typically appears during adolescence, in order to prevent gaining weight caused by overeating. However, some patients state that they 'would never 'want to vomit' and are tolerant of weight gain even if they start overeating.

We aimed to assess the presence of ASD traits in each subtype of ED and explore whether an association exists between ASD traits and EDs with or without self-induced vomiting. We retrospectively evaluated 43 females aged 15–45 years using the Eating Disorder Examination Questionnaire (EDE-Q) and Autism-Spectrum Quotient (AQ) to quantify the severity of the ED and to identify whether an ASD trait was present.

The AQ tended to be higher in the group without than in the group with self-induced vomiting. Patients with binge EDs (BED) had the highest AQ score. The results of this study suggest an association between high scores on AQ and non-vomiting. In case of absence of vomiting in EDs, the presence of ASD and a change in the treatment course must be considered. Further verification is required in the future.

Background

According to the Diagnostic and Statistical Manual of Mental Disorders, Fifth Edition (DSM-5), eating disorders (EDs) can be classified into anorexia nervosa (AN), bulimia nervosa (BN), and binge eating disorder (BED) [1, 2]. AN can then be further divided into a restricting (AN-R) type and a binge eating with self-induced vomiting (AN-BP) type. Patients frequently transition from one ED type to another, typically from the AN-R type to the AN-BP type [3]; this may be attributed to the fact that strict dietary restrictions cannot be maintained for a long time.

It is interesting that many of the common features of EDs are similar to the cognitive rigidity in the presence of changing environmental demands that is often seen in autism spectrum disorder (ASD) [4]. This may indicate a pathological link between the two disorders, with some studies indicating that 18–23% of patients with AN have comorbid ASD [5–7]. Other research has shown that scores on the Eating Disorder Examination Questionnaire (EDE-Q) were significantly and positively correlated with those on the Autism-Spectrum Quotient (AQ), 10-item version, but not with the body mass index (BMI) [8]. This correlation has also been observed in studies conducted on adults and adolescents with AN [9, 10]. Studies have shown that prognosis may be worse when EDs and ASD are comorbid [4, 5, 11].

It is necessary to assess ASD traits when deciding the treatment policy for patients with EDs. However, clinically, it is difficult to determine the ASD traits of patients with EDs. Restrictive AN is more common in younger patients, and self-induced vomiting usually appears during adolescence/young adulthood in order to prevent gaining weight caused by overeating. However, we clinically observed some patients who say that they 'would never want to vomit' and are tolerant of weight gain even if overeating began. We aimed to determine the difference between those who vomit and those who do not vomit and thought that this difference might be related to the ASD trait. Therefore, we decided to investigate whether the presence or absence of vomiting was associated with the ASD trait.

To date, many studies have discussed links between ASD and AN restricting type [8]. Given that many patients transit between ED subtypes, it is logical that research should be more expanded to other subtypes of ED. In this study, we hypothesised that the absence of self-induced vomiting may be associated with the presence of ASD and aimed to assess the presence of ASD traits in each ED. Clarifying this association helps to consider the coexistence of ASD in the clinical setting and can lead to the next detailed ASD evaluation, and as a result, helps to determine the appropriate treatment and support individually.

Methods

Procedure

The data were retrospectively sampled from outpatients from clinical records when they participated in one of three independent studies on ED were conducted at Chiba University Hospital between 2012 and 2016. The Institutional Ethics Committee of Chiba University Graduate School of Medicine approved this study (no. 3431). All subjects provided written informed consent.

Subjects were diagnosed by a psychiatrist with experience in EDs, using the DSM-IV revised criteria [12] and the DSM-5 [2]. AN, BN and BED were included if the criteria was fully met; however, one atypical ED who was chewing type was excluded from this study. Self-report questionnaires were completed by subjects at that time visited the hospital.

Subjects

The collected sample size was 43, all were female. Among them, 42 subjects were finally analysed because the chewing type was excluded. Among those 42 subjects, 23 of BN, 8 of AN-BP, 6 of AN-R and 5 of BED were included. The subjects with self-induced vomiting (BN and AN-BP) were 31, and those without self-induced vomiting (AN-R and BED) were 11 at the time of assessment. The mean age of the 42 subjects was 26.2 (± 7.8). Vomiting was assessed by both a psychiatrist and self-reported questionnaire (EDE-Q).

Measures

Relevant demographic data were collected, including age, duration of illness and BMI. ED severity was assessed using the global EDE-Q score [13], whereas autistic tendencies were assessed using the AQ [14].

Eating disorder examination questionnaire (EDE-Q)

The EDE-Q is a standardised and well-validated 36-item self-report questionnaire that measures the severity of ED symptoms and behaviours in the 28 days leading up to the survey [13]. In the questionnaire, patients are asked to rate how often they have engaged in specific ED behaviours or held ED concerns during the previous 28 days. The questionnaire generates scores for four subscales—'dietary restraint,' 'weight concern,' 'shape concern,' and 'eating concern'—together with a global score that reflects overall illness severity. The maximum global score is 6, with higher scores indicating greater severity. The optimal cut-off score is 2.5 for discriminating between those with the disorder and healthy controls [15]. Cronbach's α ranged from.78 (Eating concern at Time 1) to.92 (Shape Concern at Time 2) for women [16]. In the Japanese version, Cronbach's α coefficient was 0.94 for the global scale, 0.81 for the restricting subscale, 0.86 for the eating concern subscale, 0.88 for the shape subscale, and 0.79 for the weight subscale. It showed a significant correlation with the Eating Attitude Test-26 and the Eating Disorder Inventory-91 [17]. Considering the findings of previous studies [13, 18], the EDE-Q appears to be a psychometrically sound self-report measure for the screening of EDs.

Autism-Spectrum quotient (AQ)

The 50-item AQ was developed to provide a brief self-report measure of autistic traits in adults but was not designed to be used as a diagnostic tool despite its widespread use. The AQ consists of five domains associated with ASDs: social skills, attention switching, attention to detail and communication and imagination. Each question allows the subject to indicate 'definitely agree,' 'slightly agree,' 'slightly disagree,' or 'definitely disagree.' Approximately half the questions are worded to elicit an 'agree' response and half to elicit a 'disagree' response in neurotypical individuals. The cut-off score for ASD is 33. The internal consistency of items in each of the five domains was also calculated, and Cronbach's α coefficients were moderate-to-high (Communication = .65; Social = .77; Imagination = .65; Local Details = .63; and Attention Switching = .67) [14, 19]. In the Japanese version, the global scale was α = 0.81. The α coefficient for each individual scale was as follows: 0.78 for social skills, 0.63 for attention switching, 057 for attention to detail, 0.64 for communication, and 0.51 for imagination [19].

Statistical analysis

All data were reported as means and standard deviations or numbers (number of people) and percentages as appropriate. Demographic data were analysed by Kruskal–Wallis analysis and multiple comparisons were performed by the Steel–Dwass method. In addition, AQ scores and EDE-Q scores of patients with and without self-induced vomiting and EDE-Q scores were compared using the Mann–Whitney test, because we had assumed that the variables would not be normally distributed owing to the relatively small sample size. Assuming that BMI is a confounding factor, Mann–Whitney test was performed between anorexic group and bulimic group. Furthermore, illness duration can be a confounding factor; therefore, Kruskal–Wallis analysis was conducted to confirm this. (Correlation analysis could not be performed owing to the relatively small sample size). Finally, the ratio of the subtypes and the number of patients who exceeded the cut-off value of the AQ score was determined, and the difference in the ratio of the number of patients was examined by Fisher's exact test. We also calculated the effect size using Cramer's V. A Cramer's V > 0.10 was used as the criterion for a small effect, a value > 0.30 as a medium effect, and > 0.50 as a large effect (http://jspt.japanpt.or.jp/ebpt_glossary/effect-size.html). There was no missing value. There were some outlier values; however, all the numbers were clinically possible and were not excluded. Statistical analyses were performed using the STAT statistical package and js-STAR version 9.7.8j.

Results

Demographic analysis and clinical characteristics in subtypes of ED

The 42 female outpatients aged 12–45 years (mean 26.2 ± 7.8 years) were analysed. The sample comprised the following diagnoses: 23 with BN (54.7%), 8 with AN-BP (19.0%), 6 with AN-R (14.3%), 5 with BED (11.9%). Among these patients, only 11 did not have self-induce vomiting (i.e. had AN-R and BED) at the time of visiting the hospital. The clinical and demographic characteristics are summarised in Table 1.

As shown in Table 1, the groups were not significantly different in their age, there was a significant difference in illness duration between AN-BP and AN-R (AN-BP: 10.0 ± 6.7, AN-R: 1.9 ± 1.7). However, the AN groups (AN-BP and AN-R) had a significantly lower BMI compared with the other groups (BN and BED) (AN-R:

Table 1 Clinical profiles of the 42 patients

	BN $n = 23$ Mean (SD)	AN-BP $n = 8$ Mean (SD)	AN-R $n = 6$ Mean (SD)	BED $n = 5$ Mean (SD)	Kruskal-Wallis analyses H	Multiple Comparisons by Steel-Dwass
Illness duration (years)	6.4 (5.8)	10.0 (6.7)	1.9 (1.7)	4.6 (3.7)	8.2*	AN-BP > AN-R
BMI	20.4 (2.4)	17.0 (0.7)	15.6 (1.5)	24.3 (7.0)	26.3**	BN > AN-BP,BN > AN-R, AN-BP < BED, AN-R < BED
Age (years)	27.0 (7.0)	28.1 (7.0)	18.6 (4.8)	28.7 (11.2)	8.3*	N.S
EDE-Q						
Diagnosis	74.5 (40.8)	78.8 (39.4)	15.2 (11.5)	62.2 (45.8)	12.8**	BN > AN-R, AN-BP > AN-R
Restricting	3.4 (1.7)	5.2 (1.0)	2.4 (1.5)	4.0 (1.6)	10.7*	AN-BP > AN-R
Eating concern	3.4 (1.5)	4.9 (0.6)	2.0 (1.4)	3.8 (1.9)	10.9*	AN-BP > AN-R
Weight	4.4 (1.4)	5.4 (0.6)	2.6 (1.9)	5.2 (0.5)	10.2*	AN-BP > AN-R
Shape	4.6 (1.4)	5.1 (0.7)	2.8 (1.8)	5.3 (0.5)	6.6	N.S
Global Score	3.9 (1.3)	5.0 (0.5)	2.4 (1.6)	4.5 (0.9)	10.5*	AN-BP > AN-R
AQ						
Total score	22.1 (6.4)	25.3 (4.8)	26.0 (7.5)	32.4 (6.2)	7.6	N.S
Social skills	4.7 (2.5)	5.1 (2.6)	5.7 (3.6)	8.0 (1.0)	7.8*	N.S
Attention Switching	5.7 (1.9)	7.1 (1.6)	6.2 (1.8)	6.4 (1.5)	2.9	N.S
Attention to detail	3.5 (2.0)	5.3 (3.3)	4.0 (1.7)	7.6 (2.5)	9.4*	BN < BED
Communication	3.8 (2.3)	4.4 (1.1)	6.0 (2.1)	6.2 (1.3)	8.7*	N.S
Imagination	4.4 (2.0)	3.4 (1.8)	4.2 (1.5)	4.2 (2.2)	2.2	N.S

BN Bulimia Nervosa, *AN-BP* Anorexia Nervosa Binge Purging, *AN-R* Anorexia Nervosa Restricting, *BED* Binge Eating Disorder, *BMI* Body Mass Index, *EDE-Q* Eating Disorder Examination Questionnaire, *AQ* Autism Spectrum Quotient
**$p < 0.01$, *$p < 0.05$

15.6 ± 1.5, AN-BP: 17.0 ± 0.7; BN: 20.4 ± 2.4, BED: 24.3 ± 7.0) (H = 26.3, $p < 0.01$). There were also statistically significant differences between the AN groups and BN in terms of the EDE-Q global scores for clinical severity (AN-R: 15.2 ± 11.5; BN: 74.5 ± 40.8; and AN-BP: 78.8 ± 39.4). AN-BP tended to be higher than the other subtypes in terms of restricting, eating and weight, that were the sub-items of EDE-Q, and there was a significant difference in the comparison with AN-R (Restricting: AN-BP 5.2 ± 1.0, AN-R 2.4 ± 1.5; Eating: AN-BP 4.9 ± 0.6, AN-R 2.0 ± 1.4, Weight: AN-BP 5.4 ± 0.6, AN-R 2.6 ± 1.9).

Table 1 also shows that the average of AQ total score was highest for patients with BED (32.4 ± 6.2), followed by those with AN-R (26.0 ± 7.5), AN-BP (25.3 ± 4.8), and BN (22.1 ± 6.4). The difference between BN and BED was significant for the attention to detail score (BN: 3.2 ± 2.0, BED: 7.6 ± 2.5) (H = 9.4, $p < 0.05$).

Clinical characteristics, EDE-Q and AQ score by the presence or absence of self-induced vomiting

As observed in Table 2, two groups were formed: 31 patients with self-induced vomiting and 11without self-induced vomiting. Although there were no significant differences in age or BMI, there was a significant difference in illness duration between vomiting present group and vomiting absent group (BN, AN-BP: 7.3 ± 6.2, AN-R, BED: 3.1 ± 3.0).

There were no significant differences in the EDE-Q, except for the 'diagnosis' category, which is expected to be affected by the frequency of self-induced vomiting. The AQ total scores of those who did not self-induced vomiting were significantly higher than for those who self-induced vomiting. In particular, the scores for social and communication skills—which are subscales of the AQ—were significantly higher in the group that did not have self-induced vomiting.

There were also statistically significant differences between the vomiting and non-vomiting groups in the EDE-Q global scores for clinical severity. Two bulimic vomiting subtypes (BN and AN-BP) scored higher than non-vomiting subtypes (U = 67.5, $p < 0.01$, r = 0.46).

However, BMI was also considered to be a confounder of EDE-Q and AQ scores; therefore, the patients were divided by anorexic and bulimic, so only AN-BP to AN-R and BN to BED were analysed (Table 3).

Despite the significant differences in illness duration, BMI and age between AN-BP and AN-R, there were no differences in any of the AQ sub-items. In contrast, there was no significant difference in the illness duration, BMI and age between BN and BED. However,

Table 2 Comparison of AQ scores by the presence or absence of self-induced vomiting ($n = 42$)

	BN,AN-BP Vomiting(+)	AN-R,BED Vomiting(−)	Mann–Whitney	
	$n = 31$	$n = 11$		
	Mean (SD)	Mean (SD)	U	r
Illness duration (years)	7.3 (6.2)	3.1 (3.0)	100.5*	0.31
BMI	19.5 (2.6)	19.6 (6.5)	132.5	
Age (years)	27.3 (6.9)	23.2 (9.5)	111.0	
EDE-Q				
Diagnosis	75.6 (39.8)	36.5 (38.8)	67.5**	0.46
Restricting	3.9 (1.7)	3.1 (1.7)	116.0	
Eating concern	3.8 (1.5)	2.8 (1.8)	112.0	
Weight	4.6 (1.3)	3.7 (1.9)	123.5	
Shape	4.7 (1.3)	3.9 (1.8)	140.0	
Global Score	4.2 (1.2)	3.4 (1.7)	120.0	
AQ				
Total score	22.9 (6.1)	28.9 (7.4)	102.5	
Social skills	4.8 (2.5)	6.7 (2.9)	89.5*	0.36
Attention Switching	6.0 (2.0)	6.3 (1.6)	153.0	
Attention to detail	3.9 (2.5)	5.6 (2.7)	103.0	
Communication	4.0 (2.1)	6.1 (1.7)	71.5**	0.44
Imagination	4.2 (2.0)	4.2 (1.7)	166.0	

AN anorexia nervosa (either -R for restricting or -BP for binge eating with self-induced vomiting), *AQ* Autism Spectrum Quotient, *BMI* body mass index, *BN* bulimia nervosa, *BED* binge eating disorder, *EDE-Q* Eating Disorder Examination Questionnaire.
**$p < 0.01$ *$p < 0.05$

there was a significant difference in the social skills, attention to detail and communication in the AQ score.

In addition, illness duration could be a confounding factor for the EDE-Q and AQ scores. Therefore, we performed the multivariate analysis with 4 groups: illness duration of < 4 years for patients with and without vomiting and illness duration of ≥4 years for patients with and without vomiting. A Kruskal–Wallis analysis was conducted to confirm these groups, because illness duration of ≤4 years or more has been the common cut-off used for determining acute vs chronic EDs [20, 21].

There were 22 patients (illness duration ≥4 years) and 9 patients (illness duration < 4 years) in the vomiting group and 3 patients (illness duration ≥4 years) and 8 patients (illness duration < 4 years or less) in the non-vomiting group. The results are shown in Tables 4 and 5. Illness duration resulted in significant differences in AQ communication, EDE-Q diagnosis and age. The communication score of AQ was highest in the non-vomiting group with illness duration < 4 years, followed by the non-vomiting group with illness duration ≥4 years. The communication score of AQ in the non-vomiting group with illness duration < 4 years was significantly higher than that in the vomiting with illness duration ≥4 years.

AQ score cut-off value by ED subtype

Lastly, the ratio of the subtypes and the number of patients who exceeded the cut-off value of the AQ score were examined, and the difference in the ratio of the number of patients was examined using Fisher's exact test. Three of eight patients of BED had an AQ score above 33, which well exceeded expected value in 60% of patients with BED. By contrast, one patient with BN had an AQ ≥33 (4.3%), and this amount was below the expected value. The difference between the BN and BED groups was significant ($p = 0.02$) (Table 6).

Discussion

The aim of the current study was to examine the relationship between each subtype of EDs and ASD trait regarding the presence or absence of self-induced vomiting. We first compared the illness duration, BMI, EDE-Q scores, and AQ scores in the four groups (BN, AN-BP, AN-R, and BED). Next, the four subtypes were divided as per the presence or absence of self-induced vomiting; the illness duration, BMI, age, EDE-Q, scores and AQ scores were compared. Assuming that BMI is a confounding factor, we compared EDE-Q and AQ scores between anorexic group (AN-BP and AN-R) and bulimic group (BN and BED). Furthermore, illness duration

Table 3 Comparison AN-BP to AN-R and BN to BED (n = 42)

	Anorexia nervosa (*n* = 14)	Bulimia nervosa (*n* = 28)
	(AN-BP vs AN-R)	(BN vs BED)
	p (Mann-Whitney)	p (Mann-Whitney)
Illness duration (years)	0.00*	0.83
BMI	0.05*	0.17
Age (years)	0.01*	0.61
EDE-Q		
Diagnosis	0.00*	0.47
Restricting	0.01*	0.65
Eating concern	0.00*	0.7
Weight	0.01*	0.31
Shape	0.03*	0.25
Global score	0.00*	0.42
AQ		
Total score	0.8	0.01*
Social skills	0.6	0.00*
Attention switching	0.47	0.39
Atention to detail	0.6	0.00*
Communication	0.11	0.03*
Imagination	0.32	0.88

AN anorexia nervosa (either -R for restricting or -BP for binge eating with self-induced vomiting), *AQ* Autism Spectrum Quotient, *BMI* body mass index, *BN* bulimia nervosa, *BED* binge eating disorder, *EDE-Q* Eating Disorder Examination Questionnaire.
*p < 0.05

could be a confounding factor; therefore, we performed additional analysis to confirm it. Finally, we examined the ratio of the subtypes and the number of patients who exceeded the cut-off value of the AQ score.

We had hypothesised that patients without self-induced vomiting had a higher tendency for ASD; however, there was no difference in the AQ between AN-BP and AN-R. The significant difference in the AQ score between BN and BED was clear. Of the four ED subtypes, BED had the highest ASD trait. Even after the statistical analyses were adjusted to determine confounding factors, such as low BMI and duration of illness, the significant AQ differences in our results can be explained by the difference between BN and BED. However, this finding is not completely aligned with our hypothesis that ASD traits are correlated with a lack of vomiting. That is, for EDs of patients within or above normal weight, ASD traits were associated with a lack of vomiting in this study. In addition, when the illness duration was divided into < 4 years and ≥ 4 years, non-vomiting was common in the < 4 year group and vomiting was common in the ≥4 year group. This result supports the rationale for a 4 year cut-off to designate the chronic and acute phases. Notably, early intervention in ED (before the transition from onset to vomiting) may be necessary.

In addition, the AQ communication score was significantly higher in the group without vomiting and with < 4 years of illness duration than in the group with vomiting ≥4 years of illness duration. Second, the non-vomiting group ≥4 years of illness duration scored higher

Table 4 Multivariate analysis of AQ and EDE-Q of 4 groups in illness duration with Kruskal-Wallis analysis

AQ:Communication			statistic H = 8.38			df = 3, *p* < .05
Group	N	Mean	SD	Max	Min	Average of the rank
1	9	3.78	2.1	7	0	17.83
2	8	6.25	1.48	9	4	31.44
3	22	4.05	2.03	9	0	18.5
4	3	5.67	1.89	7	3	28

== Multiple Comparisons by Steel-Dwass == (* *p* < .05)
A2 > A3 * (T = 2.656)
Group1: < 4 years of illness duration, Vomiting(+); Group2: < 4 years of illness duration, Vomiting(−)
Group3: ≥4 years of illness duration, Vomiting(+); Group4: ≥4 years of illness duration, Vomiting(−)
N Number of subjects, *Mean* Mean value, *SD* Standard Daviation, *Max* Maximum value, *Min* Minimun value
df degrees of freedom

Table 5 Multivariate analysis of AQ and EDE-Q of 4 groups in illness duration with Kruskal-Wallis analysis

EDE-Q: Diagnosis			statistic H = 12.44			df = 3, *p* < .01
Group	N	Mean	SD	Max	Min	Average of the rank
1	9	75.44	37.27	141	21	24.78
2	8	21.38	13.9	46	4	7.75
3	22	75.68	39.9	139	10	24.84
4	3	77	47.55	132	16	23.83

== Multiple Comparisons by Steel-Dwass == (* p < .05)
A1 > A2 * (T = 3.081)
A2 < A3 * (T = 3.332)
Group1: < 4 years of illness duration, Vomiting(+); Group2: < 4 years of illness duration, Vomiting(−)
Group3: ≥4 years of illness duration, Vomiting(+); Group4: ≥4 years of illness duration, Vomiting(−)
N Number of subjects, *Mean* Mean value, *SD* Standard Daviation, *Max* Maximum value, *Min* Minimun value
df degrees of freedom

Table 6 Number and ratio of people who exceeded the AQ cut-off value by ED subtype (n = 42)

	BN	AN-BP	AN-R	BED	Fisher	Cramer's
AQ score	n (%)	n (%)	n (%)	n (%)	*χ2*	V
AQ≧33	1 (4.3)	1 (12.5)	1 (16.7)	3 (60.0)	10.4*	0.50
	3.29	1.14	0.86	0.71		
AQ≦32	22 (95.7)	7 (87.5)	5 (85.7)	2 (40.0)		
	19.71	6.86	5.14	4.29		

AN anorexia nervosa (either -R for restricting or -BP for binge eating with self-induced vomiting), *AQ* Autism Spectrum Quotient, *BN* bulimia nervosa, *BED* binge eating disorder.
*p < 0.05

than the vomiting groups. This result suggested that the non-vomiting groups tended to have a higher AQ communication score. A previous study had reported that all-or-none thinking about food and dieting was typical of patients with BED [22]. Some patients say that they 'would never want to vomit' and are tolerant of weight gain even if they start overeating. In these BED patients, the absence of self-induced vomiting means that they tend to be obese [19], and it is unclear why they do not vomit in the face of weight gain [21]. If considering the characteristics of ASD, it may be possible that some patients with BED do not vomit because another obsessive compulsion arising from ASD is stronger than the core psychopathology of the ED, i.e. fear of being fat and the failure of severe restriction leads to acceptance of weight gain. This is seen clinically in our practise with comments from patients such as 'I am scared to vomit,' 'My life is over when I am vomiting,' or 'Looking at vomit disgusts me.' In such instances, the fear or aversion to vomiting might be stronger than the desire not to gain weight. In addition, patients who were absorbed in dietary restrictions were able to postpone the desire to lose weight due to the disgust of vomiting along with the failure of restrictions, and to endure the weight gain somehow could not be explained by the psychopathology of EDs. In some cases, from the experience of vomiting once in the past, people have a strong sense to visceral sensations and/or disgust of vomiting; they are unable to forget the trauma and find it difficult to eat food because they do not want to vomit again. People with hyperaesthesia within the autism spectrum are reluctant to induce vomiting. In addition, some patients cannot eat because they are afraid of vomiting.

If there is an ASD trait, it is easy to fall into maladaptation to environment because of impairment of social skills, communication and lack of flexibility. In this study, social skills and communication scores of AQ in patients without self-induced vomiting were higher than those in patients with self-induced vomiting.

The maladaptation to environment may lead to routine behaviour, because certain routine behaviour, such as routine dietary patterns of patients, tends to reassure individuals. Environmental adjustment is the first requirement for such individuals.

For patients with EDs, it may be necessary to prioritise the identification of characteristics over the diagnosis or types. When assessing patients with EDs who never vomit, it is important to clarify the reason; i.e. determine what they are afraid of as a consequence of vomiting. Therefore, detailed assessments for appropriate recognition of each patient who does not vomit and the application of empirically derived treatments are required. Based on the above, for patients with BED with a high tendency towards ASD, environmental adjustment and psychoeducation regarding ASD may be necessary. In addition, patients should not be corrected in terms of their diet choices that are derived from sensory sensitivity (i.e. sense of smell, taste), and their feeling of disgust should not be ignored. It is also essential to take into consideration in their abnormal eating behaviour caused by the stress of their poor communication skills. For patients (AN-R and BED) who have not vomited and have illness duration of < 4 years, it is important for therapists to identify these patients' attitude towards self -induced vomiting for the evaluation of their ASD traits and to perform an early intervention before the condition becomes chronic. To the best of our knowledge, this is the first study to compare the predisposition for ASD by ED subtype and the presence or absence of self-induced vomiting.

This study had some limitations. Of note, the sample size was small, there were differences in the number of participants in each subtype. There were no data for healthy subjects to compare patient data with standard values. Besides the above, there was a large age spread. In general, it is known that AN-R is much more common in the younger ages, and self-induced vomiting usually appear later on in adolescence/young adulthood. The differences of subjects' age, BMI and illness duration may always be a confounder and should be controlled it with bigger sample size.

Symptoms of depression and anxiety disorders, irritability, emotional lability and obsessional features are frequent accompaniments in ED. Typically, these features worsen with weight loss and improve with weight regain [3]. Interest in the outside world also declines as patients become underweight, with the result that most patients become socially withdrawn and isolated. Since we did not measure anxiety or depression in this study, it is unclear how these were associated with ED and AQ scores. Since ED has a high incidence of anxiety and depression, it should be added to the evaluation index in the future study. There are still problems to be examined in the future regarding coexistence of autism trait and measurement of individual differences.

This study used only the AQ for evaluation of ASD traits. We should have used the AQ-10 in addition to the AQ because a few adolescent patients were included in our study. These are good tools for assessing the presence or absence of ASD traits in a busy clinical setting. However, the AQ is a self-completed scale and is not used to diagnose ASD. Using the Autism Diagnostic Observation Schedule (ADOS) or the Autism Diagnostic Interview (ADI) for ASD evaluation, excluding patients with extremely low body weights, and including control subjects in a larger overall sample should be done in future research [9, 21]. A future issue is to determine the clinical usefulness of using the ASD evaluation tool, which is called the gold standard such as ADOS and ADI, for ED patients whose ASD characteristics are considered to be a factor for maintaining the symptoms.

Conclusions

Our results suggest that when body weight is above normal, patients with EDs without self-induced vomiting might have a higher ASD trait than those with it. In addition, when patients with EDs are divided by illness duration, among those with shorter illness duration (< 4 years), those without self-induced vomiting might have a higher ASD trait than those with it, and the difference of ASD trait between patients who do and do not vomit could be smaller among those with longer illness duration (≥4 years).

Given these results and considering that the prevalence of higher ASD tendencies in adults with EDs might contribute to the significant treatment resistance to conventional therapies [23], it is important for therapists to determine patients' ASD trait from an early stage and to be flexible in designing treatments that are individually tailored for each patient. This study, which investigated the association between ASD traits and self-induced vomiting, could provide helpful points for future clinical research.

Abbreviations

DSM-5: the Diagnostic and Statistical Manual of Mental Disorders, Fifth Edition; EDs: Eating disorders; AN: Anorexia nervosa; BN: Bulimia nervosa; BED: Binge eating disorder; AN-R: restricting type of AN; AN-BP: binge eating with self-induced vomiting type; ASD: Autism spectrum disorder; BMI: Body Mass Index; EDE-Q: Eating Disorder Examination Questionnaire; AQ: Autism-Spectrum Quotient

Acknowledgements

The study was supported by Japan Society for the Promotion of Science (JSPS). The authors thank our research nurses Hiroko Suwabe and Hiroe Ota for all their support during this study.

Authors' contributions

Author NN designed the study and collected data. Authors RS and MN provided summaries of previous research studies. Authors KI, KY and DM conducted the statistical analysis. ES and AN supervised the study. All authors contributed to and have approved the final manuscript.

Competing interests

The authors do not have any competing interests to report.

Author details

[1]Research Center for Child Mental Development, Chiba University, 1-8-1 Inohana, Chuo-ku, Chiba 260-8670, Japan. [2]Department for School of Human and Social Sciences, Fukuoka Prefectural University, Fukuoka, Japan. [3]Centre for Psychiatry Research, Department of Clinical Neuroscience, Karolinska Institutet, Stockholm, Sweden. [4]Department of Cognitive Behavioral Physiology, Graduate School of Medicine, Chiba University, Chiba, Japan. [5]Koutokukai Sato Hospital, Yamagata, Japan. [6]Department of Psychiatry, Graduate School of Medicine, International University of Health and Welfare, Chiba, Japan. [7]Department of Psychiatry, Graduate School of Medicine, Chiba University, Chiba, Japan.

References

1. Fairburn CG, Cooper Z. Eating disorders, DSM-5 and clinical reality. Br J Psychiatry. 2018;198:8–10. https://doi.org/10.1192/bjp.bp.110.083881.
2. American Psychiatric Association. DSM-5 Development. Arlington: American Psychiatric Association; 2010. http://www.dsm5.org.
3. Fairburn C, Harrison P. Eating disorders. Lancet. 2003;361:407–16. https://doi.org/10.1016/s0140-6736(03)12378-1.
4. Tchanturia K, Smith E, Weineck F, et al. Exploring autistic traits in anorexia: a clinical study. Mol Autism. 2013;4. https://doi.org/10.1186/2040-2392-4-44.
5. Huke V, Turk J, Saeidi S, Kent A. Morgan J F: autism spectrum disorders in eating disorder populations: a systematic review. Eur Eat Disord Rev. 2013; 21:345–51. https://doi.org/10.1002/erv.2244.
6. Gillberg C, Billstedt E: Autism and Asperger syndrome: coexistence with other clinical disorders. Acta Psychiatr Scand 2001, 102 DOI:https://doi.org/10.1034/j.1600-0447.2000.102005321.x.
7. Westwood H, Mandy W, Tchanturia K. Clinical evaluation of autistic symptoms in women with anorexia nervosa. Mol Autism. 2017;8. https://doi.org/10.1186/s13229-017-0128-x.
8. Tchanturia K, Adamson J, Leppanen J, Westwood H. Characteristics of autism spectrum disorder in anorexia nervosa:A naturalistic study in an inpatient treatment programme. Autism. 2019;23:123–30. https://doi.org/10.1177/1362361317722431.
9. Nielsen S, Anckarsater H, Gillberg C, Rastam M, Wentz E. Effects of autism spectrum disorders on outcome in teenage-onset anorexia nervosa evaluated by the Morgan-Russell outcome assessment schedule: a controlled community-based study. Mol Autism. 2015;6:14. https://doi.org/10.1186/s13229-015-0013-4.
10. Stewart CS, McEwen FS, Konstantellou A, Eisler I, Simic M. Impact of ASD traits on treatment outcomes of eating disorders in girls. Eur Eat Disord Rev. 2017;25:123–8. https://doi.org/10.1002/erv.2497.
11. Huke V, Turk J, Saeidi S, Kent A, Morgan JF. The clinical implications of high levels of autism spectrum disorder features in anorexia nervosa: a pilot study. Eur Eat Disord Rev. 2014;22:116–21. https://doi.org/10.1002/erv.2269.
12. American Psychiatric Association. Diagnostic and Statistical Manual of Mental Disorders. 5th ed. Arlington: Am Psychiatric Assoc; 2013.
13. Fairburn C, Beglin S. Assessment of eating disorders: interview or self-report questionnaire? Inter J of Eat Disord. 1994;16:363–70 doi.org/10.1002/1098-108X(199412)16:4<363::AID-EAT2260160405>3.0.CO;2-%23.
14. Baron-Cohen S, Wheelwright S, Skinner R, Martin J. E C: the autism-spectrum quotient (AQ): evidence from Asperger syndrome/high-functioning autism, males and females, scientists and mathematicians. J Autism Dev Disord. 2001;31. https://doi.org/10.1023/a:1005653411471.
15. Ro R, Reas R, Stedal K. Eating disorder examination questionnaire (EDE-Q) in Norwegian adults: discrimination between female controls and eating disorder patients. Eur Eat Disord Rev. 2015;23:408–12. https://doi.org/10.1002/erv.2372.
16. Luce KH, Crowther JH. The reliability of the eating disorder examination—self-report questionnaire version (EDE-Q). Int J Eat Disord. 1999;25:349–51. https://doi.org/10.1002/(SICI)1098-108X(199904)25:3<349::AID-EAT15>3.0.CO;2-M.
17. Otani M, Tomoyo Mitsui T, Yoshida T, Komaki H, Yoshiuchi K. Reliability and validity of the Japanese version of the eating disorder examination questionnaire (EDE–Q)in patients with eating disorders (in Japanese). Japanese J Psychosom Med. 2017;157:642.
18. Jennifer S Rose, Adin Vaewsorn, Francine Rosselli-Navarra, G Terence Wilson, Weissman RS: Test-retest reliability of the eating disorder examination-questionnaire (EDE-Q) in a college sample. J Eat Disord.2013, *1* DOI:https://doi.org/10.1186/2050-2974-1-42.
19. Wakabayashi A, Tojo Y, Baron-Cohen S, Wheelwright S. The autism-Spectrum quotient (AQ) Japanese version: evidence from high-functioningclinicalgroup and normal adults. Shinrigaku Kenkyu. 2004;75:78–84. https://doi.org/10.4992/jjpsy.75.78.
20. Strober M, Freeman R, Morrell W. The long-term course of severe anorexia nervosa in adolescents: survival analysis of recovery, relapse, and outcome predictors over 10–15 years in a prospective study. Int J Eat Disord. 1997;22: 339–60. https://doi.org/10.1002/(sici)1098-108x(199712)22:4<339::aid-eat1>3.0.co;2-n

21. Woods S. Untreated recovery from eating disorders. Adolesc. 2004;39:361–71.
22. Ramacciotti CE, Coli E, Passaglia C, et al. Binge eating disorder: prevalence and psychopathological features in a clinical sample of obese people in Italy. Psychiatry Res. 2000;94:131–8. https://doi.org/10.1016/s0165-1781(00)00130-x.
23. Wallier J, Vibert S, Berthoz S, et al. Dropout from inpatient treatment for anorexia nervosa: critical review of the literature. Int J Eat Disord. 2009;42: 636–47. https://doi.org/10.1002/eat.20609.

8

The impact of the COVID-19 pandemic on individuals with eating disorders: the role of emotion regulation and exploration of online treatment experiences

L. Vuillier[1*], L. May[1,2], M. Greville-Harris[1], R. Surman[1] and R. L. Moseley[1]

Abstract

Objective: The Covid-19 pandemic has wrought disruption to everyday life and services, and emerging evidence suggests that those with eating disorders (EDs) are likely to experience marked distress and exacerbation of their symptoms. However, little is known around the most relevant factors to symptom change; whether certain emotion regulation and coping strategies are linked to better outcomes; and how people with EDs are adjusting to psychological interventions moving online.

Method: In a mixed-method design, we collected qualitative and quantitative data from 207 (76 males) self-selected UK residents with self-reported ED, who described and ranked impacts of the pandemic on their symptoms. Regression analysis examined whether emotion regulation strategies were associated with self-reported symptom change, ED symptomatology, and negative emotional states. Thematic analysis explored participants' experiences of the pandemic, particularly factors affecting their ED, coping strategies used, and experiences of psychological intervention.

Results: Most participants (83.1%) reported worsening of ED symptomatology, though factors affecting symptom change differed between specific EDs. Emotion regulation, such as having fewer strategies, poorer emotional clarity, and non-acceptance of emotions, explained nearly half of the variance in emotional distress during the pandemic. Qualitative findings indicated that difficult emotions (such as fear and uncertainty), changes to routine, and unhelpful social messages were triggering for participants during the pandemic. While some participants described employing positive coping strategies (such as limiting social media exposure), many reported using ED behaviours (among other maladaptive strategies, like alcohol use) to cope with the pandemic. Finally, loss of treatment support, feeling underserving of support and experiencing a 'detached connection' online were further exacerbating factors for these participants.

(Continued on next page)

* Correspondence: lrenshawvuillier@bournemouth.ac.uk
[1]Department of Psychology, Bournemouth University, Poole, UK
Full list of author information is available at the end of the article

(Continued from previous page)

Discussion: While our sample was self-selected and may not represent all people with EDs, our results suggest that people with EDs have been strongly affected by the pandemic. Some aspects of online treatment were found to be beneficial but our findings suggest it also needs some improvement. Our paper discusses implications for online treatment such as taking into account personal circumstances and, in a time where people have limited control over the antecedents of negative emotion, the need to develop skills to manage emotions when they arise.

Keywords: Eating disorders, Covid-19, Pandemic, Lockdown, Coping, Emotion regulation, Online therapy

Plain English summary

The Covid-19 pandemic has damaged mental health on a global scale, and emerging research suggests that people with pre-existing mental illnesses, including eating disorders (EDs), may suffer the greatest deterioration. Aiming to inform future treatment and support, the present study examined which aspects of the pandemic have been especially difficult for people with EDs, and whether certain coping strategies and ways of dealing with emotions have been associated with better wellbeing. We also explored experiences of the move to online psychological treatment. Of 207 participants surveyed online, 83.1% reported that their ED symptoms had worsened, most notably due to difficulties managing emotions like anxiety around the unknown situation, changes in routine and in physical activity. Poorer mental health was associated with having fewer emotion regulation strategies, poorer emotional clarity, and non-acceptance of emotions. Participants outlined some helpful coping strategies during this time (such as limiting social media use) as well as some more detrimental strategies (such as increased ED behaviours and alcohol use). Finally, while some aspects were found to be beneficial, our participants reported a loss of support, feeling underserving of help, and a detached connection with their therapist as barriers to a successful online treatment. Our paper discusses the clinical implications of these findings.

With the first outbreaks reported in late 2019, Covid-19 became a global pandemic with alarming speed. Many governments imposed lock-down and social distancing measures, such as those that started on 23rd March 2020 in the UK. While pandemics and periods of mass quarantine are historically linked with psychological distress and psychiatric morbidity [1–3], their impact is disproportionately felt by people living with pre-existent mental illnesses [4, 5]. Psychological services have valiantly rallied to mobilise online delivery of services [6], but the efficacy of such services and their reception with patients is thus far unknown.

One group of individuals of particular concern are those with eating disorders (EDs), long recognised as among the deadliest psychiatric illnesses [7, 8]. Recent efforts to examine the effects of the pandemic on people with eating disorders suggest a marked worsening in symptoms, most notably in restricting, binge eating, purging and pathological exercising [9–13]. Qualitative exploration of these experiences revealed that individuals with eating disorders attribute the exacerbation of their symptoms to disruption across many spheres of their lives, alongside reduced access to healthcare services [11, 14]. Changes in living situations, for instance, have meant that some people have had to move back in with their parents, which for some may mean more support towards their eating disorder, but for others more anxieties around feeling trapped, watched, or over having less influence over meal choices [11, 14]. Relatedly, being housebound during lockdown has affected access to social support networks, with individuals unable to see friends for support, and incurred changes to exercise routines, with some individuals distressed by the loss of access to gyms and others feeling compelled to exercise more due to the constant availability of online exercise classes and social pressures around it [11, 14]. Participants in these studies also highlighted social pressure in the form of triggering messages on social media, having increased their media consumption. Indeed, people during the lockdown have spent more time engaging with media online and on television [15], and others have raised concerns that greater exposure to home cooking or exercise classes may have negatively impacted individuals with EDs [16]. Finally, the lockdown has resulted in changes in food buying and eating behaviours, with participants reporting food stockpiling and resultant binge eating episodes; justifying food restriction with the reality of food insecurity [17]; or being unable to access 'safe' foods. These studies [11, 14] validated many of the concerns raised by clinical researchers [18], who also note the likelihood that the increased anxiety of this period may move individuals from a prodromal to full disease state.

The fact that this is occurring during a time of indefinite disruption to services is deeply worrying. These illnesses frequently run a protracted course [19, 20], with some evidence that this chronicity is underpinned by progressive neurobiological changes which incur treatment-resistance and impede full recovery [21]. It is paramount that changes in symptomatology are mapped and understood in order to inform emerging online paradigms and support individuals in their recovery efforts. In light of this, a valuable area of focus may be emotion regulation and coping strategies. Emotions are known to play a role in the pathology of EDs [22–24], and in this context, it is highly relevant that the pandemic has fuelled additional feelings of depression, anxiety, uncertainty and psychological distress [5, 25]. For example, many people have lost jobs or are facing unemployment, thus raising fears around an uncertain future; others may be experiencing the heightened stress and guilt associated with balancing work and childcare. Many are highly anxious about their physical health and that of their loved ones. One study conducted early in the pandemic (April–May) with a large population of people with EDs found that over 60% of participants were experiencing comorbid generalised anxiety disorder, with participants reporting substantial increase in anxiety, attributed specifically to Covid-19, since the end of 2019 [11]. Other studies reported heightened feelings of sadness, anhedonia, apathy and worthlessness [12, 13]. Identifying and regulating emotions is a known difficulty for people with EDs [23, 26], which means they may be especially poorly equipped to cope with these added difficulties. Indeed, within the same samples, substance abuse, self-injury and suicidal feelings were reported by some participants [11–13]. Some theorists suggest that eating disordered behaviours arise due to maladaptive emotion regulation strategies [23, 26], and the pandemic both increases the likelihood that these maladaptive regulation strategies will be deployed whilst simultaneously barring access to strategies which might have previously helped [18]. As such, the question arises as to which emotion regulation strategies have been used during the pandemic and whether some are associated with less exacerbation of ED behaviours. While studies have suggested that reappraisal and acceptance may be useful strategies during the pandemic [25, 27], as of yet no research has explored the relationships between emotion regulation strategies and psychological wellbeing in people living with an ED during the pandemic. It may however be the case that these emotion regulation strategies explain some of the variance in the impact of the pandemic on individuals with an ED [9, 10, 14], in which case identifying the coping strategies used by people with EDs during the pandemic and which are linked with better outcomes could help develop better treatment plans.

Given that psychological treatment seems likely to continue online for the foreseeable future, another crucial research goal lies in examining how the move to online treatment (e.g. 6) has been received. Disruption to services, routines and accountability have jeopardised recovery efforts for many people with EDs [11, 14], and even impacted the ability of individuals with past eating disorders to remain in remission [11]. In the UK, evidence-based psychological therapies, such as eating disorder focused Cognitive Behaviour Therapy (CBT-ED), are typically offered to adults with eating disorders [28]. The impact of the pandemic on treatment has varied across localities; treatment in some ED services may have been paused or reduced if there was a requirement to redeploy staff into essential areas of the NHS, whereas other services have been able to continue offering treatment by branching into telehealth, for instance video-conferencing. This kind of remote psychological treatment was already effectively employed in areas where geographical distance can make it difficult for individuals to access face-to-face healthcare [29], but does require additional considerations, such as access to adequate internet connectivity, a quiet, confidential space, and in the case of eating disorders, navigating how to conduct in-session weighing [30, 31].

While online treatment for eating disorders may become the norm, little is known at present about the patient experiences and barriers and facilitators of such treatment as deployed in the UK. A very preliminary qualitative analysis of a small group of patients with anorexia nervosa and their families [10] suggested that while some benefited from continued support in this alternative format, others were unable to tolerate seeing themselves on screens. Other concerns expressed by patients and families about online treatment included the lack of non-verbal communication; that previous homework challenges, such as eating out, would become impossible; and that virtual connection placed responsibility on patients to manage their own weigh-ins, an accountability which would be difficult for people at early stages of recovery and which might constitute an extra burden on carers. While research on the COVID-19 pandemic has flourished and there is preliminary evidence of deterioration in people with EDs [9, 10, 14], further in-depth empirical scrutiny is imperative for best supporting these individuals through the present time. The high mortality rates of EDs [7, 8], the development of treatment-resistance over time and the neurobiological changes which maintain chronicity [19–21] all underscore this crucial need for clinical and research attention to people with EDs. Accordingly, the current study had three aims. To inform clinical focus during this period, we firstly aimed to build a more comprehensive account, enabled by a mixed-methods design, of *which* factors were important during the pandemic as well as *how* these factors affected participants' experiences. As such, we built on previous research by ranking these factors in importance and exploring at a deeper, qualitative level their impacts on participants. With a more extensive and sex-balanced sample than in previous studies, we also aimed to delineate factors that might be impacted by individual differences, such as diagnosis. Second, we aimed to understand whether some emotion regulation strategies were linked to symptom changes and wellbeing outcomes for individuals affected by an ED. We also aimed to further explore this aspect with qualitative reports of the coping strategies people with an ED have used during the pandemic. Third and finally, given that previous studies offered only very sparse consideration of treatment experiences during the pandemic, we qualitatively explored participants' experiences with online treatment, hoping to inform and optimise future treatment delivery for this vulnerable population.

Methods

Participants

Participants self-reporting a current ED diagnosis (n = 222) were recruited through a participant recruitment website (Prolific, n=168) and through social media (n=54). To ensure a degree of homogeneity in treatment options, eligibility criteria required that participants be over age 18 and UK-residents for at least the prior 2 years. Recruiting participants over 18 years of age also allowed us to recruit participants as fast as possible due to the time-sensitive nature of the study. As such, we did not require additional consent from their parent or guardian, and we could use remote recruitments methods that were more suitable for an adult population. Data was excluded from participants who did not clearly specify a singular ED diagnosis (n = 3), participants with orthorexia nervosa (n = 2), ARFID (n = 2), body dysmorphia or medical issues such as reflux without a DSM-5 classified ED (n = 3), as well as participants who reported a dual diagnosis (e.g. anorexia and bulimia, n=4).[1]

The 207 participants included in the study (156 from Prolific) were those diagnosed with AN, BN, BED, or OSFED (or EDNOS if diagnosed before DSM-5) whose demographic details are shown in Table 1. Within the qualitative section, 43 participants responded to questions exploring their experience of treatment during the pandemic. Participants reported ethnicities were white British/Irish/Scottish/European (93.7%), Asian (5.3%), Black (0.5%) and Arab (0.5%).

Males and females were unevenly distributed across the four diagnostic groups ($\chi 2$ (3) = 18.8, p < .001), with female participants more likely to be found in the AN, BN or OSFED group, and males more likely to be found in the BED group.

There was no difference in duration of illness (t (219) = –.822, p = .412), mean age (t (218) = 592, p = .555) or symptom severity (t (220) = –.228, p = .820) between our samples recruited on Prolific and Social Media. There was however a significant sex difference, as we actively tried to recruit males in our Prolific sample ($\chi 2$ (1) = 23.0, p < .001).

The diagnosis groups differed significantly in age (F [3, 202] = 3.19, p = .025), and in duration of illness (F [3, 202], 2.7, p = .047) but were equally matched in EDEQ scores (p = .776).

Materials and procedure

Qualitative and quantitative data are often favourably integrated [32], for instance where researchers hope to comprehend statistical findings at a deeper, more contextual and holistic manner, and validate findings across multiple types of analysis. This motivated our decision to adopt a mixed-methods approach so as to complement quantitative data around the impact of the pandemic with insights around how it affected participants in the greater context of their lives. The impact of the pandemic on mental health and eating symptomatology was quantified with the Depression, Anxiety and Stress Scale [33], the Eating Disorder Examination Questionnaire [34] and a single numerical item in the qualitative survey. Emotion regulation strategies, as predictors of these impacts, were operationalised with the short form version of the Difficulties in Emotion Regulation Scale [35]. Richer details around the impact of the pandemic on ED symptoms, coping strategies and (if relevant) experiences of online treatment, were accrued with a short qualitative survey. The survey took approximately 45 min to complete, including additional questionnaires not reported here, and participants were rewarded with money (Prolific) or a chance to be entered in a prize draw for Amazon vouchers (social media). See supplementary material (item 1) for the detail of the measures and qualitative questions used.

Data analysis

Our three-part analysis addressed our three research questions. First (Part A), we looked at whether our participants reported a deterioration in ED symptoms due to the pandemic and then, specifically in those whose symptoms deteriorated, which of these factors were the most influential. To examine the differential importance of each variable for participants along the ED spectrum, we conducted one-way ANOVAs (diagnosis as the between-group factor) with Bonferroni-corrected post-hoc tests. To get a clearer picture of our data in this process, we computed

[1] We removed participants who reported having been given two diagnoses such as AN and BN because the DSM-5 precludes dual diagnosis. According to the DSM-5, if the person is significantly underweight, they would present with AN. As such, a diagnosis of AN would always trump a diagnosis of BN, even if the person binges and purges (in that case they would be diagnosed with AN binge purge type). We aimed to clarify with our participants these dual diagnoses when possible. This was not possible for our social media sample which was anonymous, so these four participants were removed from the analysis

Table 1 Participant demographic information

	Total	*AN*	*BN*	*BED*	*OSFED*
Total numbers (males)	*207 (76)*	*91 (29)*	*46 (14)*	*44 (28)*	*26 (5)*
Mean age (SD)	*30.0 (9.7)*	*28.7 (9.1)*	*31.8 (9.2)*	*32.6 (10.7)*	*28.8 (9.7)*
Duration of illness (SD)	*7.3 (7.5)*	*7.9 (8.0)*	*9.1 (7.9)*	*5.0 (5.4)*	*6.1 (6.8)*
In treatment (n)	*42*	*21*	*11*	*7*	*3*
Mean total EDEQ scores (SD)	*4.0 (1.1)*	*4.0 (1.2)*	*4.1 (0.9)*	*4.0 (1.1)*	*4.2 (1.1)*

non-parametric correlations between these ordinal variables (see supplementary materials, 2); in addition, thematic analysis was carried out on the qualitative responses to understand participants' experience of these pandemic-related factors in more detail.

Secondly (Part B), we used multiple linear regressions to examine whether some emotion regulation strategies were linked to better outcomes during the pandemic. While predictors were the six DERS subscales, three outcome variables were examined: the total score on the DASS (Model 1), the numerical item within the qualitative survey where participants rated the impact of the pandemic on their eating disorder behaviours (Model 2), and the total score on the EDEQ (Model 3). We used the backward method to remove all non-significant predictors. Again, qualitative descriptions of experiences of coping were analysed as part of our thematic analysis, to identify key themes exploring how participants described coping during the pandemic.

Thirdly (Part C), thematic analysis of participant's responses about treatment was carried out in order to explore participants' experiences of coping and therapeutic interventions during the pandemic.

Qualitative data for each section were imported into NVivo 12 (QSR International, 2018) software, retaining the original punctuation, spelling mistakes and grammatical errors. Thematic analysis was then carried out using Braun and Clarke's (2006) five stage process: 1) familiarisation with the data through initial reading, 2) generating initial codes, 3) collating codes into themes, 4) defining and labelling themes, and 5) selecting illustrative quotes (participant quotes were anonymised, with gender (F or M), participant code, and ED diagnostic label, presented in brackets alongside each quote).

For each part of this analysis, a data trail was kept throughout this process using concept cards. Three researchers analysed the qualitative data (MGH, LM and RS). Initial findings were then discussed within the research group to come up with a holistic set of themes. Second coding was carried out on approximately 14% of the qualitative data and any discrepancies were resolved through discussion.

The thematic analysis findings are described in each of the three sections: Experiences of the pandemic (described in Part A and comprising four main themes), coping with emotions (described in Part B and comprising two main themes), and treatment experiences (described in Part C and comprising two main themes). Figure 2 in the result section outlines all themes together as interrelated factors impacting upon ED symptomatology.

Results

Part a: overall impact of the pandemic and factors involved

Quantitative analysis

When asked about the overall impact of the pandemic on their ED, the majority of our participants (83.1%) reported that their symptoms had worsened, while 6.8% reported that their symptoms got better and 7.7% reported no change in symptoms (the remaining 2.4% failed to respond to this item). Reported changes in symptomatology did not differ between diagnostic groups ($\chi 2$ (18) = 18.8, p =.409), although see supplementary materials (3) for a breakdown per diagnoses.

Looking specifically at the participants who reported an exacerbation of ED symptomatology (n = 172), we examined which factors participants thought had had the greatest impact on their ED. There was striking heterogeneity between participants. Overall, as can be seen in Fig. 1 (and supplementary materials 4), the three most important factors were changes to routine and physical activity, and difficulties around their emotions. Non-parametric correlations between these factors were positive but weak, indicating their independence from one another.

Interestingly, the importance of some factors differed between diagnoses. This was the case for exposure to triggering messages (F(3, 171) = 3.4, p =.020) which Bonferroni-corrected posthoc tests revealed was more important for people with AN and people with OSFED than for people with BED (mean difference = 19.7, p =.005; mean difference = 18.5, p = .039, respectively). Differences in the importance of changes to food availability were marginal (F(3, 171) = 2.6, p = .056) but, in corrected posthoc comparisons, this factor was more important for people with BED than for people with AN (mean difference = 17.1; p = .013) or for people with BN (mean difference = 18.4, p = .019). Non-parametric

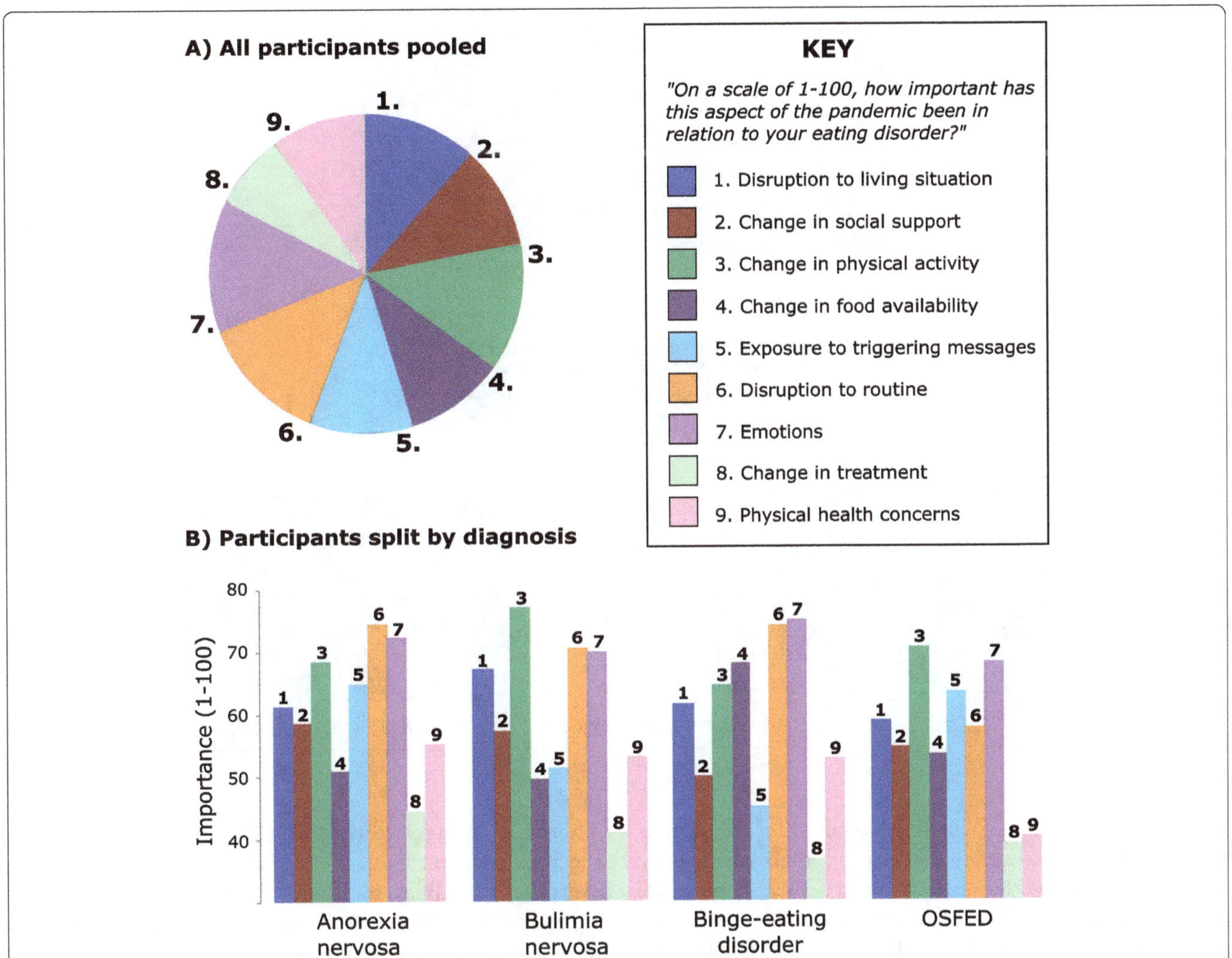

Fig. 1 Deleterious impacts of different aspects of the pandemic. Note. In all participants who reported an exacerbation of ED symptomatology, Part **a** depicts the relative importance of 9 different aspects of the pandemic to this worsening of ED symptoms. Part **b** reflects the relative importance of these different aspects when participants were categorised by diagnostic group

correlations between the 'difficulties with emotions' factor and the other factors were also illuminative in so far as suggesting which factors were most associated with strong negative emotions. For AN, corroborating the above, exposure to triggering messages was the factor most strongly correlated with emotions for participants with AN (r = .506, p < .001). The factors most strongly related to negative emotions were physical health concerns in BN (r = .637, p <.001); change in social support in BED (r = .446, p = .004); and disruption to routine in OSFED (r = .562, p = .004).

Qualitative analysis relating to overall impact of the pandemic

In free-text responses, we interpreted four main themes around experiences and impact of the pandemic. These are indicated in Fig. 2 (part A, themes 1–4) and described as follows:

Theme 1: difficult emotions Participants reported experiencing a greater level of distressing emotions during the pandemic, which had a negative impact on their ED. This mirrors our quantitative finding that difficulties with emotions were one of the main factors impacting on the deterioration of ED symptoms.

> *The pandemic situation has worsened how hopeless and depressed I feel and in turn i think my eating disorder symptoms has become a little [w] orse when my mood is low or things dont seem to be going right I tend to always turn to my eating disorder to cope. [F119, AN]*

Many participants described fear and/or uncertainty during the pandemic exacerbating their ED behaviours. Fear for the health of loved ones, fear of getting the virus, the trauma and distress of having had Covid-19 themselves, or having experienced illness or death of

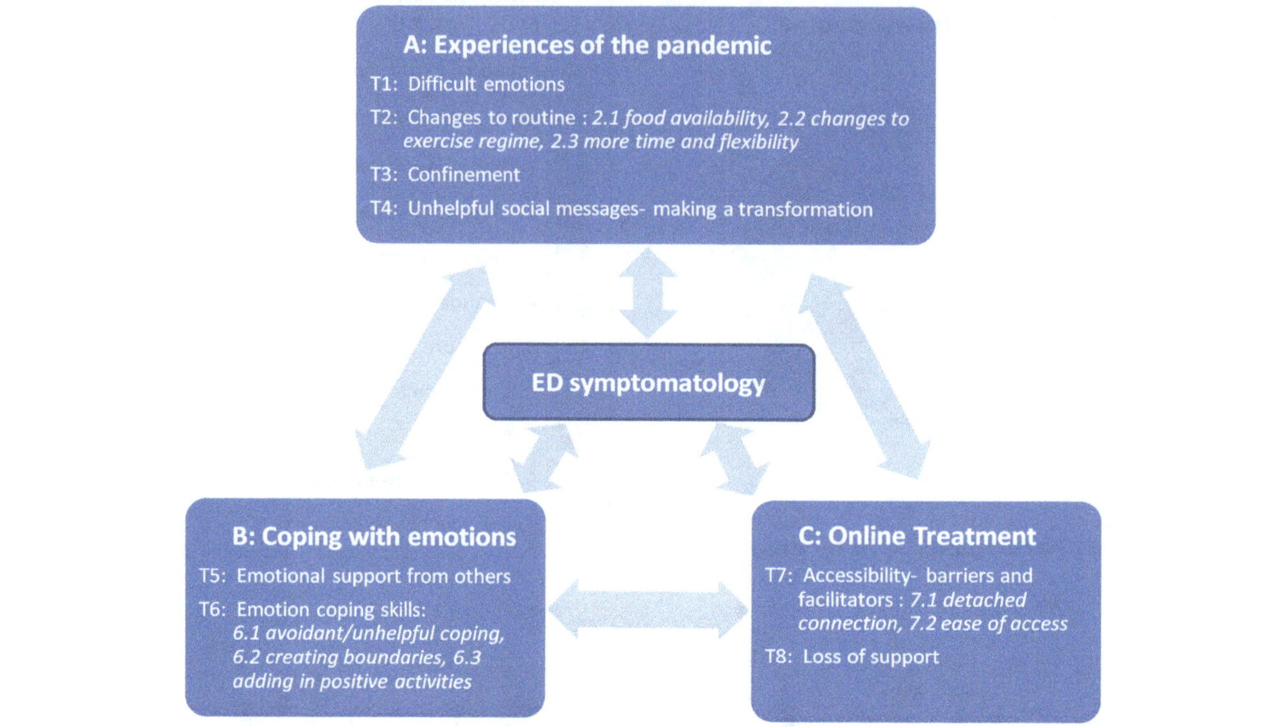

Fig. 2 Qualitative themes (T1-T8) and subthemes for experiences of the pandemic, coping with emotions and experiences of online treatment

people they knew took an emotional toll. For participants who had been furloughed, or lost their job roles or university routines, the lack of structure and purpose, lack of control and loss of income resulted in distress. Many participants reported feeling a lack of motivation, increased anxiety, and a low mood due to having their work or education taken away from them.

> *Lost all my voluntary jobs. Felt like the floor had opened up and swallowed me , felt very very lost and confused. (F17, AN):*

ED behaviours were a source of comfort for some, or allowed participants to distract themselves from the situation and their difficult feelings.

> *"restriction &b/p [binge-purge] are helpful to me as it distracts my mind from what i am worried about. i only have to focus on food related feelings which is usually easier than the difficult emotions i am avoiding" [F96, AN]*

Some participants described how changes to ED behaviours during lockdown had resulted in changes to their weight during lockdown. Inevitably weight gain added to distress levels and often further exacerbated their ED.

Theme 2: changes to routine Changes to routine during the pandemic resulted in more accessibility to food and exercise, as well as increased time and/or flexibility to engage in ED behaviours. These factors are outlined in the following three subthemes; 'food availability', 'changes to exercise regime' and 'more time and flexibility'.

Food availability. Initially during lockdown participants described anxiety about food shortages and lack of availability of their preferred or 'safe' foods. For some, food shortages resulted in reduced bingeing and purging, or encouraged restrictive eating behaviours.

> *At the very beginning due to the lack of food on the shelves at the supermarket , i did feel it was pointless trying to eat as the safe stuff was rarely available. (F17, AN)*

Greater access to food due to stockpiling increased anxiety and perceived lack of control over eating.

> *A combination of constantly being at home, with easy access to the kitchen, and doing much larger weekly shops ... has caused me a huge struggle with feelings of loss of control over food (F102, BN):*

Food availability at home caused many participants to struggle with regulating their food intake. For participants with more restrictive eating behaviours (such as those with AN), reduced access to 'safe' food was more problematic, whereas participants who struggled with binge-purge or overeating (particularly participants with BN or BED), described stockpiling and the increased access to food as home particularly triggering.

Changes to exercise regime. In line with the quantitative findings, the limitations around leaving the house and the closure of gyms resulted in reduced opportunities to exercise for many, which was particularly difficult for participants. Lack of routine exercise during lockdown led to worries about reduced energy expenditure and anxiety about how this would affect their weight and shape. This was triggering, resulting in distress, and in some cases, increased compensatory strategies.

> *I gained weight, had increased anxiety and felt out of control. My weight had been stable for the past 3 years and I gaining weight in lockdown and not having access to the gym and seeing my body change was a trigger. (F16, EDNOS)*

Changes to the ways in which participants could exercise safely, meant that exercising became a further cause of stress, rather than a way to cope. Some participants substantially increased their exercise regime at home due to more free time, or to deal with their lack of control in other areas of their lives.

More time and flexibility. As a result of the restrictions put in place during the pandemic, participants described significant reductions in their routine activities, social events or work schedule. More free time meant increased boredom and lack of distraction, which resulted in greater focus on negative thoughts, eating and weight.

> *Being inside because of covid also leaves me with so much time to spare and think about being hungry and then eating and then resenting myself and my body. There is too much time to think and nothing to distract me from obsessing about food (F115, BN)*

Working from home allowed some participants more freedom and flexibility to engage in ED behaviours. For example, by exercising during lunch, or engaging in more restriction, bingeing or purging.

> *Because I am working from home, I am able to go for runs before work and on my lunch break which is great. (F127, AN)*

Lack of value, purpose and routine resulted in lack of motivation for many. This hindered engagement in ED recovery.

> *In the initial stages of the pandemic it seemed pointless to try to manage my ED. The stress and anxiety regarding the future meant that I did not see the point in investing energy in my own physical or mental health ... (F88, BED):*

However a few participants felt that the free time was valuable for recovery, for instance they were able to focus more on healthy eating behaviours and implementing coping strategies.

Theme 3: confinement Participants who were living alone described feeling confined and isolated. The lack of social connection led participants to engage in more ED behaviours with no one there to monitor them or be accountable to.

> *It has meant that i have no one around to keep an eye on me so i can binge when i want to and then make myself sick to make myself feel better and i don't have to explain it to anyone because there is no one there to hear me ... (M44, BN)*

Although confined isolation was helpful in coping with the threat of the virus, participants who usually used activities and social interaction as ways to cope with their ED were left feeling trapped and less able to cope.

> *A usual coping mechanism before was to prevent periods of isolation when I thought Ed might surface. Haven't been able to use that strategy. [F13, AN binge purge subtype]*

In contrast many participants moved home, or spent lockdown with family, partners or friends. Participants described stress at the lack of privacy, and feeling constantly monitored by others. This resulted in distress, low mood, conflict or withdrawal.

> *... I am finding it increasingly harder to constrict as my family are able to monitor what I am eating and my every move. I have screaming matches every day with my parents which isn't good for anyone, especially my sister so I am feeling more depressed than usual. (F89, AN):*

Sometimes living with others also resulted in less control over what participants could eat, or pressure to eat certain foods, causing greater distress. These living arrangements resulted in more secrecy and attempts to hide behaviours.

> *It's meant I've had to go out of my way to hide food. For example a whole cooked chicken in my rucksack (M39, BED):*

While the support from families and friends was valued by many, some participants described the stress of family life as a trigger for their ED. Participants who were caring for others, looking after their children or working from home, described the stress and exhaustion, with no time or space to focus on caring for themselves.

> *Crazy me and husband working at home for first time, with two teenagers who are not doing school work, out of control of situation in my own home as I have to sit at a desk at home 8 hrs a day (F118, BED)*

However, some participants reported that confinement meant that they were facing fewer stress provoking situations due to lack of work and social pressure. This had reduced some of their daily stressors.

Theme 4: unhelpful social messages- making a transformation The pandemic was promoted online as a time to make a transformation, lose weight and get fit, with access to more online content promoting work outs and diets. These messages were unhelpful in promoting ED behaviours, or increasing pressure to conform to these ideals.

> *Everywhere I look there are people doing workouts or eating healthily or talking about weight gain/loss during lockdown. Theres a pressure to come out of this being amazing and self sufficient and healthy and people are promoting it. (F24, BN)*

Some participants found that their increased free time during lockdown led to them making more social comparisons on social media, which triggered their ED and negative thoughts.

> *I have spent more time on my phone and using instagram, this is harmful as i compare myself to others and this makes me feel bad about myself. [F126, AN]*

Messages about fear of gaining weight during lockdown were also triggering, exacerbating these fears in participants at a time when gyms and routine exercise were less accessible. In line with quantitative findings, triggering social media messages were mostly described by participants diagnosed with AN.

> *I have been triggered a few times from people posting things like Don't worry about gaining weight in quarantine/other body positive messages, because prior to seeing them I didn't even think that weight gain could be a potential issue of quarantine. (F15, AN)*

However, a small number of participants described how these types of messages did not affect them, as their ED was more fuelled internally.

Part B: the role of emotion regulation

Quantitative analysis

All assumptions for multiple regressions were met. Differences between diagnostic categories were slight, so for clarity we only present the regression analyses for the whole sample. The results of regression analyses split by diagnosis categories can be found in supplementary materials 5.

Model 1: DASS We found that reduced access to emotion regulation strategies (B = 3.33, p <.001), non-acceptance of emotions (B = 1.57, p = .002), and reduced emotional clarity (B = 1.50, p = .001) were significant predictors of poor mental health as measured by the DASS (*Adj.* R^2 = .472, F(3, 203) = 62.3, p <.001).

Model 2: self-reported change in symptoms We found that difficulties maintaining goals when upset (B = 0.09, p = .004) was the only significant predictor of self-reported changes in eating disorder symptoms (*Adj.* R^2 = .036, F(1, 200) = 8.54, p = .004).

Model 3: EDEQ We found that non-acceptance of emotions (B=0.07, p=.007) and difficulties maintaining goals when upset (B = 0.09, p =.001) were significant predictors of eating psychopathology (*Adj.* R^2 = .156, F(2, 204) = 20.0, p <.001).

Qualitative experiences relating to coping with emotions

We interpreted two themes relating to coping with emotions; Emotional Support, and Emotion Coping Skills (See Fig. 2, part B, themes 5 and 6). With reduced access to usual emotion regulation strategies, such as emotional support from loved ones, participants spoke about the increased use of other coping strategies.

Theme 5: emotional support from others ome participants described how supportive family members had been protective for them during the pandemic. Talking to family, partners, or friends was a key strategy for coping with their eating disorders for many participants.

> *I am also a lot more honest with my family and friends about the struggles I face so I have constant support from them when I need it. [F122, AN]*

There was a reduced amount of contact with friends or family members during lockdown and many struggled with having less connection and less emotional support from loved ones.

Not speaking to my best friends every day / not [seeing] them at all has made things worse. [F99, BN]

The lockdown also meant a loss of support group activities. However, some participants also spoke about finding new avenues for support, with some support groups moving online and this making them easier to access. There was also an increased use of recovery-focused social media use and eating disorder support websites.

I feel this pandemic has put a lot of services online that are easily accessible for help. I discovered an online zoom support group for people affected with eating disorders and this has helped me every week. I feel I can talk openly and feel less alone. My normal service has not been active during this time. [F7, AN]

In contrast, a few participants described how they did not rely on support from others and tended to deal with their difficulties on their own. For some, there was a reluctance to talk about their own issues.

Feel guilty about talking about any difficulties I have during the pandemic as there are people who are in much worse circumstances, and my difficulties are little in comparison. [F26, AN]

These participants spoke of their difficulties as feeling insignificant in comparison to the pandemic and/or not wanting to worry others at a stressful time.

Theme 6: emotion coping skills Participants discussed different strategies used to cope with emotions, both helpful and unhelpful, as outlined in three subthemes; 'avoidant or unhelpful coping strategies', 'creating boundaries to look after self', and 'adding in positive activities'.

Avoidant or unhelpful coping strategies. Some participants described drinking alcohol and increasing their use of medication, such as sleeping pills and painkillers, as a short-term escape mechanism.

I've been drinking way more than I should as a means to escape the reality for a short period of time." [M72, BED]

A few participants reported an increase in self-harm as a coping strategy; some felt as if this was their only outlet, as their other normal coping mechanisms had been restricted.

The pandemic has increased my self harm, as I've felt so restricted by the government in terms of what I can do to deal with my feelings (i.e. initially – only exercise once a day, not able to exercise with anyone else). Using healthy means to deal with difficult feelings (i.e. go for a walk, meet a friend for coffee) have been more limited and so it is really easy to go back to unhelpful ways of coping such as self harm. [F5, AN]

Participants who spoke about their increased drinking, self-medicating, and self-harm recognised these as unhelpful coping strategies.

Creating boundaries to look after self. There were several coping strategies described which were about taking positive steps to look after participants' emotional wellbeing. Getting enough sleep was one important factor for helping participants to feel able to cope with their difficulties. Some participants focused on planning appropriate meals to avoid comfort eating or takeaways. Others also put strategies into place to allow themselves to exercise for its positive effects but to use limits avoid over-exercising.

"I have been exercising more ... which, as I said, has me in two minds. More exercise can't be bad for me I'm sure, but I'm worried it will become obsessive, to stop this I've set a strict timer and forced myself to stop when the alarm goes off no matter how I feel, then I immediately go for a shower so I am not tempted to carry on." [M53, BED]

Participants also recognised that the news and social media contributed to increased anxiety and so it was important for their exposure to be limited.

I usually have a good handle on my emotions per se. I had a spike in anxiety in the beginning though. As I mentioned, this seemed to be fuelled by the media. I consequently took my usual all-or-nothing approach (which is often an issue with the eating) however it worked well with regard to abandoning the media and news. This I believe reduced my anxiety by a notable degree. [M61, BED]

Many participants also coped by limiting their time on social media, or deactivating their social media accounts completely.

So much bullshit pressure to get a lockdown body - for this reason I came off social media early on in lockdown. [F76, EDNOS]

Implementing boundaries demonstrates a helpful way to cope with distress as discussed in the earlier theme of 'unhelpful messages – making a transformation'.

Adding in positive activities. Participants recognised that unstructured time could have a negative impact on their emotional wellbeing and their eating disorders. Again, this fits with our quantitative findings in which participants rated changes to routine as having one of the greatest impacts on the worsening of the ED symptoms. Participants found that building structure, developing new routines and planning mood boosting activities were beneficial for their mood and EDs.

> *Planning what to do the next day- gives me some routine and something to actually wake up for! [F31, AN]*

There were a wide range of positive activities which helped people to cope. Participants spoke about enjoying reading and learning new skills. Having a form of creative outlet, such as oil painting, photography, was important for some participants to channel their stress and express themselves.

> *Trying to keep myself busy, I have taken up crafts as a mean to express myself and take my mind off things. [F116, AN]*

Another popular coping strategy was using different forms of writing, including gratitude diaries and stories.

> *My best and favourite it probably noting things down, whenever I come across a problem that requires a lot of thought I open a note page and jot everything ... for example, I come across a problem that gives me a lot of anxiety the best way for me to get rid of it would be to understand the situation at hand therefore I write out different notes that give me a better understanding, why its happening, whats next, best course of action for minor benefits and major benefits etc. [M59, AN]*

Participants spoke about the benefits of going outside and enjoying time with their dogs as helpful coping strategies.

> *When I feel down and want to engage in unhelpful behaviours I have asked friends to borrow their dog for a few days to help me cope. Dogs are happy 99% of the time, require walking which means I have to get out of bed and face the world, I can hug them (even though I can't hug humans outside my household which I miss) and they don't care what size my body is or what it looks like. [F5, AN]*

The range of positive activities discussed were beneficial for people's wellbeing and participants also found that keeping busy was a helpful distraction.

Part C: qualitative experiences relating to online treatment

Participants who had received some form of treatment, either by telephone or by online videoconferencing, spoke about their experiences. Participants who did not receive any treatment during the pandemic also shared their experiences on why that was the case. Themes interpreted in this part of the analysis are depicted in Fig. 2, part C, themes 7 and 8. The first theme captures aspects of remote sessions which impacted the accessibility of this support. The second theme identified an experience of loss, including those who had no support from healthcare during the pandemic and those whose experience fell short of services usual provision.

Theme 7: accessibility - barriers and facilitators

There were two subthemes reflecting some of the benefits and disadvantages to remote sessions: 'detached connection' and 'ease of access'.

Detached connection. People spoke about some of the difficulties with their experience of receiving support online and this feeling more detached.

> *I find there is something detached about online treatment in that it doesn't feel like you're really connected to the other person because at the end of the call, it's just you in the same room as you live day to day. Also, for a while my therapist used a false background that left me feeling really uneasy as it made the session feel somehow less real/professional. [M1, AN]*

For some, there was a feeling of online treatment being less safe because of not having a confidential space at home to express themselves freely. For a smaller number of participants, their anxiety about telephone or video calls meant they felt unable to engage in this support at all. Frustrations with the quality of the internet connection were an additional hindrance to participants being able to engage fully.

> *I dont feel that I can talk over video call whilst in the house with partner and children within hearing distance [F101, BED]*

Many participants spoke about the connection with the therapist as feeling less personal and more detached in comparison to face-to-face contact. This detached connection became a barrier to some participants being able to engage fully. For a few participants, there was more opportunity to hide or not disclose important information.

> *Now video meetings have started.. but I'm far less open in these sessions and hide ... what has been going on. [F13, AN-bp]*

In contrast to this detached connection, there were many participants who commented on their experience of having a strong therapeutic relationship, which allowed them to feel safe, secure, able to connect, and to feel heard and believed.

Weekly connection. Feeling heard Feeling believed [F17, AN].

For participants with a positive therapeutic relationship, this seemed to protect them from the feeling a detached connection.

Ease of access. The move to online treatment made treatment more accessible for some participants. Online treatment reduced lengthy travel times due to the large geographical regions covered by many specialist eating disorder services.

We have moved to online sessions but it is good not to have to travel an hour each way. [F62, BN]

The online aspect also reduced some of the anxiety-provoking barriers and allowed a few participants to feel more able to seek help.

Being able to have regular contact with medical professionals via telephone has made it much easier for me to seek help, as it feels much lower commitment, and gives me far less anxiety, than seeking out face-to-face treatment. [F102, BN]

Theme 8: loss of support

Participants described their experience of support during the pandemic as being of a lesser quality than their usual support. For many, the typical structure and expectations of active treatment were lost, or paused, and replaced with a less formal "check-in" chat.

I have been unable to go to my appointments, I have had some telephone sessions but they have not been as productive. [F116, AN]

Other participants spoke about a loss of treatment support. Treatment was either delayed or stopped for many. Some services were closed and there was a sense of loss at not receiving support in a time of need.

Clinics have closed. No face to face appointments. No-one to talk to. [M23 BN]

Some participants described the loss of valued support from their GP as well as their specialist ED support.

Do not get to see my GP any more. He was my lifeline and my rock. [SM22, AN]

Another factor preventing many participants from accessing treatment was strong feelings of guilt about taking up NHS time and not wanting to bother NHS services during the pandemic. One participant described feeling *"like a grotesque burden" [F39, AN].* Some participants expressed feeling undeserving of help.

I've definitely felt guilty using NHS services, i've also felt undeserving of counselling/therapy sessions. [M45, OSFED]

The hesitancy in seeking help also applied to participants who had experienced a relapse of their ED during the pandemic; participants spoke about waiting to ask for support until the end of lockdown.

I was doing well but Covid and lockdown made me think again about food. I am considering going back to the Dr's to request treatment now that we are seeing the end of lockdown, as I wish to go back to coping with my issues. [M66, BED]

In contrast, a few participants spoke about the loss of support being an opportunity for them to take more responsibility for helping themselves. For participants who spoke about having the knowledge and skills to enable themselves to get back on track, they were able to put their experience of previous therapy into practice allowing themselves to be their own therapist, despite not having access to the support of services during this time period.

It gave me a sense of direction on how to help myself as at the end of the day it's myself that needs to be able to cope with my own mental well being. [M38, AN]

The finding that a small number of participants were able to take positive steps towards looking after their mental wellbeing reflects our quantitative finding that a minority of participants reported symptom improvement or symptom maintenance.

Discussion

In a tripartite approach, the present study sought to 1) extend and crystallise former reports around the impact of COVID-19 on people with eating disorders (EDs); 2) examine emotion regulation processes and their predictive value as regards to psychological wellbeing, ED symptomatology and symptom change during the pandemic; and [3] explore the experiences of those receiving online psychological treatment. To this end we collected qualitative and quantitative data from a large sample of people with an ED. We will discuss each goal in turn, hoping that through exploring these experiences, we will elucidate pathogenic influences of the pandemic, protective interpersonal mechanisms, and factors that impede and facilitate the efficacy of remote interventions during a time of crisis.

Worsening of symptoms during the pandemic

As governments adapt to managing the threat of coronavirus, the strictest lockdown measures are hoped to slowly lift. People establish new normalities, but lessons from history and trauma studies suggest that the psychological impact of collective and individual trauma will continue for a long time to come [2, 36, 37]. Accordingly, even though our data was collected at a point (June–July, 2020) after the severest quarantine measures in the UK, most of our participants still reported a worsening in ED symptomatology since before the pandemic. It is likely that increased support will be required for a long time, so research is crucial to better understand how to help these individuals.

To assist clinicians in identifying the most appropriate targets for intervention, we explored the relative importance of factors identified in preliminary research [14] in terms of their impact on the individual's ED. Across all four diagnoses, the most marked impacts were related to difficulties with emotions, disruption to routine, and changes in physical activity schedule, all concerns which had been previously highlighted in the aforementioned literature. There was, however, striking variability between participants, a heterogeneity which might depend on situational factors and/or diagnosis, and which should be considered by clinicians.

One noticeable difference in the quantitative data suggested that people with AN or OSFED ranked triggering messages on social media as more detrimental than did people with BED. Much has been written around the association between social media use, thin idealisation, disordered eating and eating disorders [38–40]. Thin idealisation online has manifested at the present time in messages around avoiding quarantine weight gain, messages which have been suggested to be dangerous to people with EDs [18, 41]. The impact of such pernicious messages was reflected in our qualitative data, which likewise found that triggering messages led to increased pressure to eat healthily, to exercise, and to lose weight, which exacerbated ED behaviours. In accordance with the quantitative data, participants who described being triggered by social media were generally those with AN, some of whom were triggered even by ostensibly positive messages. Notably, some participants mentioned a pressure towards self-improvement and productive use of lockdown. Concerns have been raised about people with pathological perfectionism in the context of the vanishing divide between work and home, the tendency for stressful situations to increase the drive to achieve mastery, and the difficulty of these individuals to adjust self-standards despite exceptional circumstances [42]. These concerns have also been raised in the context of EDs [18], where additional risks around "self-improvement" messages lie in the social reinforcement of thin idealisation, diet and exercise. In so far as participants with AN and with OSFED appeared more affected by triggering social media, it is interesting that some studies suggest perfectionism is associated less with bingeing than with other types of eating pathology, such as restriction and purging [43–45]. In accordance with its status as a lesser known, stigmatised and misunderstood eating disorder [46–48], the particular social media usage of individuals with BED is unknown; the different impact of social media exposure on people with BED in the present study is, as such, an intriguing avenue for future research.

The role of emotion regulation

As predicted, emotion regulation was a significant predictor of our wellbeing outcomes. This was particularly the case for general mental distress (DASS scores) as an outcome variable, for which emotion regulation explained almost 50% of the variance. This is consistent with the first part of our analysis, namely the highlighting of 'difficult emotions' as one of the most impactful pandemic factors on ED symptomatology, and is wholly redolent of the theoretical stance that negative emotions and inadequate regulation strategies are central to the aetiology and maintenance of the whole spectrum of ED psychopathology [22–24, 49, 50].

Amongst all DERS subscales, lack of emotional clarity, lack of access to emotion regulation strategies, and non-acceptance of emotions were found to be the strongest significant predictors of mental distress. As pertains to this first predictor, lack of emotional clarity is characteristic of alexithymia, a personality trait characterised by an inability to identify and describe emotions. Alexithymia occurs at higher rates both in people with an ED [26] and populations more vulnerable to EDs, such as autistic people [51, 52], such that some query whether it might mediate this increased vulnerability [53]. Clarity and awareness of emotions are thought to occur early in the process of emotion regulation, such that the ability to identify feelings helps determine which strategy to use to regulate unpleasant emotions [54, 55]. Interestingly, lack of access to emotion regulation strategies was also a strong predictor of distress during the pandemic. It is possible that these two are linked, and that helping patients identify their feelings with more clarity could help them match specific negative emotions to one in an arsenal of adaptive strategies. Worryingly, maladaptive and avoidant strategies, such as ED behaviours, alcohol use, self-medicating and self-harm were common responses to difficult emotions in the pandemic, as in previous reports [11]. Unfortunately, these kind of maladaptive emotion regulation strategies are activated easily and automatically, while adaptive strategies require conscious activation [56].

Despite this, our qualitative analysis reflected that some participants *were* still able to identify and apply adaptive strategies in their lives: these included accessing social support, setting appropriate boundaries for self-care and protection, and adding adaptive strategies in the form of new structures and reinforcing activities, as implicitly aligned with behavioural activation approaches to depression [57]. Only two studies have examined the coping activities engaged in by people with EDs at this time: consistent with the importance of setting new structures and enjoyable activities highlighted by our participants, these previous studies found that among the most helpful activities for people with AN and BN were establishing routines, day planning and scheduling pleasant activities [12, 13], in addition to time with family, yoga and gentle exercise.

Non-acceptance of emotions was not explicitly mentioned by participants in our qualitative analysis but was however associated with greater distress in our quantitative analysis. The ability to accept negative emotional experiences without judgement has consistently been associated with improved wellbeing [58–60], and thus-far unpublished data collected cross-culturally by the lead author [61] found benefits of emotion acceptance above active regulation strategies (like reappraisal) during the pandemic.

Together, our findings – the increase in negative emotions; the relationships between negative emotions and ED psychopathology (as reflected numerically, statistically and explicitly stated by participants), and between regulation deficiencies and negative affect; the reported benefits from adaptive regulation strategies, and the statistical support for the advantages of emotion acceptance – highlight several clear points for therapeutic intervention to intercede the cyclic maintenance of ED psychopathology by negative emotions and maladaptive responses [22–24, 49, 50]. While clarification of emotional experience may be a crucial first step, this might be followed by attempts to increase accessibility of existing adaptive regulation strategies and develop new ones, including emotion acceptance, in response to distress. Dialectical Behaviour Therapy (DBT) for BED and BN was developed in response to patients who do not always benefit from Cognitive Behaviour Therapy (CBT)-focused treatments [62], but this and other third-wave interventions such as acceptance and commitment therapy (ACT), compassion-focused therapy (CFT) and mindfulness have wider potential in the treatment of people with EDs [63]. Their relevance in this context comes from the fact that in contrast to pure CBT which attempts to prevent strong negative emotions being activated, third wave interventions are response-focused [64]: centred around accepting, managing and finding adaptive ways to moderate the experience of strong emotions when they arise. The existing evidence suggests that CBT may be more effective than third wave therapies [63–65], but these analyses all focus on a time prior to Covid-19. Whether third wave, response-focus therapies might be useful at a time when people have limited control over the antecedents of negative emotion is an intriguing query for future researchers. Adaptions to treatment paradigms in the current climate must, however, be made with caution and based on further experimental scrutiny.

Experience of online treatment

The third strand of our analysis focused on exploring the responses of those within our UK-based sample who had been offered remote psychological interventions. Very little is presently known around the efficacy of online treatment during the present crisis, but some preliminary concerns raised by individuals and their families [10] were ratified in our analysis. Where participants in the previous study suggested that therapeutic contact online would certainly "lack something" [10], our participants also reported a feeling of "detachment"; a diminishment of the expected and desired connection with the clinician, partly due to practical difficulties, such as internet connectivity and participants being unable to find a safe and private place within their homes. Interestingly however, our participants with pre-existent therapeutic relationships seemed partly protected from this issue, and reported some benefits from maintained therapeutic contact. Likewise, the previous study [10] raised concerns around the loss of structure, the loss of more active therapeutic activities, such as homework, and the loss of accountability, for instance related to weigh-ins – concerns aligned with the comments of our participants. This allowed some of our participants to engage unchecked in ED behaviours ("I have no one around to keep an eye on me"), consistent with the ambivalence that people with EDs often feel around treatment and recovery [66, 67]. It is important to recognise that these data, and that of the previous study [10], are time-sensitive. At the point of our data collection in June–July 2020, NHS services had recently undergone mass reorganisation and deployment of staff. Though the NHS remains in a state of flux and differences are still present across localities, the importance of "business as usual" and clear, practical guidance around how to establish the same level of excellence have since been disseminated [18, 30, 31, 68, 69]. For example, with reference to issues around engagement, motivation and openness, clinicians have been recommended to thoroughly and openly explore the patient's previous experiences of and attitudes towards remote treatment; to discuss and plan the practical implementation of the therapy and develop contingency plans for issues such as connection problems; to use the full power of audiovisual technology to create openness and connection; and to, as much as possible, involve the patient as an active collaborator in therapy [18, 30, 31].

While online treatment was found to be lesser than face-to-face treatment on many aspects, some participants felt that this form of therapy demanded a "lower commitment" and was less anxiety-provoking, which confirms previous suggestions that telehealth interventions might be favoured by people with EDs due to feeling less self-conscious about their body and more in control [70]. It is however important to note that for some, using video may be upsetting, so a recent paper recommended starting with audio if the patient has concerns about seeing their own image, and/or asking them to not look at parts of their own image they find distressing, although the therapist and patient should ideally work together to accept switching to video [31]. Another important aspect concerned the convenience of online treatment which reduced lengthy travel times – currently considered as a barrier to successful treatment [71, 72]. The positive appraisals around convenience and ease of access, found in our participants and in those of the previous study [10] were actually identified as advantages of telehealth interventions prior to Covid-19 [29, 73, 74] and suggest a future for online treatment beyond the COVID-19 pandemic.

Importantly, we observed huge variation across participants' experiences, captured by the following quote "Perhaps acknowledgement of how clients differ would also help, rather than a blanket here's-how-we're-doing-it-now approach" [M61, BED]. Given comments from participants struggling with achieving space and privacy from their families, this is one among other circumstantial factors likely to have substantial impact, and which requires consideration and possible tailoring of interventions. Further investigation of the factors relating to the efficacy and acceptability of remotely-delivered evidence-based treatments is an important goal.

One last, worrying issue which emerged in our analysis was around the loss of access to other primary healthcare infrastructure (for instance, GPs) and the reticence that many participants reported around seeking help. Many reported feelings of guilt and being undeserving of treatment, which may link to the lack of self-worth underlying ED symptomatology, where low self-esteem becomes intertwined in an over-evaluation of weight and shape [75]. Internalised stigma may also contribute to these feelings [76]. However, it is possible that this is, in addition, an unintended consequence of governmental measures and communications aimed at reducing transmission and preserving medical resources to cope with Covid-19. Worrying evidence is emerging that despite increased reports of domestic violence, self-injury and suicidality, fewer individuals than would be typically expected are seeking formal help from health professionals [77]. Concerns that mental ill-health might be perceived as less important than physical health [78] seemed to be borne out in our participants. To some extent, solutions may be found in the possibility of self-referrals as an option, and in increasing awareness of the availability of online support groups, as access to these groups was identified as helpful by some participants. Research exploring the impact and perception of public health announcements may, however, be vital in ensuring that those who need to do seek help.

Limitations

While this study contributes to understanding the effect of COVID-19 on a population with pre-existent mental illness, there are several important limitations to consider. First, the time sensitivity of the study necessitated speedy and convenient recruitment of participants through social media and Prolific. While this allowed us to collect a larger and more sex-balanced sample than previous research on COVID-19 and EDs [9, 14], we relied on self-reported diagnoses. Although the EDEQ confirmed that average eating psychopathology was in the clinical range, it would have been beneficial to confirm diagnoses, which may have been especially important in our attempts to contrast different ED diagnoses. Moreover, our sample was self-selected and over 18, meaning that it is possible that it was biased towards people who may have more severe eating disorders, or who had not been able to use treatment to make change. Our sample indeed had a longer than average duration of illness in comparison to recent estimates for untreated eating disorders [79]. Therefore, it is possible that this study's sample may not be a fully generalisable representation of the entire eating disorder population, including of the younger population.

Further issues with our sample included underrepresentation of minority ethnic groups, and unequal ratio of female to male participants. Particular efforts had been made to recruit this often forgotten population, and were partially achieved in that we recruited 76 men with EDs. However as the distribution of men and women differed across specific ED diagnoses and the male sample was still comparatively underpowered, we were forced to abandon our hope to compare male and female participants with each specific type of ED pathology. Consequently, it is possible that differences between ED diagnoses, for instance in the greater importance of social media triggers for participants with AN and OSFED than for participants with BED, might be a factor of the different representation of women and men within these groups. Here, again, the paucity of data on ED in males creates the danger that in the present time, too, men with EDs may be less understood.

Finally, our cross-sectional design precludes any conclusions around the causal links between emotion regulation strategies and our wellbeing outcomes. Indeed, while extant literature supports the claim that adaptive emotion regulation strategies (such as emotion acceptance) are associated with better mental health [56, 60], it is possible that high levels of distress in our study could have led to more difficulties with emotion regulation. Longitudinal studies on the impact of emotion regulations strategies during COVID-19 could help better inform the direction of the effect.

Implications

Our findings point to several clinical implications for healthcare professionals to consider. With the likelihood that services will continue to work remotely for some time, it is crucial that services continue to deliver the most effective evidence-based treatments with its usual structure.

Our paper highlights some of the ways that reduced emotion coping skills, along with changes to routine, social contact, and living environments have impacted on people's EDs and therefore may be important areas to address within treatment. In terms of routine, we suggest that clinicians could use techniques from behavioural activation [57], which equips patients with skills to structure their day with activities which give a sense of achievement, a sense of enjoyment, and a sense of social connection.

Our findings also highlighted the importance of setting appropriate boundaries around exposure to media, alcohol, eating and exercise routines, to encourage self-care in each of these areas. These implications for treatment are consistent with other recommendations from the literature on ED during the pandemic, which have highlighted the importance of increasing value activities, social contact and placing boundaries to encourage healthy behaviours relating to eating and exercise behaviours [10, 18, 69].

For patients who use their ED as a way of coping with difficult emotions and distress, treatment may also incorporate emotion regulation skills as referenced within CBT-ED approaches [75] and discussed in further detail within DBT treatment [62]. This may include helping people to identify and label their emotions, recognise the function of their emotions, and learn adaptive strategies for coping with distressing emotions, such as emotional acceptance.

Healthcare professionals may also want to consider exploring the patient's experience of online treatment and identify potential therapy-interfering behaviours, such as our participants who identified a tendency to hold back from being open and honest in treatment sessions. A collaborative approach would allow for discussion of how potential barriers can be managed. Our findings show that the therapeutic relationship may protect from feelings of disconnection; an openness to gather in-session feedback may help patients continue to feel supported and understood, despite the connection being remote. Finally, there was a wide variation in patients' responses across our qualitative themes and it is important to tailor the treatment approach to an individual's formulation, whilst still adhering to the evidence-based approach.

Conclusion

Through a mixed-method tripartite approach, we showed that our self-selected participants with EDs have been strongly affected during the COVID-19 pandemic, and that difficulties regulating emotions was a significant predictor of their well-being. We also showed that while online treatment had some beneficial aspects, more work is needed to fully understand its impact on patients' mental health. We recommend that future research further explore the benefits of working on emotion regulation strategies as part of treatment in a post-pandemic world at a time when people have limited control over the antecedents of negative emotions.

Abbreviations

AN: Anorexia Nervosa; ARFID: Avoidant/Restrictive Food Intake Disorder; BED: Binge Eating Disorder; BN: Bulimia Nervosa; CBT-E: Enhanced Cognitive Behaviour Therapy; CBT-ED: Eating Disorder Focused Cognitive Behaviour Therapy; DASS: Depression, Anxiety and Stress Scale; DERS: Difficulties in Emotion Regulation Questionnaire; ED: Eating Disorder; EDEQ: Eating Disorder Examination Questionnaire; MANTRA: Maudsley Model of Anorexia Treatment in Adults; NHS: National Health Service; SSCM: Specialist Supportive Clinical Management

Acknowledgements

The authors would like to thank each and every participant who kindly gave their time in this study.

Authors' contributions

LV, RLM, MG and LM designed the study. RLM, LV and RS collected the data. LV and RLM analysed the quantitative data. MG, LM and RS analysed the qualitative data. LV and RLM wrote the introduction with input from all authors. LV, RLM and MG wrote the methods and result sections. LV, RLM and LM wrote the discussion with input from all authors. The author(s) read and approved the final manuscript.

Competing interests

The authors declare that they have no competing interests.

Author details

[1]Department of Psychology, Bournemouth University, Poole, UK. [2]Dorset Healthcare University NHS Foundation Trust, Poole, UK.

References

1. Holmes EA, O'Connor RC, Perry VH, Tracey I, Wessely S, Arseneault L, et al. Multidisciplinary research priorities for the COVID-19 pandemic: a call for action for mental health science. Lancet Psychiatry. 2020;7(6):547–60.
2. Usher K, Bhullar N, Jackson D. Life in the pandemic: social isolation and mental health. J Clin Nurs. 2020:1–2.
3. Pfefferbaum B, North CS. Mental health and the Covid-19 pandemic. N Engl J Med. 2020.
4. Cullen W, Gulati G, Kelly BD. Mental health in the COVID-19 pandemic. QJM. 2020;113(5):311–2.
5. Hao F, Tan W, Jiang L, Zhang L, Zhao X, Zou Y, et al. Do psychiatric patients experience more psychiatric symptoms during COVID-19 pandemic and lockdown? A case-control study with service and research implications for immunopsychiatry. Brain Behav Immun. 2020;87:100–6.
6. Wind TR, Rijkeboer M, Andersson G, Riper H. The COVID-19 pandemic: the 'black swan' for mental health care and a turning point for e-health. Internet Interv. 2020;20:100317.
7. Chesney E, Goodwin GM, Fazel S. Risks of all-cause and suicide mortality in mental disorders: a meta-review. World Psychiatry. 2014;13(2):153–60.
8. Fichter MM, Quadflieg N. Mortality in eating disorders - results of a large prospective clinical longitudinal study. Int J Eat Disord. 2016;49(4):391–401.
9. Phillipou A, Meyer D, Neill E, Tan EJ, Toh WL, Van Rheenen TE, et al. Eating and exercise behaviors in eating disorders and the general population during the COVID-19 pandemic in Australia: Initial results from the COLLATE project. Int J Eat Disord. 2020;(April):1–8.
10. Fernández-Aranda F, Casas M, Claes L, Bryan DC, Favaro A, Granero R, et al. COVID-19 and implications for eating disorders. Eur Eat Disord Rev. 2020;28:239–45.
11. Termorshuizen J, Watson H, Thornton L, Borg S, Flatt R, MacDermod C, et al. Early Impact of COVID-19 on Individuals with Eating Disorders: A survey of ~1000 Individuals in the United States and the Netherlands. medRxiv. 2020;.
12. Schlegl S, Maier J, Meule A, Voderholzer U. Eating disorders in times of the COVID-19 pandemic—results from an online survey of patients with anorexia nervosa. Int J Eat Disord. 2020;53:1791.
13. Schlegl S, Meule A, Favreau M, Voderholzer U. Bulimia nervosa in times of the COVID-19 pandemic—results from an online survey of former inpatients. Eur Eat Disord Rev. 2020.
14. Branley-Bell D, Talbot CV. Exploring the impact of the COVID-19 pandemic and UK lockdown on individuals with experience of eating disorders. Psyarxiv. 2020.
15. Dixit A, Marthoenis M, Arafat SMY, Sharma P, Kar SK. Binge watching behavior during COVID 19 pandemic: a cross-sectional, cross-national online survey. Psychiatry Res. 2020;289:113089.
16. Rodgers RF, Lombardo C, Cerolini S, Franko DL, Omori M, Fuller-Tyszkiewicz M, et al. The impact of the COVID-19 pandemic on eating disorder risk and symptoms. Int J Eat Disord. 2020;(April):1–5.
17. Power M, Doherty B, Pybus K, Pickett K. How COVID-19 has exposed inequalities in the UK food system: the case of UK food and poverty. Emerald Open Res. 2020;2:11.
18. Cooper M, Reilly EE, Siegel JA, Coniglio K, Sadeh-Sharvit S, Pisetsky EM, et al. Eating disorders during the COVID-19 pandemic and quarantine: an overview of risks and recommendations for treatment and early intervention. Eat Disord. 2020.
19. Eddy KT, Tabri N, Thomas JJ, Murray HB, Keshaviah A, Hastings E, et al. Recovery from anorexia nervosa and bulimia nervosa at 22-year follow-up. In: Journal of Clinical Psychiatry. 2017.
20. Tomba E, Tecuta L, Crocetti E, Squarcio F, Tomei G. Residual eating disorder symptoms and clinical features in remitted and recovered eating disorder patients: a systematic review with meta-analysis. Int J Eat Disord. 2019;52:759–76.
21. Treasure J, Stein D, Maguire S. Has the time come for a staging model to map the course of eating disorders from high risk to severe enduring illness? An examination of the evidence. Early Interv Psychiatry. 2015;9:173–84.
22. Treasure J, Schmidt U. The cognitive-interpersonal maintenance model of anorexia nervosa revisited: a summary of the evidence for cognitive, socio-emotional and interpersonal predisposing and perpetuating factors. J Eat Disord. 2013;1(1):13.
23. Lavender JM, Wonderlich SA, Engel SG, Gordon KH, Kaye WH, Mitchell JE. Dimensions of emotion dysregulation in anorexia nervosa and bulimia nervosa: a conceptual review of the empirical literature. Clin Psychol Rev. 2015;40:111–22.
24. Fairburn CG, Cooper Z, Shafran R. Cognitive behaviour therapy for eating disorders: a "transdiagnostic" theory and treatment. Behav Res Ther. 2003;41:509–28.
25. Restubog SLD, Ocampo ACG, Wang L. Taking control amidst the chaos: emotion regulation during the COVID-19 pandemic. J Vocat Behav. 2020; 119(May):1–6.
26. Westwood H, Kerr-Gaffney J, Stahl D, Tchanturia K. Alexithymia in eating disorders: systematic review and meta-analyses of studies using the Toronto alexithymia scale. J Psychosom Res. 2017;99:66–81.
27. Schimmenti A, Billieux J, Starcevic V. The four horsemen of fear during the COVID pandemic. Clin Neuropsychiatry. 2020;17(2):45–9.
28. Eating disorders: recognition and treatment [Internet]. National Institute of Health and Care Excellence. 2017 [cited 2020 Sep 23]. Available from: https://www.nice.org.uk/guidance/ng69.
29. Tuerk PW, Keller SM, Acierno R. Treatment for anxiety and depression via clinical videoconferencing: evidence base and barriers to expanded access in practice. Focus (Madison). 2018;16(4):363–9.
30. Murphy R, Calugi S, Cooper Z, Dalle GR. Challenges and opportunities for enhanced cognitive behaviour therapy (CBT-E) in light of COVID-19. Cogn Behav Ther. 2020;13.
31. Waller G, Pugh M, Mulkens S, Moore E, Mountford VA, Carter J, et al. Cognitive-behavioral therapy in the time of coronavirus: clinician tips for working with eating disorders via telehealth when face-to-face meetings are not possible. Int J Eat Disord. 2020;53:1132–41.
32. Guest G, MacQueen K, Namey E. Integrating qualitative and quantitative data. In: Applied Thematic Analysis: Sage; 2014. p. 187–216.
33. Lovibond PF, Lovibond SH. The structure of negative emotional states: comparison of the depression anxiety stress scales (DASS) with the Beck depression and anxiety inventories. Behav Res Ther. 1995;33:335–43. https://doi.org/10.1016/0005-7967(94)00075-U.
34. Fairburn C, Beglin S. Eating Disorder Examination Questionnaire (EDE-Q 6.0). In: Fairburn C, editor. Cognitive Behaviour Therapy and Eating Disorders. New York: Guilford Press; 2008. p. 309–14.
35. Kaufman EA, Xia M, Fosco G, Yaptangco M, Skidmore CR, Crowell SE. The difficulties in emotion regulation scale short form (DERS-SF): validation and replication in adolescent and adult samples. J Psychopathol Behav Assess. 2016;38:433–55. https://doi.org/10.1007/s10862-015-9529-3.
36. Horesh D, Brown AD. Covid-19 response: traumatic stress in the age of Covid-19: a call to close critical gaps and adapt to new realities. Psychol Trauma Theory Res Pract Policy. 2020;12(4):331–5.
37. Estes HD, Thompson RR. Preparing for the aftermath of COVID-19: shifting risk and DownstreamHealth consequences. Psychol Trauma Theory Res Pract Policy. 2020;12(1):31–2.
38. Wilksch SM, O'Shea A, Ho P, Byrne S, Wade TD. The relationship between social media use and disordered eating in young adolescents. Int J Eat Disord. 2020;53:96–106.
39. Holland G, Tiggemann M. A systematic review of the impact of the use of social networking sites on body image and disordered eating outcomes. Body Image. 2016;17:100–10.
40. Mingoia J, Hutchinson AD, Wilson C, Gleaves DH. The relationship between social networking site use and the internalization of a thin ideal in females: a meta-analytic review. Front Psychol. 2017;8:1351.
41. Shah M, Sachdeva M, Johnston H. Eating disorders in the age of COVID-19. Psychiatry Res. 2020;290:113122.
42. Flett G, Hewitt P. The perfectionism pandemic meets COVID-19: understanding the stress, distress, and problems in living for perfectionists during the Global Health crisis. J Concurr Disord. 2020;2:80–105.
43. Forbush K, Heatherton TF, Keel PK. Relationships between perfectionism and specific disordered eating behaviors. Int J Eat Disord. 2007;40(1):37–41.
44. Luo J, Forbush KT, Williamson JA, Markon KE, Pollack LO. How specific are the relationships between eating disorder behaviors and perfectionism? Eat Behav; 2013.
45. Welch E, Miller JL, Ghaderi A, Vaillancourt T. Does perfectionism mediate or moderate the relation between body dissatisfaction and disordered eating attitudes and behaviors? Eat Behav. 2009;10(3):168–75.
46. Reas DL. Public and healthcare professionals' knowledge and attitudes toward binge eating disorder: a narrative review. Nutrients. 2017;9(11):1267.
47. Chao AM, Rajagopalan AV, Tronieri JS, Walsh O, Wadden TA. Identification of binge eating disorder criteria: results of a National Survey of healthcare providers. J Nurs Scholarsh. 2019;51(4):399–407.

48. O'Connor C, McNamara N, O'Hara L, McNicholas F. Eating disorder literacy and stigmatising attitudes towards anorexia, bulimia and binge eating disorder among adolescents. Adv Eat Disord. 2016;4(2):125–40.
49. Prefit A, Cândea D, Szentagotai-Tătar A. Emotion regulation across eating pathology: a meta-analysis. Appetite. 2019;143:104438.
50. Monell E, Clinton D, Birgegård A. Emotion dysregulation and eating disorders—associations with diagnostic presentation and key symptoms. Int J Eat Disord. 2018;51:921–30.
51. Kinnaird E, Stewart C, Tchanturia K. Investigating alexithymia in autism: a systematic review and meta-analysis. Eur Psychiatry. 2019;55:80–9.
52. Tchanturia K, Adamson J, Leppanen J, Westwood H. Characteristics of autism spectrum disorder in anorexia nervosa: a naturalistic study in an inpatient treatment programme. Autism. 2019;23(1):123–30.
53. Vuillier L, Carter Z, Texeira A, Moseley R. Increased risk for eating disorders in autism spectrum conditions may derive from alexithymia. Mol Autism 2020; 11(1):1–19.
54. Barrett LF, Gross J, Christensen TC, Benvenuto M. Knowing what you're feeling and knowing what to do about it: mapping the relation between emotion differentiation and emotion regulation. Cogn Emot. 2001;15(6): 713–24.
55. Vine V, Aldao A. Impaired emotional clarity and psychopathology: a transdiagnostic deficit with symptom-specific pathways through emotion regulation. J Soc Clin Psychol. 2014;33(4):319–42.
56. Van Beveren M, Goossens L, Volkaert B, Grassmann C, Wante L, Vandeweghe L, et al. How do I feel right now? Emotional awareness, emotion regulation, and depressive symptoms in youth. Eur Child Adolesc Psychiatry. 2019;28:389–98.
57. Ekers D, Webster L, Van Straten A, Cuijpers P, Richards D, Gilbody S. Behavioural activation for depression; an update of meta-analysis of effectiveness and sub group analysis. PLoS One. 2014;9(6):e100100.
58. Aldao A, Nolen-Hoeksema S, Schweizer S. Emotion-regulation strategies across psychopathology: a meta-analytic review. Clin Psychol Rev. 2010; 30(2):217–37.
59. Kohl A, Rief W, Glombiewski JA. How effective are acceptance strategies? A meta-analytic review of experimental results. J Behav Ther Exp Psychiatry. 2012;43(4):988–1001.
60. Ford BQ, Lam P, John OP, Mauss IB. The psychological health benefits of accepting negative emotions and thoughts: laboratory, diary, and longitudinal evidence. J Pers Soc Psychol. 2018;115(6):1075.
61. Pauw L, Vu T, Sun R, Vuillier L, Milek A, Sauter D. Emotion Regulation and Wellbeing: A Cross-Cultural Study During the COVID-19 Outbreak [manuscript submitted for publication]. Dep Soc Psychol Univ Amsterdam.
62. Safer D, Telch C, Chen E, Linehan M. Dialectical behavior therapy for binge eating and bulimia: Guilford Press; 2009.
63. Linardon J, Gleeson J, Yap K, Murphy K, Brennan L. Meta-analysis of the effects of third-wave behavioural interventions on disordered eating and body image concerns: implications for eating disorder prevention. Cogn Behav Ther. 2019;48(1):15–38.
64. Linardon J, Fairburn CG, Fitzsimmons-Craft EE, Wilfley DE, Brennan L. The empirical status of the third-wave behaviour therapies for the treatment of eating disorders: a systematic review. Clin Psychol Rev. 2017;58:125–40.
65. Linardon J, Wade TD, De La Piedad GX, Brennan L. The efficacy of cognitive-behavioral therapy for eating disorders: a systematic review and meta-analysis. J Consult Clin Psychol. 2017;85(11):1080–94.
66. Gregertsen EC, Mandy W, Serpell L. The egosyntonic nature of anorexia: an impediment to recovery in anorexia nervosa treatment. Front Psychol. 2017; 8:2273.
67. Fassino S, Abbate-Daga G. Resistance to treatment in eating disorders: a critical challenge. BMC Psychiatry. 2013;13:294.
68. Matheson BE, Bohon C, Lock J. Family-based treatment via videoconference: clinical recommendations for treatment providers during COVID-19 and beyond. Int J Eat Disord. 2020:1–13.
69. Weissman RS, Bauer S, Thomas JJ. Access to evidence-based care for eating disorders during the COVID-19 crisis. Int J Eat Disord. 2020;53: 693–46.
70. Simpson S, Bell L, Knox J, Mitchell D. Therapy via videoconferencing: a route to client empowerment? Clin Psychol Psychother. 2005;12(2):156–65.
71. Linardon J, Messer M, Lee S, Rosato J. Perspectives of e-health interventions for treating and preventing eating disorders: descriptive study of perceived advantages and barriers, help-seeking intentions, and preferred functionality. Eat Weight Disord. 2020.
72. Leavey G, Vallianatou C, Johnson-Sabine E, Rae S, Gunputh V. Psychosocial barriers to engagement with an eating disorder service: a qualitative analysis of failure to attend. Eat Disord. 2011;19(5):425–40.
73. Choi NG, Wilson NL, Sirrianni L, Marinucci ML, Hegel MT. Acceptance of home-based telehealth problem-solving therapy for depressed, low-income homebound older adults: qualitative interviews with the participants and aging-service case managers. Gerontologist. 2014;54(4):704–13.
74. Langarizadeh M, Tabatabaei MS, Tavakol K, Naghipour M, Rostami A, Moghbeli F. Telemental health care, an effective alternative to conventional mental care: a systematic review. Acta Inform Medica. 2017;25(4):240.
75. Fairburn CG, Cooper Z, Shafran R, Wilson, Terence G. Eating Disorders - a Transdiagnostic Protocol. In: Barlow D. Clinical Handbook of Psychological Disorders: A Step-by-step Treatment Manual (4th Edition). Guilford Press; 2008. p. 578–614.
76. Griffiths S, Mitchison D, Murray SB, Mond JM, Bastian BB. How might eating disorders stigmatization worsen eating disorders symptom severity? Evaluation of a stigma internalization model. Int J Eat Disord. 2018;51(8): 1010–4.
77. Iob E, Steptoe A, Fancourt D. Abuse, self-harm and suicidal ideation in the UK during the COVID-19 pandemic. Br J Psychiatry. 2020:1–4.
78. Reger MA, Stanley IH, Joiner TE. Suicide mortality and coronavirus disease 2019 - a perfect storm? JAMA psychiatry; 2020.
79. Austin A, Flynn M, Richards K, Hodsoll J, Duarte TA, Robinson P, et al. Duration of untreated eating disorder and relationship to outcomes: a systematic review of the literature. Eur Eat Disord Rev. 2020.

9

What was the impact of a global pandemic (COVID-19) lockdown period on experiences within an eating disorder service? A service evaluation of the views of patients, parents/ carers and staff

Hannah Shaw[1,2*], Sarah Robertson[1] and Nadia Ranceva[1,3]

Abstract

Background: The World Health Organization declared the outbreak of COVID-19 as a global pandemic on the 11th March 2020. As a result, the UK Government imposed severe restrictions on working and social contact as part of "lockdown." Whilst the full extent of the pandemic's impact on eating disorder patients is unknown, the literature suggests that patients with pre-existing mental illness may be more vulnerable to the mental health impacts. In addition, the restrictions greatly reduced the access to mental health services and presented new challenges to service delivery. A service evaluation was carried out to explore how the COVID-19 global pandemic changed service provision in a young person's eating disorder service and how this affected patient, family and staff experiences.

Methods: An audit was carried out to explore how the lockdown period had impacted referrals and service delivery. Quantitative data was collected in an online survey and qualitative data was collected in two formats: open ended answers as part of the online survey and open-ended focus groups, structured using narrative enquiry. The 43 participants consisted of 12 patients, 19 parents/carers, and 12 staff members. Patients were under the age of 18 and had a diagnosis of an eating disorder.

Results: COVID-19 and lockdown increased the pressure on the service and changed service provision significantly. This has impacted the relational experiences for patients and their carers and staff have been faced with new challenges. Patients, parents/carers and staff all preferred face-to-face appointments over virtual options. There was no difference in service satisfaction before and during COVID-19.

(Continued on next page)

* Correspondence: Hannahshaw.hjs@gmail.com
[1]The Eating Disorder Young Person's Service, Alder Hey Children's Hospital Foundation Trust, Liverpool, UK
[2]Royal Holloway University of London, Egham, UK
Full list of author information is available at the end of the article

(Continued from previous page)

Conclusions: It is possible to provide an eating disorder service in lockdown restrictions that patients and parents report high satisfaction with. Providing face-to-face appointments at the beginning of treatment and including families in the planning should be prioritised. Staff support is crucial to be able to continue delivering high quality services. The key themes are identified, and clinical recommendations are made to guide service delivery.

Keywords: COVID-19, Eating disorders, Global pandemic, Lockdown, Parent/Carer experience, Patient experience, Service development, Service evaluation, Service satisfaction, Staff experience

Plain English summary

Online survey's and focus groups were used to find out how the COVID-19 global pandemic changed how support was provided by a young person's eating disorder service. We were interested in finding out how these changes and new ways of working were experienced by patients, families and staff. The aim was to find out how best to use the new methods to meet the needs of those accessing the service and those working for the service. Staff told us that there was an increased pressure on the service during COVID-19. We found out that patients, families and staff all preferred face-to-face appointments over virtual options (e.g. telephone calls or video calls). Although all participants told us there were significant changes to the service provided, there was no difference between the service satisfaction before and during COVID-19. This suggests that it is possible to provide an eating disorder service that patients, their families and staff are satisfied with in lockdown restrictions. However, staff must be receiving the right level of support for this to continue. Additionally, the feedback suggests that services should provide face-to-face appointments at the beginning of treatment and must ensure families are involved in the care and planning.

Background

The World Health Organization declared the outbreak of COVID-19 as a global pandemic on the 11th March 2020. On March 23rd, 2020, the UK Government imposed severe restrictions on working and social contact as part of "lockdown", which greatly reduced the access to health services, and presented new challenges to service delivery.

As a result, there are rising concerns about the detrimental impact of the pandemic on mental health [7]. Studies have found that mental health in the UK has deteriorated compared with pre COVID-19 trends [18]. The literature suggests that patients with pre-existing mental illness may be more vulnerable to the mental health impacts and at higher risk of relapse or new episodes of their disorder [20, 21]. Whilst the full extent of the pandemic's impact on eating disorder (ED) patients is unknown, emerging evidence suggests there will be a detrimental effect [2].

As a result of COVID-19, many healthcare services are only offering urgent visits and inpatient treatment for severe ED cases. Restrictions have led to the closure of day hospitals and outpatient facilities across the world and where possible, online/virtual treatments have been recommended [6]. While online and e-health measures have been developed for EDs, more research is needed to understand how they are experienced, and how to implement them effectively [1]. Patients and families will be burdened with more responsibility and self-management due to the lack of face-to-face accountability (e.g. no/less regular weigh-ins) with professionals [6]. There are also concerns that video calls could be a triggering form of communication due to the heightened awareness of bodily self which could prompt self-criticism harmful to recovery [6]. Moreover, we are yet to find out how these new ways of working impact the staff within ED services.

When lockdown restrictions were imposed, the Eating Disorder Young Person's Service (EDYS) at Alder Hey Children's Hospital had to quickly adjust to new ways of working. In order to reduce the number of patients attending the clinic, the community nursing team were engaged to carry out physical observations (lying and standing blood pressure, pulse and weight) at patients' homes. Results were then emailed to the responsible clinicians. As more infection control measures were implemented onsite, the service opened a physical monitoring clinic, where patients would come in for a 15-min physical observation appointment. All other appointments were offered virtually. Clinicians reported that patients were not responding as well to treatment when delivered in this way and as a result both mental and physical health of many patients was deteriorating. Therefore, the decision was made to re-introduce face-to-face appointments for patients deemed as high-risk in June and July.

It is crucial that we continue to support the ongoing provision of vital mental health services, whilst seeking to mitigate the negative impact of restrictions on vulnerable groups [11]. In order to understand the best way to do this, we conducted a mixed methods service evaluation aimed at exploring the impact of the pandemic on patients, family and staff experiences. This service evaluation was conducted in the EDYS at Alder Hey Children's NHS Foundation Trust.

Methods

An audit was carried out using data from the Electronic Patient Record System used by the trust to gain an understanding of how the lockdown period had impacted referrals and service delivery. A mixed method design was used to conduct a service evaluation aimed at understanding how the eating disorder service changed, and how that was experienced by staff, family, and patients. Quantitative data was collected using an online survey containing a series of questions using a five-point Likert scale ranging from strongly disagree (1) to strongly agree (5). Qualitative data was collected in two formats: open ended answers as part of the online survey and open-ended focus groups, structured using narrative inquiry.

Participants

43 participants opted to take part: 12 patients, 19 parents/carers, and 12 members of staff. All participants had experience of the service during COVID-19. As participation was based on availability, no power analysis was conducted to inform sample size. No demographic information was collected to ensure responses remained anonymous. All patients were under the age of 18 and had a diagnosis of typical or non-typical anorexia nervosa (AN), bulimia nervosa (BN) or binge-eating disorder (BED).

Procedure

This service evaluation was approved by the Clinical Audit Department at Alder Hey Children's NHS Foundation Trust. We sought consent from all participants at the start of the survey in the form of a tick box question and verbally at the beginning of each focus group.

Quantitative

We created a survey which was informed by discussions with service users at CAMHS (Child and Adolescent Mental Health Service) participation groups. Based on this feedback, we adapted the existing measure of CAMHS service satisfaction (Experience of Service Questionnaire, ESQ), recommended by CORC (Child Outcome Research Consortium). The survey consisted of two sections: experience of service during COVID-19, and experience of service before COVID-19. Only participants who stated they had been involved with the service before COVID-19 were taken to this section of the survey ($n = 29$).

We sent a short explanation about the service evaluation and the link for the relevant survey, to patients and parent/carers via text to registered numbers on the hospital record system. This was sent to staff via email.

Qualitative

We then conducted open ended focus groups structured using narrative inquiry. Narrative research begins with the premise that we tell stories about our lives [17]. Narrative interviews involve two parts: 1) an open ended exploratory question; e.g., *"what has it been like for you receiving a service/providing a service in COVID-19?"*; 2) follow up prompts based on what participants describe, in the order they describe it; e.g. *"you said that ... what did it feel like for you in the moment?", "you mentioned ... can you tell me more about what happened?"* [19]. Using this approach, we conducted three individual focus groups with groups of staff, parents, and patients. Staff attended the focus group prior to an MDT team meeting. We texted parents and patients an invitation to join the focus groups via MS teams. Focus groups were recorded and anonymously transcribed.

Analysis

Quantitative

We used Excel for descriptive statistics and JASP for inferential statistical analysis. Due to the non-parametric nature of the data, we used a Wilcoxon Signed-Rank test to determine whether there was significant difference between service satisfaction before COVID-19 and during COVID-19. Patient, parent/carer and staff scores were collated to carry out the statistical analysis as a result of the small individual sample sizes which would have led to very low power for detecting group differences.

Qualitative

Narrative analysis provides a vantage point that allows others to analyse how the storyteller constructs meaning. Storytellers depict how characters, events, interactions, and outcomes are related [13, 16]. Informed by structural and thematic traditions of narrative inquiry, we listened back to stories shared in focus groups and mapped out the key events described, and how they were experienced, into a table for patients, parents/carers and staff. The qualitative feedback received through the Qualtrics survey was also mapped into this process and overarching themes were identified through thematic analysis [3].

Results

How the lockdown period impacted the EDYS referrals and service delivery

Table 1 shows the number of referrals accepted by EDYS throughout the same time period (March – July) in

Table 1 Number of referrals accepted by EDYS from March to July in 2019 and 2020

	March – July 2019		March – July 2020	
Accepted Referrals	**n**	**%**	**n**	**%**
Urgent	7	20.59	10	34.48
Routine	27	79.41	19	65.52
Total	34	100.00	29	100.00
Paediatric Admissions	4		9	

2019, when there were no lockdown restrictions, and 2020, during the initial lockdown period. Although less referrals were accepted, more of these were triaged as urgent, meaning that patients presentations were more acute. Thus, patients had worse ED symptomology, physical health observations that were further away from the normal range and higher scores on risk assessments. There was also a marked increase in the number of admissions of ED patients to the general peadiatric ward; meaning that patients were too physically and mentally unwell to remain at home.

More recent data collected by the service (Table 2) shows that more referrals were accepted in 2020 than in 2019 over the same time period (1st January - 2nd December). It also shows that the percentage increase was larger for urgent referrals (150%) than routine referrals (129%).

Table 3 presents the number of face-to-face and virtual appointments offered by EDYS each month from December 2019 to July 2020. The data shows that on average there was an overall increase in appointments offered during lockdown (M = 402.4, SD = 37.90) compared to previous months (M = 265, SD = 37.27).

Perceptions of how young people with eating disorders are coping in COVID-19: patient, parent/carer and staff perspectives

Figure 1 shows the percentage of agreement (strongly disagree [1] to strongly agree [5]) for patient, parents/carers and staff when asked how young people with eating disorders were coping in COVID-19. Views differed between groups, with 92% of staff disagreeing that young people were coping better, 26% of parents/carers and only 16% of patients.

Table 2 Number of referrals accepted by EDYS from 1st January – 2nd December in 2019 and 2020 split by type

Year	Urgent (n)	Routine (n)	Total (n)
2019	14	107	121
2020	21	138	159
Increase in accepted referrals (%)	150	129	132

Table 3 Number of appointments offered by EDYS each month from December 2019 to July 2020 split by appointment type

2019–2020	Face-to-face (n)	Virtual (n)	Both (n)
December	222	0	222
January	288	0	288
February	285	0	285
March	Data by mode of apt not available		361
April	66	352	418
May	88	277	365
June	135	285	420
July	219	229	448
Total			2807

Self-reported types of appointments experienced in COVID-19 and staff, patient and parent/carer preferences

Most staff reported experiencing the full range of appointments but patient and parents were more likely to experience remote contact from the service (Fig. 2). Of the types of contact offered, face-to-face was the preferred type of appointment for staff, patients and parents/carers (Fig. 3). Preferences varied within groups and more patients put video calls as their first choice compared to staff and parents/carers.

Service satisfaction before and during COVID-19: a comparison

Patients satisfaction with service slightly increased during COVID-19, whilst parents/carers and staff's slightly decreased (Table 4). A Wilcoxon Signed-rank test indicated that there was no significant difference between service satisfaction before COVID-19 (Mdn = 4) and during COVID-19 (Mdn = 4), T = 26, $p = .14$, r = .43.

Qualitative

Table 5 summarises the key changes described by staff, patients and parent/carers.

Positive experiences

Continuing to provide a fantastic service

Parents and patients reported that they appreciated having a responsive, supportive multidisciplinary team that remained available. Those that received face-to-face appointments were grateful that these remained available, despite lockdown pressures. Feedback from parents stated that the service maintained integrity despite the challenges. Staff were, however, less likely to comment on and acknowledge their successes.

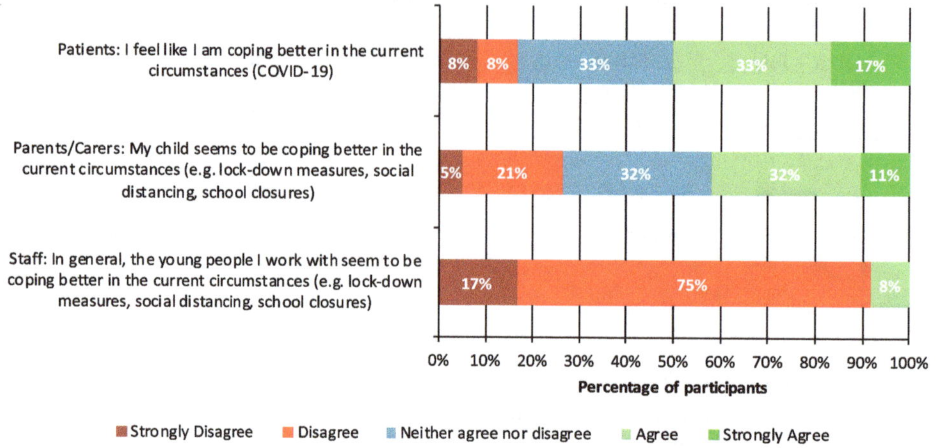

Fig. 1 Percentage of agreement (strongly disagree [1] to strongly agree [5]) for patients, parents/carers and staff on how young people with eating disorders are coping in COVID-19

Improving access

Using virtual platforms improved ease of access. Staff reported working with more autonomy, and offering more contact as they were not constrained by room availability on the hospital site. Staff felt more able to increase the number of contacts they had within the day as they had more flexibility and a variety of mediums to choose from. Patients reported enjoying using emails to contact staff, as they felt confident they received the message, and received a prompt reply. Staff reported that that their knowledge of online support available improved. Some parents reported finding it easier to meet their child's emotional needs while they were at home together. Staff reported that virtual MDTs meant they could join from anywhere and have more space in the room. Staff also described a benefit of video sessions being that they could share online resources easily.

Increasing comfort

Patients and family members reported that having a mixture of video and telephone contact reduced travel costs and left them feeling less drained. Patients commented that they also felt less tension and "build up" attending appointments. Some staff felt that having contact within their home improved relationships as people seemed to open up more within a comfortable home environment. Although some patients found it easier to open up when they were not face to face, the majority described the opposite. Patients reported

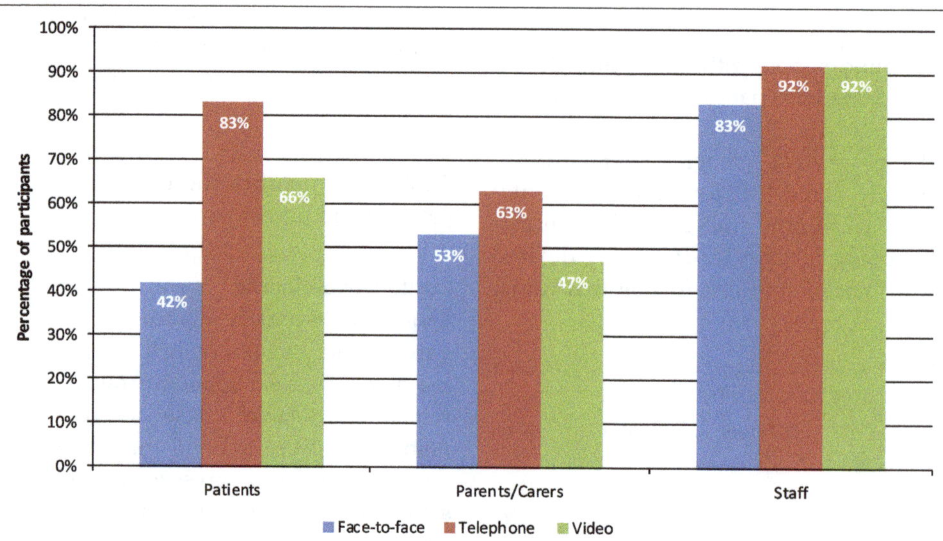

Fig. 2 Types of appointments experienced during COVID-19: self-reported by patients, parents/carers and staff

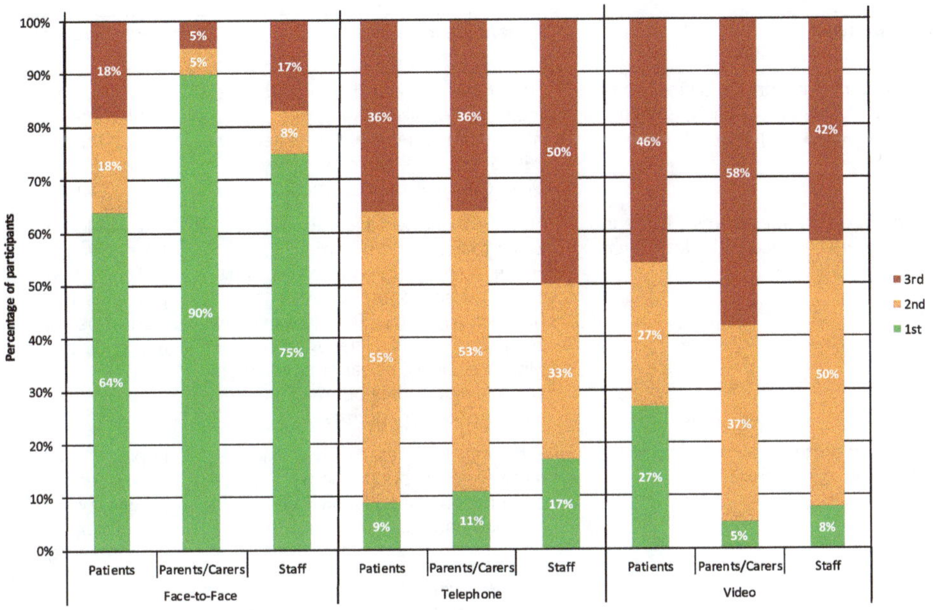

Fig. 3 Patient, parent/carer and staff ratings (1st, 2nd or 3rd) of types of appointment based on preference

enjoying a break from the pressures of "normal" life, e.g., visiting restaurants.

Negative experiences

Increased isolation and fragmentation

Family members were less likely to attend appointments with the young person which all participants reported as a major issue with lockdown restrictions. FBT did not lend itself to virtual or telephone therapy as it was hard to include everybody in the process. Endings felt more abrupt, incomplete and individuals were left feeling more anxious about relapse. Staff also reported reduced capacity to monitor physical health in the community as other sites were not in full operation. At the beginning, there was only one practitioner on site which practitioners found very "lonely". Practitioners said they found it harder to make decisions about risk, or care plans, when there was nobody else on site. Staff that remained working from home described being left with "strong feelings" at the end of a difficult day, which could leave them feeling stressed in a place they could usually relax.

Altered relational experiences

The restrictions changed the experience of relationships and contacts. Staff and patients reported finding it difficult to wear PPE and talk in face-to-face sessions. Patient reported preferring not to wear PPE, and finding the video sessions easier as they did not have to talk through a mask.

Using technology impacted on the quality of experience within services. Staff, patients and parents/carers all preferred having some face-to-face contact. Patients found it frustrating if they experienced technological difficulties whilst sharing their feelings as it was difficult enough to "open up" and "share". Staff found it hard not having access to a printer to give out material for people to take away. Patients said that in some ways the video sessions felt "less real", and that they also felt under less

Table 4. Median Scores of patient, parent/carer and staff service satisfaction before COVID-19 and during COVID-19

Topic of Item	Patient		Parents & Carers		Staff		All participants	
	Before	During	Before	During	Before	During	Before	During
The help provided in general	4	4.5	5	5	4	4	5	4
Information provided about the service and help available	4	4.5	4.5	4	4	4	4	4
Accessibility of appointments/groups	5	4	4.5	4	4	3.5	4	4
Ease of contacting the team	4	4.5	4.5	4	4	4	4	4
Enough going on for the young person to get involved in	4	4	4.5	4	4	2.5	4	4
Total	4	4.5	4.5	4	4	4	4	4

Table 5 Summary of Key Changes

Changes Described	Staff experience	Patient's experience	Parent's/Carer's experience
Experiencing "lockdown" restrictions.	Having one clinician onsite- difficult to fit face to face contacts in. Lonely, isolating. Missed colleagues support.	Have more space and time to focus on recovery. Feel like missing out on less in general life. Relief avoiding restaurants. Less distractions, more time to think. More exposure to social media.	Fantastic team response, always available and responsive despite lockdown.
Moving to virtual video consultations.	Feels inappropriate for high risk. Those in good recovery engaged well. Not limited by room availability.	Travel avoided which can be tiring. Easier to access from home. Harder to open up on a screen. Can't see body language. Feels easier to hide how actually doing. Feels less genuine. Technological difficulties are a barrier. Miss face-to-face as easier to open up. Would enjoy choice but may choose easier option for anorexia.	Mix would be good to limit demands of travel. Difficult when IT and connection problems. Face-to-face needed to build trust in beginning. Affected discharge and ending – felt abrupt, left with high anxiety.
Having telephone appointments.	Feels inappropriate for high risk cases. Less effective. Raised staff anxieties.	Felt family were less involved and received less support. Shorter consultations. Need family to be involved and a bigger part of it.	Impractical. Family sessions don't involve family. Sessions much shorter. Feel left on own with anxieties. Feel more responsibility to communicate what is not visible e.g., child's response.
Using emails for contact.		Enjoyed being able to ensure messages got to practitioners and enjoyed quick response.	
Being restricted to one parent in the session.	Asking one parent to relay information to another parent not effective. Need whole family for family treatment.	Wished parents had more support. Parents need family sessions for themselves and to help recovery. Parents essential to recovery.	
Accessing/ Offering support from home environment.	Difficult. Much rather be on site. Isolating. Can be left with strong feelings on own, at home. Very hard managing childcare at the same time. Miss travel to switch off.	More comfortable. Easier to leave if want to. Less afraid of practitioners and consequences of not adhering to meal plan. Feel intimidated to ask for something else as feels like how the service is provided is not within the services control.	Able to give more support to child, more supervision. Better meet their needs. Feels more intense in lockdown. No respite. Harder if can't get food in shops. More to deal with.
Virtual MDTs.	Good to have more space on own, not limited by room size. Easier to access and attend. IT issues make more challenges. Not seeing people's faces hard to pick up cues. Affects feeling of team working. Easily distracted by laptops.		

pressure from services if they were not being seen. Patients reported feeling like they could easily get out of the situation if they wanted to by hanging up. This was positive in some ways, but others reported that they needed a "check in" and "eyes on" to resist the demands of anorexia. Some patients described feeling like they needed to be "uncomfortable to get comfortable again." Whilst patients may have opted *not* to come in if they had a choice, they acknowledged that it was necessary to experience the feelings they did in sessions to make a full recovery.

Families and patients reported that telephone consultations were more likely to be shorter. All participants felt telephone sessions were least effective. Staff commented that having face-to-face sessions was vital at the beginning of a patient's journey, when individuals needed more intensive input. Patients described struggling to open up with people they first met online, as it was hard to trust someone without meeting them. Patients and parents described feeling like it was not always clear if they were allowed face-to-face contact, or not. Patients said they would avoid asking for something different to what was offered as they did not want to put pressure on the NHS.

Some staff found that working virtually affected their role and made the work less satisfying. Others reported that it affected team support and morale. For a new member joining the team, it was a harder experience being inducted and understanding processes. Virtual MDTs could go on for longer as it was harder to read the cues of attendees and know when to stop. Virtual MDTs were described as being more task orientated, although staff commented this was likely impacted by increased service pressures too.

Increased acuity and more pressure

Parents reported finding it more intense offering support to their child whilst working from home, and without the support from school. Staff were generally much more likely to comment on the increased pressure on the service. Staff reported having more presenting risk in the cases that were referred during lockdown. They also report missing the travel time to "switch off" and have a break from work. Many staff reported working longer hours from home and over working. Staff talked about increased pressure managing their home life during a pandemic, in particular, having to care for their own children from home whilst providing a clinical service. One staff member reported that the childcare provision during the pandemic did not align with the hours of service provision.

Patients felt it was unfair that "pubs could open" but mental health services were not prioritised. Patients and their parents described struggling with a lack of routine and structure. Patients also said they found they were more likely to spend time on their phones and be exposed to social media which hindered their recovery.

Discussion

This is the first mixed methods study exploring how patients, families and staff are experiencing the new ways of working driven by COVID-19 in a young person's eating disorder service. Although there was no difference in service satisfaction before COVID-19 and during COVID-19, face-to-face was the preferred type of appointment for patients, parents/carers and staff.

In our focus groups, we observed a marked difference in the views of staff, parents and patients. Staff and parents have different insights into a child's experience of treatment in an eating disorder service. Staff are more likely to have experienced the service prior to lockdown and may be judging and evaluating the service based on how it has run before. Parents may be experiencing the service for the first time and are likely grateful for the support from any service during lockdown as many healthcare providers stopped offering treatments. It is also likely that the parents that took part in the focus group were more likely to be engaging well with the service, and virtual treatments, as they provided feedback through virtual platforms. However, staff saw a broader spectrum of presentations, and were able to comment on the challenges they faced with engagement in treatment and risks that were difficult to manage. Staff also faced different challenges in running a service, which children and families were unaware of. It could be that this stress and pressure influenced evaluations of the service.

Despite inviting all patients open to the service and their parents/carers, the small sample size is an important limitation of the study that must be noted. As the study intended to capture the impact of a global pandemic lockdown period on experiences within an eating disorder service, a change in government restrictions meant we were unable to extend the recruitment window. As restrictions lifted, changes to service provision were reversed and face-to-face appointments were no longer limited to high-risk patients. Given the small sample size, the conclusions of this paper should be treated with caution and further research should be conducted to validate the findings. Future research should be broken down into diagnostic groups (e.g. AN, BN and BED) so that differences can be reported and discussed. This is another limitation of the current study, but as diagnostic labels are not always used in treatment at this service, it was felt it would have been inappropriate to ask patients and parents/carers this as part of the survey. As the caseload of patients registered with EDYS is relatively small, it is common for there to be only one patient of a certain age or gender at one point in time. Therefore, collecting basic demographics could have violated ethical approval, as clinicians analysing the data may have been able to identify which patient had submitted the response. However, including this information would add value to future research. We also recognise there is likely to be a self-selection bias with regards to the sample, as those who are in the later stages of treatment are more likely to have the time and motivation to respond. However, staff will be seeing patients at all stages of their recovery and their answers reflect this. This may explain the disparity between staff, parent's and patient's perceptions of how young people are coping in lockdown. The key changes to service provision were centred on the restriction measures implemented by the government and the use of virtual services to provide treatment. Below we will outline the key themes identified before making clinical recommendations to guide service delivery.

Locking down but ramping up

Despite being forced to minimise direct patient contact, the service saw an increase in inpatient admissions and referrals, during and following lockdown. This implies that the pandemic is not only having a negative impact on those who already have an eating disorder as suggested by Branley-Bell and Talbot [2], but is also increasing the likelihood of young people developing an ED. Patients reported having less distractions and more exposure to social media was a negative consequence of the lockdown restrictions on recovery; which is commensurate with other recent research [2, 6]. Parents/carers expressed concerns about obtaining food from the shops and described the experience of caring for a child with an eating disorder as more intense. All participants described a frustration with the government guidelines. In particular, patients felt it was unfair that "pubs could open" but mental health services widely could not. Despite limitations, there was a considerable increase in the number of appointments offered by EDYS during lockdown in comparison to the previous months. Staff reported that they had more flexibility to offer appointments with the new ways of working, but also reported overworking and finding it harder to manage risk. Staff commented on the difficulties of limiting service provision, whilst dealing with more acute presentations. At a time of increased need, and more presenting risk, service delivery was compromised.

The Silver lining

Online/virtual treatments were recommended to reduce the risk of viral transmission [6] and as a result, EDYS had to quickly adopt remote consultations. Only 42% of patients that took the survey had experienced face-to-face appointments. Despite most individuals favouring face-to-face contact, having the flexibility to use different mediums improves ease and access. Appointments would no longer be limited by room availability or parent/carer availability. Attending appointments from home can also reduce treatment burden through reducing travel and limiting the associated costs (e.g. public transport fares, petrol, and parking). Furthermore, using emails would not previously have been part of practice, but was greatly valued by patients. Staff reported an improved knowledge of online support available for the young people they were seeing, which may continue to benefit current and future patients. Service satisfaction did not change during COVID-19 despite the significant changes to service provision.

Timing is everything

Given the evidence for intensive interventions at the early stages of an ED [5, 8], it is unsurprising that all participants felt face-to-face contact was crucial at the beginning of treatment. Staff felt that virtual appointments were inappropriate for high risk patients given the difficulty of adequately assessing physical and mental health risks remotely [12]. In line with this, patients felt they needed the face-to-face contact to resist the demands of their ED. At the right time, virtual appointments can be effective and act as a step down. ED services must carefully assess when it is appropriate to start using virtual interventions for their patients, on a case to case basis. Introducing virtual methods when they are deemed as effective can also increase availability of rooms for the cases where face-to-face contact is vital. It should also be considered, that the absence of face-to-face appointments before discharge, left parents feeling like endings were abrupt, leaving them with more anxieties about the cease in support. Careful consideration of the implementation of virtual methods will maximise the chance of them providing a positive addition.

Learning from the losses

A lack of time to prepare, made changes to services more challenging. In this sample, patients and their carers felt there was a lack of support for whole families during restrictions. Given that FBT is advocated as the evidence-based intervention for child and adolescent eating disorders [15], it is important that services ensure that the family are not forgotten. As it was generally felt that FBT was less effective virtually, careful planning must go into how services can involve and support families moving forward. Despite lockdown measures easing, staff reported still being restricted to one parent per session. A balance of risks should be considered as families are within the same "bubble" and pose limited additional risk, whereas the reduction in treatment effectiveness could be life threatening. Future research must aim to understand how best to adapt treatments, such as FBT, for virtual delivery to ensure that it is safe and effective [10].

Over time, access to technology has improved but many individuals still struggle to navigate this without guidance. All participants reported issues with connectivity, which had a negative impact on engagement in sessions. As virtual interventions are also only accessible to patients and families who have the relevant devices, there is a risk of services becoming less inclusive. Being aware of the barriers to accessing services virtually and at home is of paramount importance.

Restrictions also involved limiting the number of clinicians allowed onsite, leaving staff feeling lonely and isolated, which has also been found in other studies [4, 14]. Staff reported missing the support of their colleagues and were left with strong feelings to manage alone; whether that be in the hospital or at home. Staff found it harder to make decisions about risk or care plans when there was nobody present to discuss this with. This must be considered alongside other challenges of working remotely, such as the ability to switch off and stay well. While the service kept running and remained effective, we must wonder at what cost? Staff were less likely to comment on their successes and described working extra hours, whilst struggling to manage caring commitments at home. The negative psychological effects of the pandemic include higher rates of burnout, PTSD, anxiety and depression in NHS staff [9]. It is now even more important to look after the health and wellbeing of NHS Staff, as called for in the NHS People Plan (2020–2021).

Conclusions

The Covid-19 global pandemic and the associated lockdown restrictions increased the pressure on a young person's specialist eating disorder service in the UK. The service saw more acute presentations in those referred and more referrals following the lockdown. The elevated levels of risk felt harder to manage with restrictions to service provision. Despite the significant changes to service delivery, an eating disorder service that children and parents report high satisfaction with can still be offered during lockdown restrictions. Email contact with practitioners improved responsiveness and was perceived as a positive change. Virtual and telephone appointments increased flexibility within the service and improved autonomy for practitioners. However, the quality of the relational experience is altered online and through virtual mediums. In the context of appointment types, patient choice must be carefully considered, as individuals may want to resist pressure and providing face-to-face appointments is necessary in the treatment of acute anorexia. Including parents/carers in treatment plans is essential and appointments with multiple people in a room need to be prioritised for family-based treatments. A mixture of appointment types is likely to be the most effective in the treatment of eating disorders in young people. Those providing services may face new and intense pressures, putting practitioners at an increased risk of burnout. Multiple practitioners on site are required to support decision making about risk and to share ideas to deliver MDT working. Supporting NHS staff is a vital part of continuing to deliver high quality NHS services.

Abbreviations

ED: Eating Disorders; EDYS: Eating Disorder Young Person's Service; FBT: Family-based Therapy; ESQ: Experience of Service Questionnaire; CAMH S: Child and Adolescent Mental Health Service

Acknowledgements

Not applicable.

Authors' contributions

All authors were involved in conceiving the presented idea and designing the project. H.S. developed the online survey's with support from N.R. and S.R. Focus groups were carried out by H.S. and S.R., then transcribed by S.R. Qualitative data was analysed and written up by S.R. and quantitative data by H.S. H.S. wrote the manuscript with support from N. R and S.R. All authors provided critical feedback throughout and helped shape the research, analysis and manuscript. The author(s) read and approved the final manuscript.

Competing interests

The authors declare that they have no competing interests.

Author details

[1]The Eating Disorder Young Person's Service, Alder Hey Children's Hospital Foundation Trust, Liverpool, UK. [2]Royal Holloway University of London, Egham, UK. [3]Vilnius University, Vilnius, Lithuania.

References

1. Anastasiadou D, Folkvord F, Lupiañez-Villanueva F. A systematic review of mHealth interventions for the support of eating disorders. Eur Eat Disord Rev. 2018;26(5):394–416.
2. Branley-Bell D, Talbot CV. Exploring the impact of the COVID-19 pandemic and UK lockdown on individuals with experience of eating disorders. J Eat Disord. 2020. [Preprint].
3. Braun V, Clarke V. Using thematic analysis in psychology. Qual Res Psychol. 2006;3(2):77–101.
4. Brooks SK, Webster RK, Smith LE, Woodland L, Wessely S, Greenberg N, Rubin GJ. The psychological impact of quarantine and how to reduce it: rapid review of the evidence. Lancet. 2020;28(10227):912–20.
5. Currin L, Schmidt U. A critical analysis of the utility of an early intervention approach in the eating disorders. J Ment Health. 2005;14(6):611–24.
6. Fernández-Aranda F, Casas M, Claes L, Bryan DC, Favaro A, Granero R, Gudiol C, Jiménez-Murcia S, Karwautz A, Le Grange D, Menchón JM. COVID-19 and implications for eating disorders. Eur Eat Disord Rev. 2020;28(3):239.
7. Fiorillo A, Gorwood P. The consequences of the COVID-19 pandemic on mental health and implications for clinical practice. Eur Psychiatry. 2020; 63(1):E32. https://doi.org/10.1192/j.eurpsy.2020.35.
8. Fukutomi A, Austin A, McClelland J, Brown A, Glennon D, Mountford V, Grant N, Allen K, Schmidt U. First episode rapid early intervention for eating disorders: a two-year follow-up. Early Intervention in Psychiatry. 2020;14(1): 137–41.
9. Greenberg N, Docherty M, Gnanapragasam S, Wessely S. Managing mental health challenges faced by healthcare workers during covid-19 pandemic. BMJ. 2020;368. https://doi.org/10.1136/bmj.m1211.
10. Hambleton A, Le Grange D, Miskovic-Wheatley J, Touyz S, Cunich M, Maguire S. Translating evidence-based treatment for digital health delivery: a protocol for family-based treatment for anorexia nervosa using telemedicine. J Eat Disord. 2020;8(1):1–2.
11. Holmes EA, O'Connor RC, Perry VH, Tracey I, Wessely S, Arseneault L, Ballard C, Christensen H, Silver RC, Everall I, Ford T. Multidisciplinary research priorities for the COVID-19 pandemic: a call for action for mental health science. Lancet Psychiatry. 2020;7(6):547–60.
12. Keshen A, Helson T, Ali S, Dixon L, Tregarthen J, Town J. Efficacy and acceptability of self-monitoring via a smartphone application versus traditional paper records in an intensive outpatient eating disorder treatment setting. Eur Eat Disord Rev. 2020;28(4):473–9.
13. Kierans C. Narrating kidney disease: the significance of sensation and time in the emplotment of patient experience. Cult Med Psychiatry. 2005;29(3): 341–59.
14. Lai J, Ma S, Wang Y, Cai Z, Hu J, Wei N, Wu J, Du H, Chen T, Li R, Tan H. Factors associated with mental health outcomes among health care workers exposed to coronavirus disease 2019. JAMA Network Open. 2020; 3(3):e203976-.
15. Lock J, Le Grange D. Family-based treatment: where are we and where should we be going to improve recovery in child and adolescent eating disorders. Int J Eat Disord. 2019;52(4):481–7.
16. Lapum J, Angus JE, Peter E, Watt-Watson J. Patients' narrative accounts of open-heart surgery and recovery: authorial voice of technology. Soc Sci Med. 2010;70(5):754–62.
17. Marks DF, Yardley L, editors. Research methods for clinical and health psychology. UK: SAGE Publications; 2004.
18. Pierce M, Hope H, Ford T, Hatch S, Hotopf M, John A, Kontopantelis E, Webb R, Wessely S, McManus S, Abel KM. Mental health before and during the COVID-19 pandemic: a longitudinal probability sample survey of the UK population. Lancet Psychiatry. 2020;7(10):883–92.
19. Wengraf T. Interviewing for life-histories, lived situations and ongoing personal experiencing using the Biographic-Narrative Interpretive Method (BNIM): The BNIM Short Guide bound with The BNIM Detailed Manual; 2011.
20. Yao H, Chen JH, Xu YF. Rethinking online mental health services in China during the COVID-19 epidemic. Asian J Psychiatr. 2020;50:102015.
21. Zhu Y, Chen L, Ji H, Xi M, Fang Y, Li Y. The risk and prevention of novel coronavirus pneumonia infections among inpatients in psychiatric hospitals. Neurosci Bull. 2020;25:1–4.

10

Physiological, emotional and neural responses to visual stimuli in eating disorders

Victoria Burmester*, Esme Graham and Dasha Nicholls

Abstract

Background: Overconcern with food and shape/weight stimuli are central to eating disorder maintenance with attentional biases seen towards these images not present in healthy controls. These stimuli trigger changes in the physiological, emotional, and neural responses in people with eating disorders, and are regularly used in research and clinical practice. However, selection of stimuli for these treatments is frequently based on self-reported emotional ratings alone, and whether self-reports reflect objective responses is unknown.

Main body: This review assessed the associations across emotional self-report, physiological, and neural responses to both food and body-shape/weight stimuli in people with anorexia nervosa (AN), bulimia nervosa (BN) and binge eating disorder (BED). For food stimuli, either an aversive or lack of physiological effect was generated in people with AN, together with a negative emotional response on neuroimaging, and high subjective anxiety ratings. People with BN showed a positive self-rating, an aversive physiological reaction, and a motivational neural response. In BED, an aversive physiological reaction was found in contrast to motivational/appetitive neural responses, with food images rated as pleasant. The results for shape/weight stimuli showed aversive responses in some physiological modalities, which was reflected in both the emotional and neural responses, but this aversive response was not consistent across physiological studies.

Conclusions: Shape/weight stimuli are more reliable for use in therapy or research than food stimuli as the impact of these images is more consistent across subjective and objective responses. Care should be taken when using food stimuli due to the disconnect reported in this review.

Keywords: Emotional, Physiological, Neuroimaging, Anorexia nervosa, Bulimia nervosa, Binge eating disorder, Shape/weight, Food, Visual stimuli, Images

Plain English summary

Images of food and body shape are extremely salient to people with eating disorders (ED). These images cause changes to occur in physiological measures, such as heart rate, and in neural function, as seen on brain scans. Because such images are used in clinical practice, it is important that they induce reliable physiological and neural responses. However, images used in treatment are usually selected based on patients' subjective emotional ratings or by clinicians using variable criteria. It is important to know how well patients' subjective ratings correlate with physiological and neural measures.

This review looks at the responses of people across ED diagnoses (anorexia nervosa, bulimia nervosa and binge-eating disorder) and compares subjective ratings, physiological and neural responses to food and body shape images. For food stimuli, emotional responses were mixed, but overall emotional ratings for these images did not

* Correspondence: v.burmester@imperial.ac.uk
Division of Psychiatry, Department of Brain Sciences, Imperial College London, Du Cane Road, London W12 0NN, UK

reflect the changes that were seen physiologically or in neuroimaging. Images of body shapes resulted in participants providing negative emotional ratings, with physiological and neural measures also reflecting negative emotion.

This suggests that body shape images are potentially more useful in clinical practice and research than food images, as emotional ratings better represent the changes seen both in brain scans and physiological tests.

Background

Eating disorders (ED) are defined by negative thoughts and behaviours towards eating, body-shape and weight, leading to disturbance of eating behaviour. The main ED diagnoses are anorexia nervosa (AN), bulimia nervosa (BN) and binge eating disorder (BED) [1, 2]. The transdiagnostic model of ED suggests that overconcern with shape, weight and food is central to maintenance of all ED and that clinical features are maintained by common underlying psychopathology, including food, weight, and shape overconcern [3].

The impact of overconcern is manifest as attentional bias. Beck and Clark's information-processing model reveals the importance of attentional biases for information that is seen as threatening to the individual; this is thought to be the basis of anxiety [4]. Such attentional bias has been shown to be present in those with ED [5], effects that differ in healthy controls, reinforcing the role of salient visual stimuli in ED psychopathology. Looking at attentional bias to a range of stimuli is key to understanding the effects of visual stimuli on those with ED pathology and its translation into physiological, emotional, and neural responses. Understanding these responses can help inform clinical practice involving imagery, such as cognitive behavioural therapy (CBT) and virtual reality (VR) based treatments [6, 7].

Attentional bias has been measured using a range of different tasks. The Stroop Colour and Word Test (Stroop) requires participants to read a list of colours printed in incongruent coloured ink, such that the word "red", might be coloured blue, and subsequent delay in colour-naming constitutes attentional bias [8]. Performance on the Stroop by women with ED showed they were slower to name colour words related to food and body image than healthy controls [9, 10]. This was replicated for food words in those with AN and BN, who were slower naming food than neutral words and slower than the control group [11]. These early findings have been extended using the dot probe, which involves participants looking at two images or words on a screen and responding as quickly as possible to a probe that appears in place of one; the response time indicates potential bias [12]. Rieger et al. found a bias towards words connoting a large physique and away from those representing a small physique in those with ED [13]. For eating, weight, and shape images, patients with ED were quicker to respond to the probe when it appeared in the same location as negative eating and neutral weight stimuli, indicating an attentional bias is present to these stimuli [5]. No effect, though, was found for shape stimuli [5]. However, in those with AN, attentional bias towards shape stimuli is found when an image is shown of the participant's own body but did not produce attentional bias in participants with BN, suggesting attentional biases differ among ED diagnoses [14]. The spatial cueing task is similar to the dot probe; a cue picture is presented on one side of a fixation cross; a dot then appears on the same or opposite side of the picture that the participant must respond to [15]. Participants with BED preferentially identified food words in a clarification task [16] faster than weight-matched controls, and also demonstrated attentional bias to food stimuli via a stimulus engagement effect [17]. This bias was heightened when viewed in the context of real-world stimuli, with BED participants focusing gaze on food items significantly more than controls [18].

The strong attentional bias demonstrated by these studies emphasises the importance of visual stimuli for those with ED pathology and reinforces its current use in therapeutic practice. However, as highlighted by Giel et al.'s review of responses to pictorial food stimuli in those with ED, there is not always consistency for food stimuli in the responses seen and there is often a disconnect between subjective and objective responses [19]. The present review builds on the previous findings of Giel et al. by including new papers looking at food stimuli and additionally assesses responses to body shape stimuli that have been shown to be important in those with ED, to provide further clarity on relationships that exist across these measures of emotion.

Emotions involve a range of processes including affective, cognitive, and physiological responses, so these different aspects should be considered together [20]. The processing of emotions alters physiological states via the autonomic nervous system, with activity in the anterior cingulate and amygdala associated with generating a physiological response to emotions [21]. This has been demonstrated in healthy individuals whose self-reported valence and arousal measures correlated with physiological measures [22, 23] and is relevant to ED populations that have high levels of alexithymia [24]. Subjective ratings of images are frequently used to guide therapeutic practice and as salient stimuli for research studies, so understanding relationships among subjective emotional ratings and their objective physiological and neural response correlates is important for both therapeutic and research endeavours.

Scope and inclusion criteria

This narrative review compares emotional responses to images of food and of weight/shape among subjects with ED in comparison with healthy controls, measured by subjective ratings, physiological arousal, and neural responses. The aim was to summarise the findings; provide clarification on outcomes; examine associations across emotional, physiological, and neuroimaging responses to ED-relevant stimuli; assess which stimuli result in the greatest responses in people with ED and explore the implications for treatment. Studies looking at participants diagnosed with or reporting symptomology of AN, BN, BED, and atypical variants previously diagnosed as "eating disorder not specified", now termed "other specified feeding and eating disorders" were included [25]. Studies looking at participants with ED symptomology were included, but studies looking at participants with avoidant restrictive food-intake disorder were excluded. All ages, genders and ethnicities were included.

Emotional ratings for stimuli are gained by self-report through all studies used. Studies of peripheral autonomic physiological responses were included but research examining hormonal changes or changes in salivation was not. Physiological response is examined through changes in the startle-blink reflex, facial-electromyographic activity (EMG), skin conductance response (SCR), heart rate (HR) and posturographic destabilisation. Neural imaging data were gained by examining functional magnetic resonance imaging (*f*MRI) whilst participants viewed salient images. Only studies using *f*MRI were used to assess neural responses as this form of imaging is able to demonstrate reward activation, unlike event related potentials that only show cortical activation. Additionally, a lack of studies using alternative imaging forms was found.

Studies were found by using the databases Pubmed and Google Scholar. The search terms used for finding papers were: eating disorder, anorexia nervosa, bulimia nervosa, binge eating disorder, physiological, emotional, neurological, or neural, visual stimuli, food images or stimuli, body image or stimuli, shape image or stimuli, weight image or stimuli.

Twenty-nine papers were included in the review and these are considered in two sections: food (Table 1) and body/weight images (Table 2).

Food stimuli

Physiological responses

Startle-blink and postauricular reflexes The startle-blink response increases when viewing threatening and unpleasant images and decreases while viewing pleasant images or exposed to appetitive cues [28, 41, 42]. The startle-blink reflex is also thought to infer a motivational state, with rodent studies showing a decreased startle blink to food and water [43]. In healthy controls, food images usually have appetitive properties and so should result in a reduced startle-blink reflex due to a motivational and pleasant response [28]; it was thought the opposite effect would be seen in those with ED.

In people with AN, food images produced similar startle-blink responses to those of positive and negative images, and were significantly different from neutral images, indicating that food images affected individuals with AN [26]. Food images also received arousal ratings similar to those of negative images [26], suggesting an association between physiological and emotional ratings to food images in those with AN, with a negative affect being seen. By contrast, a separate study, found that the startle-blink reflex to food images in people with AN was not significantly different from neutral cues or from those of healthy controls [27]. Food images were self-rated as highly anxiety provoking, demonstrating a disconnect between emotional and physiological responses in AN groups [27].

Mauler et al. looked at the startle-blink reflex in women with BN and healthy controls using positive, negative, neutral, and food images [28]. In those with BN, the startle-blink reflex for food images was significantly greater than for healthy controls. A potentiated startle-blink reflex for food images was also seen when compared to positive and neutral images within the BN group, suggesting that food images prompted negative affect in those with BN; this conflicted with verbal ratings of food images as pleasant and interesting in this group. However, when compared to the control group, those with BN rated food images as more disgusting and fearful, indicating that an association with physiological responses may be present [28]. Interestingly, when the startle-blink reflex was examined in a group with BN, no significant startle-blink response was seen [27]. Although, when subgroup analysis was performed for those with BN who were medication-free, a significantly reduced startle-blink reflex to food images versus neutral images was seen [27], indicating that food images may have evoked the appetitive motivational response; however, negative self-rated emotional responses to the same stimuli undermine this argument [27]. Additionally, the reduced startle-blink reflex suggests that selective serotonin reuptake inhibitors (SSRI) attenuate the startle blink response.

This difference in emotional ratings was also observed in those exhibiting binge or restrictive eating patterns: those with binge eating behaviours rated food images as more pleasant than those with restrictive behaviours [29]. Participants with binge-eating behaviours exhibited a larger startle-blink reflex for food images than both control and restrained eaters, indicating a greater

Table 1 Summary of physiological responses to food stimuli

	Participants	Image type	Physiological outcome	Result of food stimuli
Racine et al. 2016 [26]	• 19 AN females	• Positive images • Negative images • Neutral images • Food images	• Startle blink response	• Potentiated startle response > neutral
Friederich et al. 2006 [27]	• 15 AN female • 15 BN female • 30 HC female	• Food images • Body images • Positive images • Neutral images • Aversive images	• Startle blink response	• BN startle inhibition > neutral • No significantly different response in AN
Mauler et al. 2006 [28]	• 32 BN women • 32 HC women	• Unpleasant images • Neutral images • Pleasant images • Food images	• Startle blink response • Corrugator EMG • HR • SCR	• BN potentiated startle > control • BN increased corrugator activity > HC
Drobes et al. 2001 [29]	• 23 controls • 13 with restrained eating • 19 with binge behaviours • 21 food deprived subjects	• Unpleasant images • Pleasant images • Food images • Neutral images	• Startle blink response • HR • SCR	• Binge group potentiated startle response • Binge group greater startle response > control • Elevated HR for both binge and restrained
Suissa Rocheleau et al. 2019 [30]	• 18 controls • 19 with binge eating symptoms • 19 with dietary restriction symptoms • 23 with restriction and binge eating symptoms	• Food images • Pleasant images • Aversive images • Neutral images	• Startle blink response	• Higher self-reported craving correlated with a larger startle reflex • Binge and restrictive behaviours caused decreased startle reflex to food cues
Soussignan et al. 2009 [31]	• 16 AN females • 25 HC females	• Food images	• Facial EMG • SCR • HR	• AN decreased zygomatic activity
Racine et al. 2017 [32]	• 67 male and female participants who completed the eating disorder examination questionnaire	• Food images • Neutral images • Aversive images • Pleasant images	• Startle probe • Post auricular reflex • Facial EMG	• High eating disorder cognitions had increased corrugator activation > neutral • Increased post auricular reflex in those with binge eating behaviours > those without
Overduin et al. 1997 [33]	• 11 female restrained eaters • 13 female controls	• Neutral images • Food images • Body images	• SCR • HR • Startle reflex • Facial EMG	• Decreased corrugator activity in restrained > unrestrained eaters for food images • No other group differences seen
Leehr et al. 2016 [34]	• 16 Overweight women with BED • 23 Overweight women without BED • 22 Healthy controls	• High calorie food images • Non-food images	• Facial EMG	• Increased corrugator activator for all groups > non food
Svaldi et al. 2010 [35]	• 22 females with BED • 22 female controls with BMI over 25	• Food images	• HR and SCR	• Decreased HR and SCR > non-food in those with BED

negative affect and aversive emotional reaction [29]. Similar responses were seen in those with BN [28], which is expected, given the overlap in diagnostic features. The conflict between self-rated emotional and physiological responses may be explained by the use of a non-clinical sample [29]. Subjects in this study were healthy volunteers with no prior ED diagnosis who were chosen according to their scores on the eating disorders

Table 2 Summary of physiological responses to body stimuli

	Participants	Stimuli	Physiological outcome	Result of body shape stimuli
Oretga-Roldan et al. 2014 [36]	• 30 females with BN • 30 HC	• Image of own body • Startle noise	• Startle reflex • ECG • SCR	• Increased skin conductance response in BN > HC • Decreased startle reflex in those with BN > HC
Friederich et al. 2006 [27]	• 15 AN female • 15 BN female • 30 HC	• Food images • Body images • Positive images • Neutral images • Aversive images	• Startle blink response	• No startle reflex potentiation of body > neutral in either BN or AN
Herbert et al. 2013 [37]	• 35 healthy females screened for ED risk	• Body words • Neutral words	• Startle blink response • HR	• No difference in startle modulation between body and neutral words • HR differed significantly between body and neutral words • Correlation between women with high body dissatisfaction and increased startle response to body > neutral words
Spresser et al. 2012 [38]	• 53 females who took the eating disorder inventory	• Picture of participants own face altered to different levels of weight gain	• Startle blink response	• Startle responses to self-image predicted more variance in drive for thinness and body dissatisfaction scores
Vocks et al. 2007 [39]	• 28 female HC • 7 females with BN • 5 females with AN • 9 females with EDNOS	• Viewing own body image in a mirror	• HR • SCR	• Increase in SCR when viewing own body image in both HC and ED group
Overduin et al. 1997 [33]	• 11 female restrained eaters • 13 female controls	• Neutral images • Food images • Image of own Body	• SCR • HR • Startle reflex • Facial EMG	• No difference in EMG or startle reflex for body shape image • Increased SCR recovery time to body shape seen in both restrained and unrestrained eaters • Increased heart rate acceleration to body image in both restrained and unrestrained eaters
Forghieri et al. 2016 [40]	• 18 female HC • 10 females with AN • 3 females with BN • 4 females with EDNOS	• Neutral image • Looking at a mirror • Image of participants thin ideal body image	• Static posturography	• Increased body sway in ED group > HC when viewing own body image and ideal body image • Increased body sway for own body image and ideal > neutral image

inventory (EDI) and split into restrained and binge eaters. Given that these individuals do not have formal ED diagnoses and only show patterns of restraint and binging behaviour, results cannot be applied to a clinical population [29]. Nonetheless, these findings suggest that responses in healthy populations with ED behaviours are similar to those with an ED diagnosis.

In another non-clinical sample of women reporting dietary restraint and binge-eating symptoms, food images resulted in a decreased startle-blink reflex, suggesting a more appetitive than aversive physiological response [30]. This reduced startle-blink reflex correlated with a greater self-reported craving, supporting the appetitive response theory [27]. In contrast to the startle-blink reactions, the postauricular reflex is a muscular reaction that occurs behind the ear and is elicited by a pleasant, startling stimulus [44]. Similarly, the postauricular reflex was found to be significantly larger to food images relative to neutral images in a non-clinical cohort with binge eating, suggesting that food was experienced as positive by those who binge eat [32]. No correlations, however, were seen between the startle-blink reflex and valence or arousal ratings for images [30], meaning a difference may exist between "liking" and "wanting" responses to food images. "Wanting" and "liking" are distinct neural processes: wanting is the process of incentive salience attributed towards a reward, whereas liking is an affective state arising from pleasure and no motivation for reward is required to induce it [45].

In summary, startle-blink reflex research presents a very mixed result with both potentiated and decreased startle-blink responses seen to food images, so provides little clarity on the responses generated to these images. However, the physiological response generated, frequently opposed the self-rated responses to these images indicating a decoupling between these responses.

Facial-electromyographic activity Facial electromyographic activity (EMG) allows direct examination of facial responses to images by measuring muscle change and so is a physiological marker of emotional valence [33]. Increased corrugator activity is seen in response to frowning whereas zygomatic activity is seen with smiling [28, 33].

Individuals with AN had less zygomatic muscle activity when viewing food images than healthy controls, indicating reduced smile activity to these images [31]. Food pictures were rated as less pleasant by this group, so here a similarity between emotional and physiological response was seen [31].

In people with BN, viewing visual food cues resulted in significantly increased corrugator muscle use compared to pleasant images; this was not seen in controls [28]. A larger startle-blink reflex was also seen in this BN group, reinforcing the proposition that food images result in negative affect. These images were rated as pleasant; given that both physiological measures have the same aversive result, the lack of association between emotional and physiological responses is emphasised [28]. This increased corrugator activity to food images was also demonstrated in those with high eating-disorder cognitions compared to low on the eating disorder examination questionnaire, this was correlated with reduced pleasantness ratings of food within this group [32]. In restrained eaters both food and neutral images resulted in reduced corrugator activity, suggesting a pleasant response to these images, these images elicited emotional responses of arousal and craving in both restrained and unrestrained eaters [33]. However, as this study was only performed in those with restrained eating and not a diagnosed ED, the conclusions that can be made from this are limited.

People with BED, together with overweight and normal weight controls, rated food stimuli on wanting and liking scales adapted from Berridge [34]. Individuals with BED rated food higher on these scales than overweight individuals and heathy controls [34]. This is in contrast to the EMG data, where food stimuli evoked greater aversion for all groups, demonstrated by increased activation of the corrugator [34].

In summary, EMG data provide mixed physiological responses for food images, except for congruent negative responses in those with AN. For BN and BED, the picture is more complex, with food images inducing negative physiological responses in opposition to the self-rated pleasant scores.

Heart rate and skin conductance response The skin conductance response (SCR) is an indirect measure of sympathetic nervous system activity, with the size of the response seen related to the level of arousal [23]. Heart rate (HR) is also a measure of autonomic arousal, with a deceleration in HR often seen for affective stimuli [23]. SCR and HR have been found to increase when smoking addicts were presented with smoking-related cues, but only SCR was found to increase in those with alcohol addiction [33]. However, there is mixed evidence as to whether a fear/phobic response results in HR deceleration or acceleration [46], making it difficult to interpret the response from this measure. Heart rate variability (HRV) is thought to be an important measure of emotional regulatory ability, and differences in HRV correlate with the capacity to regulate emotional responses [47]. HRV has also been found to be an index of self-regulatory strength, which is important for adaptive behaviour, and increased HRV is typically seen as beneficial [48]. This illustrates the problem of using HR as a physiological measure of emotion, as studies frequently do not consider HRV and the impact this has on emotional regulation.

In people with BED, SCR and HR were lower when viewing high calorie as opposed to low calorie images, suggesting that food images may have had a potentially soothing effect, despite being viewed as forbidden [35]. In restrained eaters HR response to food images was greater than seen in controls with restrained eaters also rating these images as more pleasant [29]. SCR and HR in restrained eaters, binge eaters, controls, and food-deprived participants were greater for pleasant and unpleasant images than for neutral [29]. Increases in HR when viewing food images may have been due to elevated arousal given the pleasant nature of the images, suggesting that an association may exist between physiological and emotional response. Alternatively, increased HR may represent fear or anxiety, suggesting a dissociation between self-report and physiological measures, and highlighting another limitation of HR as a physiological measure. Conversely, no difference in HR was seen between restrained and unrestrained eaters to food or non-food images, despite different emotional ratings for these images [33]. These negative findings could potentially be explained by the use of a non-clinical population, but this lack of change was also seen between those with BN and healthy controls across food, pleasant, unpleasant, and neutral cues [28]. This lack of association could be attributed to the short viewing window for images, with changes after 12 s no longer being measured [33]. As changes in HR due to emotion are typically slower, longer measurement durations are needed to capture them, particularly if the individual has low HRV.

In summary, in those with BED, high-calorie food images may be soothing due to the decreased HR and SCR seen. The lack of response frequently demonstrated in people who exhibit restrained or binge-eating behaviours makes general conclusions difficult.

Neural response studies

When viewing food images, activation was seen in the anterior cingulate cortex (ACC), dorsolateral prefrontal cortex (DLPFC) and medial orbitofrontal cortex (OFC) in people with AN, but not in healthy controls [49–51] (Table 3). Activation of the DLPFC and ACC is

Table 3 Neural responses to food stimuli in people with AN

	AN Participants	HC participants	Stimuli	AN > HC	AN < HC
Uher et al. 2004 [50]	16	19	Colour pictures of food > non-food images Emotional aversive > neutral images	M.OFC, ACC	LI parietal, L occipital, posterior cerebellum
Brooks et al. 2011 [49]	18	24	Food > non-food images	DLPFC, cerebellum, R precuneus	Bilateral insula
Kim et al. 2012 [51]	18	20	High calorie food images > non-food images	L anterior insula, superior frontal gyrus, ACC, cerebellum	n/a

R right, *L* left, *DLPFC* dorsolateral prefrontal cortex, *OFC* orbitofrontal cortex, *ACC* anterior cingulate cortex, *M* medial, *S* superior, *I* inferior

suggestive of an attempt to control and restrict an emotional and appetitive response due to the role these areas play in cognitive control [49, 52], and may accord with the restrictive eating patterns typically seen in this group. An emotional impact to these images can be inferred from the neural activation seen, as the medial OFC and ACC are involved in processing of emotional information [50]. This finding is supported by activation present in the DLPFC, which is implicated in emotional processing [49]. When people with anxiety were shown emotional stimuli, activation was seen in the DLPFC [52], so food stimuli may have generated a similar negative emotional reaction in those with AN. Despite a response that may suggest negative emotion, increased amygdala activation compared to controls was not seen for food images. Amygdala activation is seen in response to threatening stimuli [53], so it is unexpected that food images did not produce this response given the aversive emotional and physiological response previously reported. The fear network involves activation of the amygdala, PFC, ACC, insular cortex, striatum, and hippocampus, and so may be activated in those with AN to food stimuli, but this is unclear due to the lack of amygdala activation [54].

These studies also demonstrate that activation of top-down control may be present to food images, with top-down control playing a role in response inhibition to stimuli [55]. This may help explain the restrictive behaviour shown towards food by those with AN.

In people with BN, activation of the ACC, medial OFC and DLPFC occurred when viewing food images [49, 50, 56] (Table 4), suggesting these stimuli had an emotional impact and, given DLPFC activation, this may be interpreted as a negative emotional response [49]. Activation of somatosensory and motor areas was also shown to be increased in this group compared to healthy controls due to activation of the supplementary motor area, precentral gyrus and caudate [49], pointing towards an appetitive response also being present. However, hypoactivation of these areas was also seen in those with

Table 4 Neural responses to food stimuli in people with BN

	BN participants	HC participants	Stimuli	BN > HC	BN < HC
Uher et al. 2004 [50]	10	19	Colour pictures of food > Non-food images Emotional aversive > neutral images	ACC, MOFC	L lateral and anterior parietal, LI parietal, L occipital, posterior cerebellum
Schienle et al. 2009 [56]	14	38	High calorie food images > disgust inducing images> neutral images	Insula and ACC	n/a
Brooks et al. 2011 [49]	8	24	Food > non-food	DLPFC, postcentral gyrus, caudate, precentral gyrus, supplementary motor area	bilateral superior temporal gyrus, bilateral insula, and visual cortex
Spangler et al. 2011 [59]	12	12	Computer generated thin and large body image Scrambled image	Pregenual ACC	n/a
Kim et al. 2012 [51]	20	20	High calorie food images > non-food images	Anterior Insula, R middle frontal gyrus and cerebellum	n/a
Skunde et al. 2016 [57]	28	29	Visual food stimuli > household item stimuli	No differences seen	No differences seen

R right, *L* left, *DLPFC* dorsolateral prefrontal cortex, *OFC* orbitofrontal cortex, *ACC* anterior cingulate cortex, *M* medial, *I* inferior

BN and a high severity of binge eating [57]. So, though there is uncertainty about the somatosensory and motor response, there is evidence that differences may be accounted for by symptom severity. Activation in the ACC and insula are suggestive of an appetitive response, and this correlated with increased arousal ratings to food [56]. There is evidence that the insula is involved in perceiving the salience of signals, which leads to a subjective state of arousal [56, 58], so activation of the insula in response to food images should correlate with a physiological response indicating arousal. This has been seen in those with binge-eating characteristics, a feature of BN, suggesting that activation of these areas indicates arousal. Hypoactivation of the visual and occipital cortex was present in people with BN compared to controls, suggesting attention may be being diverted away from food stimuli [49, 50], correlating with a negative emotional response and indicating an aversive response. However, this contrasts with increased arousal findings, so increased insular activity may be due to its primary gustatory role, rather than the arousal of these images.

Insula and ACC activity also play a crucial role in the salience network, this network identifies relevant salient stimuli in order to guide behaviours [60]. This increased insula activity compared to HC for food images may suggest enhanced salience responses to food imagery in those with BN which coincides with the increased attention shown to these images.

Activation of the OFC as well as the ACC in those with BED, suggested an appetitive response to food stimuli occurs [56, 61] (Table 5). The OFC is the secondary gustatory cortex and so activation is expected in response to food images. It is also thought to be involved in reward sensitivity [56], with increased OFC activity potentially suggesting greater food motivation [62]. In people with BED, increased reward sensitivity to food images was self-reported so these findings correlate with neural responses. However, due to the limited studies available for BED it is difficult to draw firm conclusions.

Summary of food stimuli

For food images, a dissociation exists between self-reported and physiological response in people with ED. This dissociation is present across a range of physiological measures and across ED pathologies. A difference in emotional response to images across ED diagnoses exists, with food images rated as more pleasant by those with BN and BED compared to those with AN. This is in contrast to the physiological response, which appears to be relatively consistent across all three groups that display aversive physiological responses to food images. The neuroimaging findings support the dissociation with negative emotional processing seen in those with AN, whereas motivational and appetitive responses appear to dominate in BN and BED.

Body shape and weight

Physiological response

Startle-blink reflex There is a dissociation across ED diagnoses between emotional responses and the startle-blink reflex. When people with BN viewed a video of their own body, they had a smaller startle-blink reflex than that of healthy controls, despite those with BN having rated these images as more unpleasant [36]. A reduced startle-blink reflex for those with BN was also present during a noise-only trial with no image stimulus, which may be interpreted as a sense of alertness throughout the trial due to the knowledge that they would be viewing images of their own body at a later point [36]. This is reinforced by the elevated attention paid to these trials in attentional bias studies by this patient group [5, 63]. However, the startle-blink reflex when viewing own-body image for those with BN was smaller than the noise-only trial. This finding cannot be explained by vigilance and is contrary to the emotional ratings where own-body image evoked unpleasant feelings and greater arousal [36], suggesting a dissociation between emotional and physiological responses. A further study in those with BN observed no change in the startle-blink reflex between viewing body-shape and neutral images, despite high anxiety ratings towards the images [27]. This pattern did not change once those taking SSRI were excluded, unlike with food images [27]. These findings are replicated in people with AN, with no change in the startle-blink reflex observed for body-shape images, despite similarly high anxiety ratings [27].

In healthy women screened for their risk of ED, no difference was seen in the startle-blink response between

Table 5 Neural responses to visual stimuli in people with BED

	BED participants	HC participants	Stimuli	BED > HC	BED < HC
Schienle et al. 2009 [56]	17	38	High calorie food images > disgust inducing images > neutral images	MOFC	n/a
Geliebter et al. 2015 [61]	10	10	Food > non-food images Food > non-food spoken word	Dorsal ACC	n/a

ACC anterior cingulate cortex, *MOFC* medial orbito frontal cortex body and neutral words [37]. However, an association was found with women who reported high body dissatisfaction, but not drive for thinness or BN, and a larger startle-blink response for body shape compared to neutral words. Body-shape words were rated as more negatively valenced and higher for arousal, with significantly greater differences in ratings seen for those with higher EDI scores [37]. Emotional ratings and startle-blink responses were recorded in response to self-photos that had been edited to represent a large and XL shape [38]. XL-shape images resulted in a startle-blink response that significantly predicted more variance in EDI body dissatisfaction and drive for thinness scales than emotional self-report. No significance was seen for the BN subscale rating [38]. In line with previous studies of the differences between self-report and physiological data, these results suggested that the startle reflex response may be a better predictor of ED behaviour than self-reported emotional ratings, which have potential reporting bias [38].

In summary, startle-blink reflex studies show little change between neutral and body-shape images, despite these images being consistently rated as more unpleasant. However, the startle-blink reflex was found to be a better predictor of ED pathology than self-report in one study, so further research is needed to explore this discrepancy.

HR, SCR and posturographic destabilisation In women with BN, a larger SCR was seen compared with healthy controls when viewing a video of their own body [36]. Unlike startle-blink responses [36], this correlated with more unpleasant feelings and arousal in this group, which suggests an aversive response was present in those with BN to images of self. Despite those with BN demonstrating greater negative emotions across a greater range of cognitions compared with healthy controls, no significant difference in SCR was seen in those with ED compared with healthy controls when looking at their own body in a mirror [39]. An association was seen between the physiological and emotional reaction, as SCR increased when looking at self in the mirror in this group [39]. However, this increase in SCR was the same as in healthy controls, so the value of this association is decreased.

In both restrained and unrestrained eaters, self-image resulted in greater negative arousal, as longer SCR recovery times were seen [33]. However, there was no difference in SCR between these groups and no difference in emotional rating was seen between restrained and unrestrained eaters [33]. This points towards the response to body-shape images being aversive to those with normal eating patterns as well as those with disordered eating, and would explain the lack of significant effect seen in the startle-blink reflex [33].

A potentiation of the cardiac defence response is seen with a HR acceleration-deceleration pattern found in those with BN when exposed to own-body images [36]. The same response was also seen in both restrained and unrestrained eaters when shown pictures of self [33]. This pattern suggests an aversive response occurs coinciding with the negative emotional ratings reported towards these images [36].

Postural control is affected by psychological states, with anxiety mediated by visual stimuli resulting in increased body sway [40]. A group of patients with ED and healthy controls were shown their own image reflected in a mirror as well as the image of a thin ideal model [40]. The ED group experienced greater body sway when looking at both images compared with the healthy controls, representing postural destabilisation [40]. This suggests that, in those with ED, images of self and a thin ideal are anxiety provoking and may induce a quasi-phobic state that is not seen in healthy controls.

In summary an aversive physiological response is present in those with ED to body-shape stimuli based on their autonomic responses; This correlates with negative self-rating of the same images.

Neuroimaging response

In those with AN, neuroimaging evidence supports an association between emotional and neural response. In females with AN, increased amygdala activation was seen to body-shape and weight stimuli [53, 64–66] (Table 6). These neural responses correlated with self-reported negative affect towards these images [37] and correspond with responses in previous emotional and physiological studies [36]. Amygdala activation is also correlated with unpleasantness ratings of XL-shape images of self, reinforcing the association between emotional and neural response in people with AN [53]. Along with amygdala activation, activation of other brain areas involved in the fear network was also seen [54] suggesting that this network is activated when body images are viewed. Activation in areas known to have a role in emotion: medial-prefrontal cortex (PFC), DLPFC and limbic system, was demonstrated to self-images, supporting the finding of a negative emotional response [52, 53, 64, 67, 69]. Right cingulate hyperactivation, an area directly involved in negative emotional processing, was also found when those with AN reported negative affect towards these images reinforcing the association between neural and emotional responses [65].

Areas of hypoactivation compared to controls were demonstrated. These were mainly in the lateral PFC and inferior parietal lobe [50, 65, 68, 69], which were interpreted by the author as decreased capacity for attention

Table 6 Neural responses to body shape stimuli in people with AN

Author	AN Participants	HC participants	Stimuli	AN > HC	AN < HC
Seeger et al. 2002 [66]	3	3	Distorted image of self > distorted image of other > abstract colour image	R amygdala, brainstem, R gyrus fusiformis	n/a
Wagner et al. 2003 [67]	15	11	Distorted image of self > distorted image of other > abstract colour image	DLPFC and intraparietal sulcus	n/a
Uher et al. 2005 [68]	13	18	Line drawing of body shape > line drawing of houses	n/a	R parietal, R and lateral fusiform gyrus
Sachdev et al. 2008 [69]	10	10	Images of self > grey screen	n/a	Insula, PFC and occipital lobe
			Image of other > grey screen	MPFC	n/a
Miyake et al. 2010 [64]	24 total 12 restrictive 12 binge purge subtype	12	Negative body image words > neutral words Negative emotional words > neutral words	Amygdala, L MPFC, DLPFC and LI parietal	n/a
Vocks et al. 2010 [65]	13	27	Self-image	n/a	LI parietal lobe, M temporal gyrus, L uncus, parahippocampal
			Image of other	R amygdala, bilateral para hippocampal, L uncus, L hippocampus, R posterior cingulate	n/a
Miyake et al. 2010 [53]	22	11	Distorted own body image	Amygdala, MPFC, DLPFC	n/a
			Distorted image of other	R amygdala	
Castellini et al. 2013 [52]	18	19	Own body image normal > distorted	frontal gyrus, M temporal gyrus, DLPFC	n/a

R right, *L* left, *DLPFC* dorsolateral prefrontal cortex, *OFC* orbitofrontal cortex, *ACC* anterior cingulate cortex, *M* medial, *S* superior, *I* inferior

being present, and that decreased visual processing may be occurring in an attempt to avoid stimuli with a negative emotional impact [65]. Hypoactivation of these areas also suggests decreased bottom-up processing of these images as well as increased top-down control with activation of the PFC, which may be due to the aversive nature of these stimuli [55].

In contrast to *f*MRI studies of AN groups, only one study demonstrated increased amygdala activation in response to body-shape stimuli in individuals with BN [64]

Table 7 Neural responses to body shape stimuli in people with BN

	BN participants	HC participants	Stimuli	BN > HC	BN < HC
Uher et al. 2005 [68]	9	18	Line drawings of body shapes > line drawing of houses	n/a	R and lateral fusiform gyrus
Miyake et al. 2010 [64]	12	12	Negative body image words > neutral words Negative emotional words > neutral words	R amygdala, L ventro MPFC	n/a
Vocks et al. 2010 [65]	15	27	Own body	n/a	RI parietal, right middle frontal
			Image of other	Bilateral postcentral gyrus and bilateral hippocampal	n/a
Miyake et al. 2010 [53]	11	11	Own distorted body image	R occipital and R parietal	MPFC, DLPFC, amygdala
			Distorted body image of other	R occipital and R parietal	n/a
Spangler et al. 2011 [59]	12	12	Distorted image of self > distorted image of other > abstract image	Pregenual ACC	n/a

R right, *L* left, *MPFC* medial prefrontal cortex

(Table 7), suggesting that these stimuli were less threatening to those with BN. However, as activation of the ACC and ventromedial PFC—centres involved in the processing of emotional information—was seen, an emotional response was still evoked to body-shape images [59, 64]. The negative emotional properties of these neural activations were confirmed by activation of the limbic system in conjunction with self-reported negative emotional affect to these images [65]. Once again, increased top-down processing is seen to body-shape images suggesting an aversive nature and inhibition of focus towards these images [55].

Summary of body-shape stimuli

Viewing self-image resulted in an increase of negative emotions across all ED diagnoses with no distinct variations seen, emphasising the importance of body shape and weight in ED maintenance and pathology. The physiological impact was mixed, with little clarity provided by the current evidence base. A lack of physiological response was seen in startle-blink reflex, whereas SCR and HR suggest aversive responses that are associated with negative emotional affect. In neuroimaging, a consistent aversive and negative emotional impact was seen. This suggests a consistent association across emotional, physiological, and neural responses to body image and is supported by findings of postural destabilisation.

Methodological issues

Methodological issues may account for inconsistent physiological responses to both food and body-shape images. In some studies, participants selected the imagery used, whereas other studies provided images. Some studies obtained participant ratings of image salience, some studies used images selected for their valence by volunteers with both ED diagnoses and healthy controls [27, 65], and other studies did not measure the valence or salience of images. A lack of replication of findings was also present in studies using the same physiological measure, limiting the strength of the conclusions that can be formed. This lack of replication was particularly prevalent in neuroimaging studies with a wide range of activation areas indicated. A large overlap of activation areas with healthy controls was seen for body-shape stimuli and suggests that these results may be continuous between healthy individuals and those with ED.

SSRI attenuate the startle-blink reflex [43], and given that this was not controlled for in several studies [26, 29], the startle-blink reflex to food images may be underestimated and the validity of results weakened. SSRI have also been shown to have an impact on HRV and HR, and so may have attenuated other physiological measures [70, 71]. A decrease in HRV was seen in those with anxiety and depression taking an antidepressant compared with those who were not [71]. The same effect may be present in those with ED taking SSRI, which could impact capacity to regulate emotional responses. As use of SSRI was not consistently controlled for, this may invalidate the physiological responses seen: serotonin pathways have a role in both autonomic regulation and modulation of emotion [72], so use of SSRI has the potential to modulate both these behaviours, further propagating the dissociation between subjective and emotional responses.

Inconsistent levels of ED pathology across this literature also reduce the validity of results and limit comparisons. Several studies rely on participants presenting ED symptoms but no formal diagnosis, whereas clinical thresholds in other studies vary widely. The use of broad diagnostic categories can also lead to mixed results, since binge-eating behaviour can occur in some patients with AN.

The majority of studies only had female participants, despite binge eating prevalence being comparable in males and females [73]. This greatly reduces the applicability of these findings to the wider ED population, as males typically present with less shape and weight concern, so the responses to these stimuli may be very different from females and need to be examined separately [74].

Conclusions

This narrative review draws together emotional, physiological, and neural responses that studies have demonstrated in using food and body-shape/weight stimuli in people with ED. The pattern for food stimuli is inconsistent, with differing responses seen to these stimuli amongst the ED pathologies and a dissociation across the emotional, physiological, and neural modes of response measurement. Body-shape and weight stimuli induce more consistent emotional, physiological, and neural responses across all the ED groups than food stimuli, with greater associations seen across all three modalities.

People with AN have mixed responses to food images. Food images are consistently rated as anxiety provoking and generate a negative emotional impact. This was seen in the neuroimaging findings, with activation of areas indicating negative emotional processing; however, no amygdala activation was seen, which would be expected given the high anxiety ratings. The physiological response is also quite varied with some studies indicating an aversive response is present, while in others no effect was seen for the stimuli.

Body-shape and weight stimuli consistently induce a negative emotional self-reported affect, produce an aversive physiological response, and result in activation of areas associated with processing negative emotions.

Additionally, amygdala activation was observed to these stimuli in people with AN, indicating that these stimuli do not just evoke negative emotions but are also perceived as threatening to the individual. However, this association is weakened by the physiological response findings: several startle-blink studies found no significant differences in the startle-blink response, so this association relies on data from HR, SCR, and posturographic destabilisation research.

In individuals with BN, a dissociation exists in the emotional, physiological, and neural response. Aversive physiological responses were seen in both startle-blink and facial EMG to food stimuli, despite often being rated as pleasant. This was also seen in the neural response, with activation in areas associated with processing negative emotion. Further neural activation was seen, suggesting an appetitive response associated with greater arousal ratings, but this was not present in physiological studies.

Conversely for BED, an association does appear to exist but only between the neural and emotional response. A motivational and reward response was seen in neuroimaging that correlated with food images being consistently rated as more pleasant and with higher reward. However, this appetitive response was not seen physiologically, where an aversive response appears to be present as demonstrated by increased startle-blink reflex and corrugator activity. Unfortunately, this cannot be compared across all three measures for those with BED due to a lack of appropriate neuroimaging studies comparing individuals with BED to healthy controls.

Associations across neural, physiological, and subjective emotional responses

In healthy individuals, there are several proposed mechanisms for the associations across neural, physiological measures, and emotional responding. HRV, which was earlier discussed as a measure of emotional regulation, has been found to be correlated with the medial-PFC activation during emotional activation [75]. Further correlation for HRV was also found to the caudate nucleus, the mid-left insula, and the periaqueductal grey matter [75]. These areas are part of the medial visceral network, indicating that this pathway is involved in the emotional and cognitive control of the autonomic response. The ventro-medial PFC has also been further implicated in controlling cardiovascular responses to emotional stimuli [76], with problems in the ventro-medial PFC shown to cause altered responses to these stimuli, which may be the case in those with ED. Substantial evidence also exists to support the role the amygdala plays in controlling autonomic nervous system responses to fear stimuli with increased amygdala responses correlating with both increased SCR and HR [77, 78].

Abnormal amygdala responses to fearful stimuli have been shown to be present in several psychiatric disorders [79], this may also be the case in ED, and offers an explanation for the dissociated responses seen due to the role the amygdala plays in autonomic control. Another possible explanation is the effect that physiological impacts of ED have on neural function, with malnutrition resulting in widespread changes throughout the brain and in some instances causing decreased grey matter [80]. Altering of the OFC and insula also appears to take place in ED, suggesting that altered reward processing is present [80]. Given the role neural function plays in autonomic control of emotions it is logical that this could lead to a decoupling of the subjective and objective responses in people with ED that impact neural structures.

There are several other possible explanations for the lack of association across neural, physiological, and subjective emotional responses frequently seen in those with ED. The high rates of alexithymia that are present in those with ED might result in a decoupling between self-reported emotional responses and physiological responses. This decoupling was demonstrated when those with alexithymia were put under the stressful scenario of giving an impromptu speech [81]. Given that food and body-shape images may induce negative feelings and stressful responses, a similar decoupling response may have been present in these studies. Another possible explanation is that emotional responses are not always coherent, even within a healthy population [82], so the differences seen may be due to normal emotional responses within the population. The motivational conflict hypothesis offers an additional explanation for the lack of association seen for those with binge-eating behaviours by suggesting that the eating behaviours seen are associated with both positive and negative reactions towards food [32]. So it may be this mixed response results in both positive and negative subjective and objective responses. Blunting of the startle-blink reflex in those with AN to fear stimuli offers might explain why no potentiation of the startle-blink reflex was frequently seen [83]. A lack of association between subjective and objective responses to affective images was demonstrated in those with AN, so the lack of correspondence may not be cue dependent but instead point to a more general dissociation seen in those with AN [84]. There is potential that this may also be the case in other ED offering an explanation for the differing results reported in this review.

Implications for clinical practice

The associations and dissociations described in this review have implications for clinical practice. Images are increasingly being used in both VR [7] and imagery-based CBT [6]. In order for these treatment methods to be effective, the impact these stimuli have on participants needs to be understood. The subjective ratings of the patient and their objective responses often oppose each other, with stimuli inducing an aversive or motivational self-report response but having the opposite impact, or no impact, physiologically and neurally. Substantial negative impact was found for self-image across all modalities, which is particularly important for mentalisation practices. Food stimuli may be less appropriate to use in therapy and may require careful consideration for research due to the differing responses seen and inconsistency in impact. In VR, repeated food image exposure has been used in order to decrease negative emotions [85], but in those with BN and BED, motivational and appetitive responses were shown to these images alongside negative affect, suggesting some dissonance in responses.

Research has shown that alexithymia has a negative impact on treatment outcomes, with poorer responses to therapeutic interventions seen [86]. This may be due to the decoupling that is seen in alexithymia, with a decreased awareness of emotional cues and responses potentially reducing the ability to engage successfully in psychotherapy [87]. This decoupling is similar to the lack of association present between the subjective and objective responses. Those patients who display a high lack of association, therefore, may also have worse treatment outcomes and be less successful in therapeutic engagement. Thus, the findings of this review have important implications for treatment outcomes.

In order to increase the validity of studies, images are initially shown to a group of patients who rate the images to ensure that they are salient. However, given that there may be a dissociation between these subjective emotional ratings and the objective physiological and neural responses, the images selected may not have the desired impact. This needs to be considered when using imagery in trials, as it may impact findings. Motivational conflict present may also have important treatment indications as it means both positive and negative feelings or reactions towards food/body-shape need to be treated and addressed by clinicians [32].

In summary, body-shape and weight stimuli appear to consistently generate more aversive responses in people with ED than food stimuli, suggesting that these images may have greater salience for patients with ED. Given the increased consistency between subjective and objective responses to these images, greater reliance can be made on self-reported responses to these stimuli when considering their use in therapy and research.

Limitations

Several limitations are present in the existing literature. The majority of studies only focused on females and as evidence exists that men and women differ in their response to emotional stimuli [88], research reported in this review may not be generalisable. In addition, there was a large heterogeneity in the stimuli used, the physiological measures and the emotional valence ratings that reduces the validity of this review's findings. This, combined with the lack of comparison across all three measures in the majority of studies, provides a significant limitation to the strength of conclusions that can be drawn. The small sample sizes consistently used in studies using *f*MRI also greatly limits the validity of their findings.

Food and body-shape importance depends on individual cultural beliefs, and this was not always considered in studies. Body-shape studies were mainly focused on self-image, so the impact of images of others is still relatively unknown. Due to the lack of response seen in startle-blink studies for body-shape stimuli, the physiological findings are limited to HR and SCR, which are less reliable measures. This review is further limited by the measures that were focused on: by only examining neural imaging studies using *f*MRI, other neuroimaging measures were excluded. Several physiological measures were also excluded, such as hormonal changes, and the responses seen in these measures may differ from the conclusions drawn in this review.

Abbreviations

ACC: Anterior cingulate cortex; AN: Anorexia nervosa; BED: Binge eating disorder; BN: Bulimia nervosa; CBT: Cognitive Behavioural Therapy; DLPFC: Dorsolateral prefrontal cortex; ED: Eating disorders; EDI: Eating Disorders Inventory; EMG: Electromyographic; fMRI: Functional magnetic resonance imaging; HR: Heart rate; HRV: Heart rate variability; OFC: Orbitofrontal cortex; PFC: Prefrontal cortex; SCR: Skin conductance response; SSRI: Selective serotonin reuptake inhibitor; VR: Virtual reality

Acknowledgements

We would like to thank the Imperial college CAMH research team for their support throughout writing this paper.

Authors' contributions

VB conceived the review, EG and VB were involved in its design, with interpretation and first manuscript drafting performed by EG. All authors revised and contributed to manuscript writing. The authors read and approved the final manuscript.

Competing interests

The authors declare that they have no competing interests.

References

1. National Institute for Health and Care Excellence (NICE). *Eating disorders: recognition and treatment: NICE Guideline [NG69] | Guidance | NICE.* 2017. Available from: https://www.nice.org.uk/guidance/ng69/chapter/Context [Accessed May 8, 2020].
2. Fairburn CG, Walsh BT. Atypical eating disorders (eating disorder not otherwise specified). In: Fairburn CG, Brownell KD, editors. Eating disorders and obesity: a comprehensive handbook. 2nd ed. New York: Guilford Press; 2002. p. 171–7.
3. Fairburn CG, Cooper Z, Shafran R. Cognitive behaviour therapy for eating disorders: a "transdiagnostic" theory and treatment. Behav Res Ther. 2003; 41(5):509–28.
4. Beck AT, Clark DA. An information processing model of anxiety: Automatic and strategic processes. Behaviour Research and Therapy. 1997;35(1): 49–58. Available from: https://doi.org/10.1016/S0005-7967(96)00069-1.
5. Shafran R, Lee M, Cooper Z, Palmer RL, Fairburn CG. Attentional bias in eating disorders. Int J Eat Disord. 2007;40(4):369–80.
6. Tatham M. The role of imagery-based techniques in cognitive–behavioural therapy for adults with eating disorders. *Clinical Psychology Review.* 2011; 31(7): 1101-1109. Available from: doi:https://doi.org/10.1016/j.cpr.2011.06.008.
7. Perpiñá C, Botella C, Baños RM. Virtual reality in eating disorders. *European Eating Disorders Review.* 2003;11(3): 261-278. Available from: doi:https://doi.org/10.1002/erv.520.
8. Stroop JR. Studies of interference in serial verbal reactions. *Journal of Experimental Psychology.* 1935;18(6): 643-662. Available from: doi:https://doi.org/10.1037/h0054651.
9. Ben–Tovim DI, Walker MK, Fok D, Yap E. An adaptation of the Stroop test for measuring shape and food concerns in eating disorders: A quantitative measure of psychopathology? Intern J Eating Dis. 1989;8(6):681–7.
10. Cooper MJ, Fairburn CG. Selective processing of eating, weight and shape related words in patients with eating disorders and dieters. British J Clin Psyc. 2011:31(3):363–5.
11. Stormark KM, Torkildsen Ø. Selective processing of linguistic and pictorial food stimuli in females with anorexia and bulimia nervosa. *Eating Behaviors.* 2004; 5(1): 27-33. Available from: doi:https://doi.org/10.1016/j.eatbeh.2003.07.002.
12. MacLeod C, Mathews A, Tata P. Attentional bias in emotional disorders. *Journal of Abnormal Psychology.* 1986;95(1):15-20. Available from: doi:https://doi.org/10.1037/0021-843X.95.1.15.
13. Rieger E, Schotte DE, Touyz SW, Beumont PJV, Griffiths R, Russell J. Attentional biases in eating disorders: A visual probe detection procedure. *International Journal of Eating Disorders.* 1998; 23(2):199–205. Available from: doi:https://doi.org/10.1002/(SICI)1098-108X(199803)23:23.0.CO;2-W.
14. Blechert J, Ansorge U, Tuschen-Caffier B. A body-related dot-probe task reveals distinct attentional patterns for bulimia nervosa and anorexia nervosa. *Journal of Abnormal Psychology.* 2010;119(3): 575-585. Available from: doi:https://doi.org/10.1037/a0019531.
15. Posner MI, Snyder CR, Davidson BJ. Attention and the detection of signals. *Journal of Experimental Psychology: General.* 1980;109(2): 160-174. Available from: doi:https://doi.org/10.1037/0096-3445.109.2.160.
16. Feustel TC, Shiffrin RM, Salasoo A. Episodic and lexical contributions to the repetition effect in word identification. *Journal of Experimental Psychology: General.* 1983;112(3): 309-346. Available from: doi:https://doi.org/10.1037/0096-3445.112.3.309.
17. Schmitz F, Naumann E, Trentowska M, Svaldi J. Attentional bias for food cues in binge eating disorder. *Appetite.* 2014;80: 70-80. Available from: doi: https://doi.org/10.1016/j.appet.2014.04.023.
18. Popien A, Frayn M, von Ranson KM, Sears CR. Eye gaze tracking reveals heightened attention to food in adults with binge eating when viewing images of real-world scenes. *Appetite.* 2015;91: 233-240. Available from: doi: https://doi.org/10.1016/j.appet.2015.04.046.
19. Giel KE, Teufel M, Friederich H, Hautzinger M, Enck P, Zipfel S. Processing of pictorial food stimuli in patients with eating disorders—a systematic review. Int J Eat Disord. 2011;44(2):105–17.
20. Hagemann D, Waldstein SR, Thayer JF. Central and autonomic nervous system integration in emotion. *Brain and Cognition* 2003;52(1): 79-87. Available from: doi:https://doi.org/10.1016/S0278-2626(03)00011-3.
21. Critchley HD, Eccles J, Garfinkel SN. Chapter 6 - interaction between cognition, emotion, and the autonomic nervous system. *Handbook of Clinical Neurology.* 2013;117: 59-77. Available from: doi:https://doi.org/10.1016/B978-0-444-53491-0.00006-7.
22. Lang PJ, Greenwald MK, Bradley MM, Hamm AO. Looking at pictures: affective, facial, visceral, and behavioral reactions. *Psychophysiology.* 1993;30(3): 261-273. Available from: doi:https://doi.org/10.1111/j.1469-8986.1993.tb03352x.
23. Bradley MM, Codispoti M, Cuthbert BN, Lang PJ. Emotion and motivation I: defensive and appetitive reactions in picture processing. *Emotion.* 2001;1(3): 276-28. Available from: doi:https://doi.org/10.1037/1528-3542.1.3.276.
24. Nowakowski ME, McFarlane T, Cassin S. Alexithymia and eating disorders: a critical review of the literature. *Journal of Eating Disorders.* 2013;1(1): 21. Available from: doi:https://doi.org/10.1186/2050-2974-1-21.
25. American Psychiatric Association. *Diagnostic and Statistical Manual of Mental Disorders (DSM-5®).* American Psychiatric Pub; 2013.
26. Racine SE. Emotional ratings of high- and low-calorie food are differentially associated with cognitive restraint and dietary restriction. *Appetite.* 2018;121: 302-308. Available from: doi:https://doi.org/10.1016/j.appet.2017.11.104.
27. Friederich H, Kumari V, Uher R, Riga M, Schmidt U, Campbell IC, et al. Differential motivational responses to food and pleasurable cues in anorexia and bulimia nervosa: a startle reflex paradigm. *Psychological Medicine.* 2006; 36(9): 1327-1335. Available from: doi:https://doi.org/10.1017/S0033291706008129.
28. Mauler BI, Hamm AO, Weike AI, Tuschen-Caffier B. Affect regulation and food intake in bulimia nervosa: emotional responding to food cues after deprivation and subsequent eating. *Journal of Abnormal Psychology.* 2006;115(3): 567-579. Available from: doi:https://doi.org/10.1037/0021-843X.115.3.567.
29. Drobes DJ, Miller EJ, Hillman CH, Bradley MM, Cuthbert BN, Lang PJ. Food deprivation and emotional reactions to food cues: implications for eating disorders. *Biological Psychology.* 2001;57(1-3): 153-177. Available from: doi: https://doi.org/10.1016/S0301-0511(01)00093-X.
30. Suissa-Rocheleau L, Benning SD, Racine SE. Associations between self-report and physiological measures of emotional reactions to food among women with disordered eating. *International Journal of Psychophysiology.* 2019;144: 40-46. Available from: doi:https://doi.org/10.1016/j.ijpsycho.2019.08.004.
31. Soussignan R, Jiang T, Rigaud D, Royet JP, Schaal B. Subliminal fear priming potentiates negative facial reactions to food pictures in women with anorexia nervosa. *Psychological Medicine.* 2010;40(3): 503-514. Available from: doi:https://doi.org/10.1017/S0033291709990377.
32. Racine SE, Hebert KR, Benning SD. Emotional Reactivity and Appraisal of Food in Relation to Eating Disorder Cognitions and Behaviours: Evidence to Support the Motivational Conflict Hypothesis. *European Eating Disorders Review.* 2018; 26 (1): 3–10. Available from: doi: https://doi.org/10.1002/erv.2567.
33. Overduin J, Jansen A, Eilkes H. Cue reactivity to food-and body-related stimuli in restrained and unrestrained eaters. *Addictive Behaviors.* 1997;22(3): 395-404. Available from: doi:https://doi.org/10.1016/S0306-4603(97)80002-0.
34. Leehr EJ, Schag K, Brinkmann A, Ehlis A, Fallgatter AJ, Zipfel S, et al. Alleged approach-avoidance conflict for food stimuli in binge eating disorder. *PLoS One.* 2016;11(4): e0152271 Available from: doi:https://doi.org/10.1371/journal.pone.0152271
35. Svaldi J, Tuschen-Caffier B, Peyk P, Blechert J. Information processing of food pictures in binge eating disorder. *Appetite.* 2010;55(3): 685-694. Available from: doi: https://doi.org/10.1016/j.appet.2010.10.002.
36. Ortega-Roldan B, Rodríguez-Ruiz S, Perakakis P, Fernandez-Santaella MC, Vila J. The emotional and attentional impact of exposure to one's own body in bulimia nervosa: a physiological view. *PloS one.* 2014;9(7): e102595. Available from: doi:https://doi.org/10.1371/journal.pone.0102595.
37. Herbert C, Kübler A, Vögele C. Risk for eating disorders modulates startle-responses to body words. *PloS one.* 2013;8(1): e53667. Available from: doi: https://doi.org/10.1371/journal.pone.0053667.
38. Spresser CD, Keune KM, Filion DL, Lundgren JD. Self-report and startle-based measures of emotional reactions to body image cues as predictors of drive for thinness and body dissatisfaction in female college students. *Body Image.* 2012;9(2): 298-301. Available from: doi:https://doi.org/10.1016/j.bodyim.2011.12.005.
39. Vocks S, Legenbauer T, Wächter A, Wucherer M, Kosfelder J. *What happens in the course of body exposure?:* emotional, cognitive, and physiological reactions to mirror confrontation in eating disorders. *Journal of Psychosomatic Research.* 2007;62(2): 231-239. Available from: doi:https://doi.org/10.1016/j.jpsychores.2006.08.007.

40. Forghieri M, Monzani D, Mackinnon A, Ferrari S, Gherpelli C, Galeazzi GM. Posturographic destabilization in eating disorders in female patients exposed to body image related phobic stimuli. *Neuroscience Letters.* 2016; 629: 155-159. Available from: doi:https://doi.org/10.1016/j.neulet.2016.07.002.
41. Vrana SR, Spence EL, Lang PJ. The startle probe response: a new measure of emotion? *Journal of Abnormal Psychology.* 1988;97(4): 487-491. Available from: doi:https://doi.org/10.1037/0021-843X.97.4.487.
42. Koch M, Schmid A, Schnitzler H. Pleasure-attenuation of startle is disrupted by lesions of the nucleus accumbens. *Neuroreport.* 1996;7(8): 1442-1446. Available from: doi:https://doi.org/10.1097/00001756-199605310-00024.
43. Schmid A, Koch M, Schnitzler HU. Conditioned pleasure attenuates the startle response in rats. *Neurobiology of Learning and Memory.* 1995;64(1): 1-3. Available from: doi:https://doi.org/10.1006/nlme.1995.1037.
44. Benning SD, Patrick CJ, Lang AR. Emotional modulation of the post-auricular reflex. Psychophysiology. 2004;41(3):426–32.
45. Berridge KC. 'Liking' and 'wanting' food rewards: brain substrates and roles in eating disorders. *Physiology & Behavior.* 2009;97(5): 537-550. Available from: doi:https://doi.org/10.1016/j.physbeh.2009.02.044.
46. Hare RD, Blevings G. Defensive responses to phobic stimuli. *Biological Psychology.* 1975;3(1): 1-13. Available from: doi: https://doi.org/10.1016/0301-0511(75)90002-2.
47. Appelhans BM, Luecken LJ. Heart rate variability as an index of regulated emotional responding. *Review of General Psychology.* 2006;10(3): 229-240. Available from: doi:https://doi.org/10.1037/1089-2680.10.3.229.
48. Segerstrom SC, Nes LS. Heart rate variability reflects self-regulatory strength, effort, and fatigue. Psychol Sci. 2007;18(3):275–81.
49. Samantha J. Brooks, Owen G. ODaly, Rudolf Uher, Hans-Christoph Friederich, Vincent Giampietro, Michael Brammer, et al. differential neural responses to food images in women with bulimia versus anorexia nervosa. *PLoS ONE.* 2011; 6(7): e22259.. Available from: doi:https://doi.org/10.1371/journal.pone.0022259.
50. Uher R, Murphy T, Brammer MJ, Dalgleish T, Phillips ML, Ng VW, et al. Medial prefrontal cortex activity associated with symptom provocation in eating disorders. *American Journal of Psychiatry.* 2004;161(7): 1238-1246. Available from: https://doi.org/10.1176/appi.ajp.161.7.1238.
51. Kim KR, Ku J, Lee J, Lee H, Jung Y. Functional and effective connectivity of anterior insula in anorexia nervosa and bulimia nervosa. *Neuroscience Letters.* 2012;521(2): 152-157. Available from: doi:https://doi.org/10.1016/j.neulet.2012.05.075.
52. Castellini G, Polito C, Bolognesi E, D'Argenio A, Ginestroni A, Mascalchi M, et al. Looking at my body. Similarities and differences between anorexia nervosa patients and controls in body image visual processing. *European Psychiatry.* 2013;28(7): 427-435. Available from: doi:https://doi.org/10.1016/j.eurpsy.2012.06.006.
53. Miyake Y, Okamoto Y, Onoda K, Kurosaki M, Shirao N, Okamoto Y, et al. Brain activation during the perception of distorted body images in eating disorders. *Psychiatry Research: Neuroimaging.* 2010;181(3): 183-192. Available from: doi:https://doi.org/10.1016/j.pscychresns.2009.09.001.
54. Shin LM, Liberzon I. The neurocircuitry of fear, stress, and anxiety disorders. Neuropsychopharmacology. 2010;35(1):169–91.
55. Chambers CD, Garavan H, Bellgrove MA. Insights into the neural basis of response inhibition from cognitive and clinical neuroscience. Neurosci Biobehav Rev. 2009;33(5):631–46.
56. Schienle A, Schäfer A, Hermann A, Vaitl D. Binge-eating disorder: reward sensitivity and brain activation to images of food. *Biological Psychiatry.* 2009;65(8): 654-661. Available from: doi:https://doi.org/10.1016/j.biopsych.2008.09.028.
57. Skunde M, PhD, Herzog W, MD, Walther S, PhD, Simon JJ, PhD, Wu M, PhD, Friederich H, MD, et al. neural signature of behavioural inhibition in women with bulimia nervosa. *Journal of Psychiatry and Neuroscience.* 2016;41(5): E69-E78. Available from: doi:https://doi.org/10.1503/jpn.150335.
58. Critchley HD, Mathias CJ, Dolan RJ. Fear conditioning in humans: the influence of awareness and autonomic arousal on functional neuroanatomy. *Neuron.* 2002;33(4): 653-663. Available from: doi:https://doi.org/10.1016/s0896-6273(02)00588-3.
59. Spangler DL, Allen MD. An fMRI investigation of emotional processing of body shape in bulimia nervosa. *International Journal of Eating Disorders.* 2012;45(1): 17-25. Available from: doi:https://doi.org/10.1002/eat.20899.
60. Menon V, Uddin LQ. Saliency, switching, attention and control: a network model of insula function. Brain Struct Funct. 2010;214(5–6):655–67.
61. Geliebter A, Benson L, Pantazatos SP, Hirsch J, Carnell S. Greater anterior cingulate activation and connectivity in response to visual and auditory high-calorie food cues in binge eating: preliminary findings. *Appetite.* 2016; 96: 195-202. Available from: doi:https://doi.org/10.1016/j.appet.2015.08.009.
62. Bruce AS, Holsen LM, Chambers RJ, Martin LE, Brooks WM, Zarcone JR, et al. Obese children show hyperactivation to food pictures in brain networks linked to motivation, reward and cognitive control. Int J Obes. 2010;34(10): 1494–500.
63. Cooper MJ, Fairburn CG. Selective processing of eating, weight and shape related words in patients with eating disorders and dieters. *British Journal of Clinical Psychology.* 1992;31(3): 363-365. Available from: doi:https://doi.org/10.1111/j.2044-8260.1992.tb01007.x.
64. Miyake Y, Okamoto Y, Onoda K, Shirao N, Okamoto Y, Otagaki Y, et al. Neural processing of negative word stimuli concerning body image in patients with eating disorders: an fMRI study. *NeuroImage.* 2010;50(3): 1333-1339. Available from: doi:https://doi.org/10.1016/j.neuroimage.2009.12.095.
65. Vocks S, Busch M, Grönemeyer D, Schulte D, Herpertz S, Suchan B. Neural correlates of viewing photographs of one's own body and another woman's body in anorexia and bulimia nervosa: an fMRI study. *Journal of Psychiatry & Neuroscience: JPN.* 2010;35(3): 163-176. Available from: doi: https://doi.org/10.1503/jpn.090048.
66. Seeger G, Braus DF, Ruf M, Goldberger U, Schmidt MH. Body image distortion reveals amygdala activation in patients with anorexia nervosa–a functional magnetic resonance imaging study. *Neuroscience Letters.* 2002; 326(1): 25-28. Available from: doi:https://doi.org/10.1016/s0304-3940(02)00312-9.
67. Wagner A, Ruf M, Braus DF, Schmidt MH. Neuronal activity changes and body image distortion in anorexia nervosa. *Neuroreport.* 2003;14(17): 2193-2197. Available from: doi:https://doi.org/10.1097/00001756-200312020-00012.
68. Uher R, Murphy T, Friederich H, Dalgleish T, Brammer MJ, Giampietro V, et al. Functional Neuroanatomy of body shape perception in healthy and eating-disordered women. *Biological Psychiatry.* 2005;58(12): 990-997. Available from: doi:https://doi.org/10.1016/j.biopsych.2005.06.001.
69. Sachdev P, Mondraty N, Wen W, Gulliford K. Brains of anorexia nervosa patients process self-images differently from non-self-images: an fMRI study. *Neuropsychologia.* 2008;46(8): 2161-2168. Available from: doi:https://doi.org/10.1016/j.neuropsychologia.2008.02.031.
70. Licht CMM, de Geus, Eco J. C., van Dyck R, Penninx, Brenda W. J. H. Longitudinal Evidence for Unfavorable Effects of Antidepressants on Heart Rate Variability. *Biological Psychiatry.* 2010; 68 (9): 861–868. Available from: doi: https://doi.org/10.1016/j.biopsych.2010.06.032.
71. Licht CM, de Geus EJ, Zitman FG, Hoogendijk WJ, van Dyck R, Penninx BW. Association between major depressive disorder and heart rate variability in the Netherlands study of depression and anxiety (NESDA). Arch Gen Psychiatry. 2008;65(12):1358–67.
72. Agorastos A, Kellner M, Stiedl O, Muhtz C, Wiedemann K, Demiralay C. Blunted autonomic reactivity to pharmacological panic challenge under long-term escitalopram treatment in healthy men. Int J Neuropsychopharmacology. 2015;18:5.
73. Striegel-Moore R, Rosselli F, Perrin N, DeBar L, Wilson GT, May A, et al. Gender difference in the prevalence of eating disorder symptoms. *International Journal of Eating Disorders.* 2009; 42 (5): 471–474. Available from: doi: https://doi.org/10.1002/eat.20625 .
74. Darcy AM, Doyle AC, Lock J, Peebles R, Doyle P, Le Grange D. The eating disorders examination in adolescent males with anorexia nervosa: how does it compare to adolescent females? Int J Eat Disord. 2012;45(1):110–4.
75. Lane RD, McRae K, Reiman EM, Chen K, Ahern GL, Thayer JF. Neural correlates of heart rate variability during emotion. *NeuroImage.* 2009; 44 (1): 213–222. Available from: doi: https://doi.org/10.1016/j.neuroimage.2008.07.056.
76. Hänsel A, von Känel R. The ventro-medial prefrontal cortex: a major link between the autonomic nervous system, regulation of emotion, and stress reactivity? BioPsychoSocial Medicine. 2008;2(1):1–5.
77. LeDoux JE. Emotion circuits in the brain. Annu Rev Neurosci. 2000;23(1): 155–84.
78. Williams LM, Barton MJ, Kemp AH, Liddell BJ, Peduto A, Gordon E, et al. Distinct amygdala–autonomic arousal profiles in response to fear signals in healthy males and females. NeuroImage. 2005;28(3):618–26.
79. Yang TT, Simmons AN, Matthews SC, Tapert SF, Bischoff-Grethe A, Frank GKW, et al. Increased amygdala activation is related to heart rate during emotion processing in adolescent subjects. *Neuroscience Letters.* 2007; 428 (2): 109–114. Available from: doi: https://doi.org/10.1016/j.neulet.2007.09.039.
80. Frank GK. Advances from neuroimaging studies in eating disorders. CNS Spectrums. 2015;20(4):391.

81. Eastabrook JM, Lanteigne DM, Hollenstein T. Decoupling between physiological, self-reported, and expressed emotional responses in alexithymia. *Personality and Individual Differences.* 2013; 55 (8): 978–982. Available from: doi: https://doi.org/10.1016/j.paid.2013.08.001.
82. Mauss IB, Levenson RW, McCarter L, Wilhelm FH, Gross JJ. The tie that binds? Coherence among emotion experience, behavior, and physiology. Emotion. 2005;5(2):175.
83. Brockmeyer T, Pellegrino J, Maier C, Münch HM, Harmer CJ, Walther S, et al. Blunted emotion-modulated startle reflex in anorexia nervosa. Int J Eat Disord. 2019;52(3):270–7.
84. Erdur L, Weber C, Zimmermann-Viehoff F, Rose M, Deter H. Affective responses in different stages of anorexia nervosa: results from a startle-reflex paradigm. Eur Eat Disord Rev. 2017;25(2):114–22.
85. Clus D, Larsen ME, Lemey C, Berrouiguet S. The use of virtual reality in patients with eating disorders: systematic review. *Journal of Medical Internet Research.* 2018;20(4): e157. Available from: doi:https://doi.org/10.2196/jmir.7898.
86. Speranza M, Loas G, Guilbaud O, Corcos M. Are treatment options related to alexithymia in eating disorders? Results from a three-year naturalistic longitudinal study. Biomed Pharmacother. 2011;65(8):585–9.
87. Grabe HJ, Frommer J, Ankerhold A, Ulrich C, Gröger R, Franke GH, et al. Alexithymia and outcome in psychotherapy. Psychother Psychosom. 2008; 77(3):189–94.
88. Poláčková Šolcová I, Lačev A. Differences in male and female subjective experience and physiological reactions to emotional stimuli. *International Journal of Psychophysiology.* 2017;117: 75-82. Available from: doi: https://doi.org/10.1016/j.ijpsycho.2017.04.009.

11

Treatment of compulsive exercise in eating disorders and muscle dysmorphia

Jordan Andre Martenstyn[1,2*], Stephen Touyz[2] and Sarah Maguire[2,3]

Abstract

Background: Compulsive exercise is a core feature of both eating disorders and muscle dysmorphia. Earlier models of treatment recommended complete abstinence from exercise in eating disorder populations, but recent guidelines advocate for the gradual inclusion of healthier forms of exercise into an overall treatment plan where appropriate. Given the association between problematic exercise behaviour and poorer prognosis, there has been a recent upsurge in the number of treatment interventions for compulsive exercise in eating disorders. However, no systematic review has been published summarising this existing treatment literature. The aim of this review is to determine the efficacy of existing treatments for compulsive exercise in eating disorders and muscle dysmorphia.

Methods: A systematic review will be conducted according to the Preferred Reporting Items for Systematic Reviews and Meta-Analyses (PRISMA) guidelines. Five electronic databases (PsycInfo, MEDLINE, Embase, Web of Science, and Scopus) will be searched from database inception until November 2020. We will include studies that: (a) sampled adolescents and/or adults with either an eating disorder or muscle dysmorphia; (b) assessed changes in compulsive exercise from pre- to post-intervention; and (c) used a standardised instrument to measure compulsive exercise or related constructs. We will include studies with a comparison group (e.g., randomised controlled trials) and without a comparison group (e.g., pilot studies and case studies) to provide a comprehensive overview of the literature. One reviewer will screen all titles and abstracts against eligibility criteria, with 20% of excluded articles cross-referenced by another reviewer. Full texts will be obtained for articles deemed relevant or where inclusion was uncertain, and will be screened by both reviewers. We will also evaluate the quality of the included studies using a modified Downs and Black (J Epidemiol Community Health 52:377–384, 1998) assessment checklist.

Discussion: Results from this review will help to determine the most efficacious treatment components for compulsive exercise in eating disorders and muscle dysmorphia. We hope that our results will help inform clinical practice guidelines in recommending targeted interventions for the treatment of compulsive exercise.

Keywords: Compulsive exercise, Exercise addiction, Eating disorders, Muscle dysmorphia, Bigorexia, Treatment, Intervention

* Correspondence: jordan.martenstyn@sydney.edu.au
[1]Clinical Psychology Unit, School of Psychology, The University of Sydney, Sydney, Australia
[2]InsideOut Institute for Eating Disorders, The Boden Collaboration for Obesity, Nutrition, Exercise and Eating Disorders, The University of Sydney, Sydney, Australia
Full list of author information is available at the end of the article

Background

Excessive exercise has long been considered an important feature of eating disorder psychopathology, mentioned in the earliest recorded medical description of anorexia nervosa [20]. In people with eating disorders, unhealthy exercise is associated with poorer prognosis, including lower quality of life [52], longer inpatient hospitalisations [46], greater suicidal behaviour [45], and increased risk of relapse [6]. There is growing agreement that unhealthy exercise and related constructs are best defined based on one's qualitative relationship with exercise, rather than the quantitative amount of exercise performed, as what constitutes 'excessive' exercise will differ depending on age, fitness, and health status [8, 37]. However, to date, there is no consensus on what constitutes problematic exercise in the context of eating disorders [37]. Indeed, an array of terminology has been used to describe the unhealthy relationship with exercise often observed in people with eating disorders, such as compulsive exercise [4, 11, 25], exercise addiction [1, 17, 51], exercise dependence [3, 22], and obligatory exercise [47]. While these terms are often used interchangeably, they reflect different conceptualisations of problematic exercise behaviour: either as a behavioural addiction like gambling (exercise addiction), a dependence to exercise similar in nature to a substance dependence disorder (exercise dependence), or a behaviour that one feels obligated to perform, even in the absence of a pleasurable reward (obligatory exercise). A recent Delphi study indicated that 60% of international experts in the treatment of eating disorders preferred the term *compulsive exercise*, although it must be noted that 60% agreement did not meet their threshold for consensus (≥ 85% agreement) or near consensus (≥ 75% agreement [37]). Results from this Delphi study are consistent with other research positing that compulsive exercise offers the most theoretically sound construct to define problematic exercise in the context of eating disorders [27, 29, 43].

Compulsive exercise describes a highly driven and rigid urge to exercise, combined with a perceived inability to stop exercising, despite awareness of the risk of harm from continued exercise [49]. Estimates of the prevalence of compulsive exercise range from 16.7 to 85.3% in adolescents with eating disorders [16] and 31.9 to 80.0% in adults with eating disorders [9, 44]. Given this high crossover, the most recent clinical practice guidelines on eating disorders published by The Royal Australian and New Zealand College of Psychiatrists emphasised the importance of screening for compulsive exercise when assessing someone with a suspected eating disorder [23].

Earlier models of treatment recommended complete abstinence from exercise in underweight women for which weight restoration was the main treatment goal [21]. However, several reviews have demonstrated that performing structured exercise under supervision does not interfere with weight restoration in women with anorexia nervosa [30, 36, 53]. In fact, some exercise interventions in women with anorexia nervosa led to greater weight gain compared with those who did not exercise [5, 48]. In light of this evidence, current practice adopts a more nuanced approach, advocating for the gradual reintroduction of safe exercise into an eating disorder treatment program where appropriate [7, 10, 37].

Unhealthy exercise is also a core feature of muscle dysmorphia, an illness characterised by an intense preoccupation that one is not big enough or sufficiently muscular, despite often being significantly larger and more muscular than the average person [40, 41]. Although this phenomenon has been recognised in bodybuilding communities under the term *bigorexia* since the 1980s, it did not receive scientific attention until Pope et al. [41] identified nine bodybuilders (out of a larger sample of 108 bodybuilders) who had irrational beliefs that they were too small. Given this psychiatric presentation, the disorder was aptly labelled reverse anorexia [41]. However, it was later renamed as muscle dysmorphia and a set of diagnostic criteria was proposed that placed the compulsive need to exercise at the crux of muscle dysmorphia symptomology [40]. Although the literature on muscle dysmorphia is still in its infancy, it was recently included in the fifth edition of the Diagnostic and Statistical Manual of Mental Disorders as a specifier of body dysmorphic disorder [2], which has helped to spur additional research.

Compulsive exercise has been highlighted in the original diagnostic criteria for muscle dysmorphia [40] and a number of recent case studies on people with the disorder [31, 32]. This centrality of compulsive exercise may explain why the majority of studies on muscle dysmorphia have sampled adult male bodybuilders (e.g., [14, 26, 28, 38]). Murray et al. [33] found that men with muscle dysmorphia reported significantly greater compulsive exercise ($d = 2.6$) than male gym-goers without muscle dysmorphia and similar scores on three subscales of the Compulsive Exercise Test (avoidance and rule-driven behaviour, exercise rigidity, and mood improvement) when compared against men with anorexia nervosa. Men with muscle dysmorphia were also found to share other common features with men suffering from anorexia nervosa, including comparable weight and shape concern, appearance intolerance, and functional impairment [33]. However, it is unclear whether these concerns are similar in magnitude between men with muscle dysmorphia and women with anorexia nervosa. There is also evidence that disordered eating confers a risk factor for the development of muscle dysmorphia; Pope et al. [40] found that 22% of men with muscle dysmorphia previously met diagnostic criteria for anorexia nervosa, while Olivardia et al. [38] reported that 29% of men with muscle dysmorphia had a past diagnosis of any eating disorder. Given this intersection between muscle dysmorphia and eating disorders, some authors have argued that muscle dysmorphia should be nosologically classified as an eating disorder that captures the drive for muscularity more frequently associated with males [34, 35].

Although men with muscle dysmorphia are often admired for their self-control in maintaining strict exercise and diet practices [18], there is more to this disorder than meets the eye. Men with muscle dysmorphia report quality of life scores that are 1.7–2.6 standard deviations below community norms, indicating significant impairment to quality of life [39]. This same study also found that men with muscle dysmorphia are almost three times as likely to have attempted suicide compared to men with body dysmorphic disorder unrelated to muscularity [39], highlighting the importance of evidence-based treatment approaches.

In the past few years, there has been a rapid upsurge in the number of treatment interventions for compulsive exercise in eating disorders (e.g., [12, 24]). The majority of these studies sampled people with diagnosed anorexia nervosa (AN), bulimia nervosa (BN), eating disorder not otherwise specified (EDNOS; DSM-IV), or other specified feeding or eating disorder (OSFED; DSM-V). However, to our knowledge, no systematic review has been published summarising the existing treatment literature in eating disorder samples. One such review is urgently needed to identify the common treatment components (e.g., psychoeducation, cognitive challenging, sport therapy) driving effects across existing interventions. As compulsive exercise is also a defining characteristic of muscle dysmorphia [40], and this disorder shares many features with other eating disorders, specifically anorexia nervosa, suggesting that effective treatment components may be similar across the groups, we decided to make both eating disorders *and* muscle dysmorphia the focus of this review. Although significantly less treatment research has been conducted on muscle dysmorphia samples compared to eating disorder samples [19, 50], there is still scope to explore whether insight can be gained from the extant literature into the treatment of compulsive exercise in muscle dysmorphia.

The primary aim of this systematic review is to determine the efficacy of existing treatments for compulsive exercise in eating disorders and muscle dysmorphia. A secondary aim is to evaluate the methodological quality of included studies. We hope that findings from this review will inform evidence-based guidelines for the treatment of compulsive exercise in disorders defined by maladaptive preoccupations with body image.

Methods

Eligibility criteria

Our systematic review will be conducted according to the Preferred Reporting Items for Systematic Reviews and Meta-Analyses (PRISMA) guidelines and studies will be selected for inclusion in this review according to the criteria outlined below.

Study designs

Eligible studies must assess changes in compulsive exercise from pre- to post-intervention. This comprises studies that include a comparison group (e.g., randomised controlled trials) and those that do not include a comparison group (e.g., pilot studies and case studies). If data are reported for the same intervention across multiple studies, for example, a pilot study and a subsequent randomised controlled trial, only data from the randomised controlled trial will be extracted for narrative synthesis. Literature reviews, theoretical articles, and conference abstracts will be excluded.

Participants

We will include studies that sampled adolescents, defined as age above 10 years [42], and/or adult participants of both sexes who have been diagnosed with either an eating disorder or muscle dysmorphia. These clinical diagnoses must be determined using established diagnostic criteria, such as the Diagnostic and Statistical Manual of Mental Disorders (DSM) or the International Classification of Diseases (ICD). The list of possible eating disorder diagnoses includes AN, BN, binge eating disorder, EDNOS (DSM-IV), and OSFED (DSM-V). Although muscle dysmorphia is included in the DSM-V as a specifier of body dysmorphic disorder [2], it was not officially included in earlier versions of the DSM or any version of the ICD. Thus, we will also include studies carried out prior to publication of the DSM-V that used the diagnostic criteria for muscle dysmorphia outlined in Pope et al. [40]. Studies that used clinical cut-off scores from questionnaires to infer the presence of an eating disorder or muscle dysmorphia without a corresponding clinical interview will be excluded. Likewise, studies that sampled participants based on a self-reported diagnosis and not a formal diagnosis from a relevant medical professional will also be excluded. The presence of comorbidities (e.g., depression, generalised anxiety disorder, or obsessive-compulsive disorder) will not be used to determine inclusion or exclusion.

Interventions

Studies that used any type of biopsychosocial treatment and reported longitudinal changes in compulsive exercise will be considered for inclusion in this review. These interventions may consist of, but may not be limited to, cognitive-behavioural therapy, psychoeducation, sport therapy, structured exercise programs, physical exercise and dietary therapy, exposure and response prevention, pharmacotherapy, and multi-component strategies. Both individual and group interventions will be included. We will not place restrictions on the treatment setting, for example, inpatient, outpatient, self-help app, and web-based interventions are eligible for inclusion. There will also be no restrictions on the length of treatment or the number of treatment sessions provided over the course of the intervention.

Outcomes of interest

The primary outcome of interest in this review is changes in compulsive exercise from pre- to post-intervention. Although compulsive exercise is the preferred term to describe problematic exercise behaviour in patients with eating disorders, its use did not reach consensus in a recent Delphi study [37]. Thus, a number of other related terms will also be included as primary outcomes, including exercise addiction, exercise dependence, and obligatory exercise (see Appendix for the full list of terms used in the search strategy). We will only include studies that measured compulsive exercise or a related construct using a standardised instrument, such as the Compulsive Exercise Test [49], Exercise Addiction Inventory [17], or Obligatory Exercise Questionnaire [47]. We will exclude studies that only reported on the quantity or frequency of exercise performed without assessing the corresponding qualitative relationship with exercise. Secondary outcomes of interest in this review are changes in weight, eating disorder psychopathology, and other relevant psychological outcomes (e.g., mood and anxiety).

Search strategy and study selection

The following five electronic databases will be searched from database inception until November 2020: (1) PsycInfo, (2) MEDLINE, (3) Embase, (4) Web of Science, and (5) Scopus. These particular databases were chosen in consultation with an experienced university librarian who specialises in systematic reviews in the psychological sciences. To find additional eligible studies, the reference lists of included articles will be manually searched. Studies citing relevant articles will also be reviewed using the 'cited by' function in Google Scholar. We will conduct manual searches for unpublished and ongoing randomised controlled trials in international registers (e.g., www.clinical-trials.gov). If a relevant conference abstract is returned without a corresponding full text article, publications of the lead author will be searched. Papers are required to be peer-reviewed and written in English for inclusion in this review. We did not place restrictions on the date of publication or the geographical location where the research was conducted.

We developed a preliminary search strategy in PsycInfo that was modified in response to suggestions from the aforementioned university librarian. The final search strategy (see Appendix) comprised three clusters of terms relating to: (a) unhealthy exercise behaviour (e.g., compulsive exercise, exercise addiction, and obligatory exercise); (b) diagnostic labels for eating disorders (e.g., anorexia, bulimia, and binge eating disorder) and muscle dysmorphia; and (c) study design (e.g., intervention, treatment, and protocol).

One reviewer (JM) will screen all titles and abstracts against the eligibility criteria after removing duplicates and full texts will be obtained for papers deemed relevant or where inclusion was uncertain. Another reviewer (PA) will cross-review 20% of excluded papers, selected at random. Both reviewers (JM and PA) will review all obtained full texts against the eligibility criteria. Queries regarding eligibility of articles will be resolved through discussion with a third reviewer (SM).

Data extraction

Data from included articles will be extracted by one author (JM) and checked for accuracy by a second reviewer (PA). The following information will be extracted from each article: (a) study characteristics (title, lead author, year of publication, country, and language); (b) participant characteristics (sample size, age and sex distribution, ethnicity, socioeconomic status, type of disorder, diagnostic classification system, baseline body mass index, comorbidities, duration of illness, dropout rates); (c) study methodology (type of study, study setting, intervention description, comparison group description, length of intervention, and number of treatment sessions); (d) compulsive exercise assessment (questionnaire name, questionnaire domains reported, and assessment time points); and (e) study results (statistical measures used, and primary and secondary outcomes results reported across all time points).

Quality assessment

The methodological quality of included studies will be appraised using a modified version of the Downs and Black [13] criteria, as amended by Ferro and Speechley [15] to encompass a broad range of study designs. This modified quality checklist excluded items specific to randomised controlled trials, such as those items assessing randomisation, dropouts, blinding, and intervention integrity. The amended quality checklist had 15 items, as opposed to the original 27, and dichotomously scored items as 0 (unable to determine/no) or 1 (yes). The amended checklist assesses four domains: (1) reporting (seven items), (2) external validity (three items), (3) internal validity (four items), and (4) statistical power (one item). Scores from these four domains can be summed to determine an overall quality score for each study. The maximum checklist score for each study is 15 with higher scores (quality score > 10) indicative of greater methodological quality [15].

Two reviewers (JM and PA) will independently score all included studies after data extraction has been completed. Inter-rater agreement will be calculated using the kappa statistic. Large discrepancies in quality evaluation will be resolved through discussion with a third reviewer (SM).

Data synthesis

Results for this review will be reported using narrative synthesis. Meta-analysis was considered but is likely not feasible taking into account the heterogeneity of study designs, intervention approaches, compulsive exercise instruments, and assessment intervals. Studies receiving a higher overall quality score will be weighted more in the narrative synthesis than studies with a lower overall quality score.

Dissemination

Findings from this review will be published in a peer-reviewed scientific journal and may be presented by the lead author (JM) at national and international conferences. Data extracted from individual articles will be made available with the full manuscript.

Discussion

The aim of this systematic review is to summarise the efficacy of existing treatments for compulsive exercise in eating disorders and muscle dysmorphia. Building upon the consensus that targeted interventions are needed to address compulsive exercise in eating disorder populations [37], there has been a rapid upsurge in the number of treatment interventions. It will be useful to determine the most promising treatment components in these interventions to help inform future clinical practice guidelines.

There are a number of strengths of our method. We will include a broad range of samples (adolescents and adults), treatment approaches (e.g., CBT, sport therapy, and multi-component strategies), and study designs (e.g., randomised controlled trials, pilot studies, and case studies) to provide a complete overview of the literature. Secondly, we will conduct a detailed quality assessment of all included studies using an established assessment checklist [13], as amended by Ferro and Speechley [15] to apply to a broad range of study designs. Thirdly, we decided to review treatment interventions for muscle dysmorphia, in addition to eating disorders, as compulsive exercise is a core feature of both groups of disorders and there is a high rate of diagnostic cross-over between these illness groups. Finally, to facilitate transparency, the full search strategy that will be used to find relevant studies has been made available (see Appendix) and all data extracted from included studies will be published with the final manuscript.

The main limitation of this review is the heterogeneity in questionnaires used to assess problematic exercise behaviour. As a consequence, not all included studies will measure compulsive exercise per se, but may measure other related constructs like exercise addiction or exercise dependence. However, considering the theoretical overlap between these constructs, we do not expect substantial differences in results between studies as a function of the choice of exercise behaviour questionnaire. Moreover, due to large variations in treatment approaches, exercise questionnaires, study designs, and assessment intervals, we do not anticipate that a meta-analysis will be feasible. We also anticipate that few, if any, randomised controlled trials will be returned for samples of patients with muscle dysmorphia. Nonetheless, a systematic review of the literature is still warranted to test this supposition and highlight areas for future research in this burgeoning field of clinical psychology.

Appendix

PsycInfo Search Strategy

1. (compulsive exercise*).ti,ab,mp
2. (exercise addiction).ti,ab,mp
3. (exercise dependence).ti,ab,mp
4. (excessive exercise*).ti,ab,mp
5. (unhealthy exercise*).ti,ab,mp
6. (obligatory exercise).ti,ab,mp
7. (driven exercise).ti,ab,mp
8. (rigid exercise). ti,ab,mp
9. (exercise abuse).ti,ab,mp
10. (exercise pathology).ti,ab,mp
11. (pathological exercise).ti,ab,mp
12. overexercis*.ti,ab,mp
13. over-exercis*.ti,ab,mp
14. overtraining.ti,ab,mp
15. OTS.ti,ab,mp
16. or/1–15
17. (eating disorder*).ti,ab,mp
18. ED.ti,ab,mp
19. (disordered eating).ti,ab,mp
20. anorexia.ti,ab,mp
21. bulimia.ti,ab,mp
22. (binge eating).ti,ab,mp
23. (eating disorder not otherwise specified).ti,ab,mp
24. EDNOS.ti,ab,mp
25. (other specified feeding or eating disorder).ti,ab,mp

26. OSFED.ti,ab
27. (muscle dysmorphi*).ti,ab,mp
28. bigorexia.ti,ab,mp
29. (reverse anorexia).ti,ab,mp
30. (body dysmorph*).ti,ab,mp
31. exp. eating disorders/
32. exp. anorexia nervosa/
33. exp. bulimia/
34. exp. binge eating disorder/
35. exp. body dysmorphic disorder/
36. or/17–35
37. treatment.ti,ab,mp
38. intervention.ti,ab,mp
39. therap*.ti,ab,mp
40. program*.ti,ab,mp
41. protocol.ti,ab,mp
42. regimen.ti,ab,mp
43. exp. treatment/
44. exp. intervention/
45. or/37–44
46. 16 and 36 and 45

Acknowledgments
We would like to thank Phillipa Hay for her guidance during the brainstorming phase of this research project and Thomas Goodfellow who assisted with the search strategy. We are also thankful for Phillip Aouad who has offered to help with reviewing relevant articles for inclusion.

Authors' contributions
JM and SM developed the systematic review topic. JM wrote the manuscript. JM and SM edited the manuscript. All authors read and approved the final manuscript. SM and ST provided supervision.

Competing interests
The authors declare that they have no competing interests.

Author details
[1]Clinical Psychology Unit, School of Psychology, The University of Sydney, Sydney, Australia. [2]InsideOut Institute for Eating Disorders, The Boden Collaboration for Obesity, Nutrition, Exercise and Eating Disorders, The University of Sydney, Sydney, Australia. [3]Sydney Local Health District, NSW Health, St Leonards, Australia.

References

1. Adams J, Kirkby RJ. Excessive exercise as an addiction: a review. Addict Res Theory. 2002;10(5):415–38. https://doi.org/10.1080/1606635021000032366.
2. American Psychiatric Association. Diagnostic and statistical manual of mental disorders: DSM-5™. 5th ed. Arlington: American Psychiatric Publishing, Inc.; 2013.
3. Blaydon MJ, Lindner KJ. Eating disorders and exercise dependence in triathletes. Eat Disord. 2002;10(1):49–60. https://doi.org/10.1080/106402602753573559.
4. Bratland-Sanda S, Mathisen T, Sundgot-Borgen J, Rosenvinge J. Defining compulsive exercise in eating disorders: acknowledging the exercise paradox and exercise obsessions. J Eat Disord. 2019;7(1):8. https://doi.org/10.1186/s40337-019-0238-2.
5. Calogero RM, Pedrotty KN. The practice and process of healthy exercise: an investigation of the treatment of exercise abuse in women with eating disorders. Eat Disord. 2004;12(4):273–91. https://doi.org/10.1080/10640260490521352.
6. Carter J, Blackmore E, Sutandar-Pinnock K, Woodside B. Relapse in anorexia nervosa: a survival analysis. Psychol Med. 2004;34:671–9. https://doi.org/10.1017/S0033291703001168
7. Cook BJ, Wonderlich SA, Mitchell JE, Thompson R, Sherman R, McCallum K. Exercise in eating disorders treatment: systematic review and proposal of guidelines. Med Sci Sports Exerc. 2016;48(7):1408–14. https://doi.org/10.1249/MSS.0000000000000912.
8. Dalle Grave R. Features and management of compulsive exercising in eating disorders. Phys Sportsmed. 2009;37:20–8. https://doi.org/10.3810/psm.2009.10.1725.
9. Dalle Grave R, Calugi S, Marchesini G. Compulsive exercise to control shape or weight in eating disorders: prevalence, associated features, and treatment outcome. Compr Psychiatry. 2008;49(4):346–52. https://doi.org/10.1016/j.comppsych.2007.12.007.
10. Danielsen M, Ro O, Bjørnelv S. How to integrate physical activity and exercise approaches into inpatient treatment for eating disorders: fifteen years of clinical experience and research. J Eat Disord. 2018;6(1):34. https://doi.org/10.1186/s40337-018-0203-5.
11. Dittmer N, Jacobi C, Voderholzer U. Compulsive exercise in eating disorders: proposal for a definition and a clinical assessment. J Eat Disord. 2018;6(1):42. https://doi.org/10.1186/s40337-018-0219-x.
12. Dittmer N, Voderholzer U, Mönch C, Cuntz U, Jacobi C, Schlegl S. Efficacy of a specialized group intervention for compulsive exercise in inpatients with anorexia nervosa: a randomized controlled trial. Psychother Psychosom. 2020;89(3):161–73. https://doi.org/10.1159/000504583.
13. Downs SH, Black N. The feasibility of creating a checklist for the assessment of the methodological quality both of randomised and non-randomised studies of health care interventions. J Epidemiol Community Health. 1998; 52(6):377–84. https://doi.org/10.1136/jech.52.6.377.
14. Fabris MA, Longobardi C, Prino LE, Settanni M. Attachment style and risk of muscle dysmorphia in a sample of male bodybuilders. Psychol Men Masculinity. 2018;19(2):273–81. https://doi.org/10.1037/men0000096.
15. Ferro MA, Speechley KN. Depressive symptoms among mothers of children with epilepsy: a review of prevalence, associated factors, and impact on children. Epilepsia. 2009;50(11):2344–54. https://doi.org/10.1111/j.1528-1167.2009.02276.x.
16. Fietz M, Touyz S, Hay P. A risk profile of compulsive exercise in adolescents with an eating disorder: a systematic review. Adv Eating Disord. 2014;2(3): 241–63. https://doi.org/10.1080/21662630.2014.894470.
17. Griffiths MD, Szabo A, Terry A. The exercise addiction inventory: a quick and easy screening tool for health practitioners. Br J Sports Med. 2005;39(6):e30. https://doi.org/10.1136/bjsm.2004.017020.
18. Griffiths S, Mond JM, Murray SB, Touyz S. Positive beliefs about anorexia nervosa and muscle dysmorphia are associated with eating disorder symptomatology. Aust N Z J Psychiatry. 2015;49(9):812–20. https://doi.org/10.1177/0004867415572412.
19. Griffiths S, Murray SB. Muscle dysmorphia: clinical presentation and treatment strategies. In: Clinical handbook of complex and atypical eating disorders. New York: Oxford University Press; 2018. p. 235–52.
20. Gull WW. Anorexia nervosa (apepsia hysterica, anorexia hysterica). Obes Res. 1868;5(5):498–502. https://doi.org/10.1002/j.1550-8528.1997.tb00677.x.
21. Hausenblas HA, Cook BJ, Chittester NI. Can exercise treat eating disorders? Exerc Sport Sci Rev. 2008;36(1):43–7. https://doi.org/10.1097/jes.0b013e31815e4040.
22. Hausenblas HA, Downs DS. Exercise dependence: a systematic review. Psychol Sport Exerc. 2002;3(2):89–123. https://doi.org/10.1016/S1469-0292(00)00015-7.
23. Hay P, Chinn D, Forbes D, Madden S, Newton R, Sugenor L, et al. Royal Australian and new Zealand College of Psychiatrists clinical practice guidelines for the treatment of eating disorders. Aust N Z J Psychiatry. 2014; 48(11):977–1008. https://doi.org/10.1177/0004867414555814.
24. Hay P, Touyz S, Arcelus J, Pike K, Attia E, Crosby RD, et al. A randomized controlled trial of the compuLsive exercise activity TheraPy (LEAP): a new approach to compulsive exercise in anorexia nervosa. Int J Eat Disord. 2018; 51(8):999–1004. https://doi.org/10.1002/eat.22920.
25. Lichtenstein MB, Hinze CJ, Emborg B, Thomsen F, Hemmingsen SD. Compulsive exercise: links, risks and challenges faced. Psychol Res Behav Manag. 2017;10:85–95. https://doi.org/10.2147/prbm.S113093.
26. Longobardi C, Prino LE, Fabris MA, Settanni M. Muscle dysmorphia and psychopathology: findings from an Italian sample of male bodybuilders. Psychiatry Res. 2017;256:231–6. https://doi.org/10.1016/j.psychres.2017.06.065.

27. Meyer C, Taranis L. Exercise in the eating disorders: terms and definitions. Eur Eat Disord Rev. 2011;19(3):169–73. https://doi.org/10.1002/erv.1121.
28. Mitchell L, Murray SB, Hoon M, Hackett D, Prvan T, O'Connor H. Correlates of muscle dysmorphia symptomatology in natural bodybuilders: distinguishing factors in the pursuit of hyper-muscularity. Body Image. 2017; 22:1–5. https://doi.org/10.1016/j.bodyim.2017.04.003.
29. Mond JM, Hay PJ, Rodgers B, Owen C. An update on the definition of "excessive exercise" in eating disorders research. Int J Eat Disord. 2006;39(2): 147–53. https://doi.org/10.1002/eat.20214.
30. Moola FJ, Gairdner SE, Amara CE. Exercise in the care of patients with anorexia nervosa: a systematic review of the literature. Ment Health Phys Act. 2013;6(2):59–68. https://doi.org/10.1016/j.mhpa.2013.04.002.
31. Murray SB, Griffiths S. Adolescent muscle dysmorphia and family-based treatment: a case report. Clin Child Psychol Psychiatry. 2015;20(2):324–30. https://doi.org/10.1177/1359104514521639.
32. Murray SB, Maguire S, Russell J, Touyz SW. The emotional regulatory features of bulimic episodes and compulsive exercise in muscle dysmorphia: a case report. Eur Eat Disord Rev. 2012a;20(1):68–73. https://doi.org/10.1002/erv.1088.
33. Murray SB, Rieger E, Hildebrandt T, Karlov L, Russell J, Boon E, et al. A comparison of eating, exercise, shape, and weight related symptomatology in males with muscle dysmorphia and anorexia nervosa. Body Image. 2012b;9(2):193–200. https://doi.org/10.1016/j.bodyim.2012.01.008.
34. Murray SB, Rieger E, Touyz SW, De la Garza García Lic Y. Muscle dysmorphia and the DSM-V conundrum: where does it belong? A review paper. Int J Eat Disord. 2010;43(6):483–91. https://doi.org/10.1002/eat.20828.
35. Murray SB, Touyz SW. Muscle dysmorphia: towards a diagnostic consensus. Aust N Z J Psychiatry. 2013;47(3):206–7. https://doi.org/10.1177/0004867412452018.
36. Ng LW, Ng DP, Wong WP. Is supervised exercise training safe in patients with anorexia nervosa? A meta-analysis. Physiotherapy. 2013;99(1):1–11. https://doi.org/10.1016/j.physio.2012.05.006.
37. Noetel M, Dawson L, Hay P, Touyz S. The assessment and treatment of unhealthy exercise in adolescents with anorexia nervosa: a Delphi study to synthesize clinical knowledge. Int J Eat Disord. 2017;50(4):378–88. https://doi.org/10.1002/eat.22657.
38. Olivardia R, Pope HG Jr, Hudson JI. Muscle dysmorphia in male weightlifters: a case-control study. Am J Psychiatr. 2000;157(8):1291–6. https://doi.org/10.1176/appi.ajp.157.8.1291.
39. Pope CG, Pope HG, Menard W, Fay C, Olivardia R, Phillips KA. Clinical features of muscle dysmorphia among males with body dysmorphic disorder. Body Image. 2005;2(4):395–400. https://doi.org/10.1016/j.bodyim.2005.09.001.
40. Pope HG, Gruber AJ, Choi P, Olivardia R, Phillips KA. Muscle dysmorphia: an underrecognized form of body dysmorphic disorder. Psychosomatics. 1997; 38(6):548–57. https://doi.org/10.1016/S0033-3182(97)71400-2.
41. Pope HG, Katz DL, Hudson JI. Anorexia nervosa and "reverse anorexia" among 108 male bodybuilders. Compr Psychiatry. 1993;34(6):406–9. https://doi.org/10.1016/0010-440x(93)90066-d.
42. Sawyer SM, Azzopardi PS, Wickremarathne D, Patton GC. The age of adolescence. Lancet Child Adolesc Health. 2018;2(3):223–8. https://doi.org/10.1016/s2352-4642(18)30022-1.
43. Scharmer C, Gorrell S, Schaumberg K, Anderson D. Compulsive exercise or exercise dependence? Clarifying conceptualizations of exercise in the context of eating disorder pathology. Psychol Sport Exerc. 2020;46:101586. https://doi.org/10.1016/j.psychsport.2019.101586.
44. Shroff H, Reba L, Thornton LM, Tozzi F, Klump KL, Berrettini WH, et al. Features associated with excessive exercise in women with eating disorders. Int J Eat Disord. 2006;39(6):454–61. https://doi.org/10.1002/eat.20247.
45. Smith AR, Fink EL, Anestis MD, Ribeiro JD, Gordon KH, Davis H, et al. Exercise caution: over-exercise is associated with suicidality among individuals with disordered eating. Psychiatry Res. 2013;206(2–3):246–55. https://doi.org/10.1016/j.psychres.2012.11.004.
46. Solenberger SE. Exercise and eating disorders: a 3-year inpatient hospital record analysis. Eat Behav. 2001;2(2):151–68. https://doi.org/10.1016/s1471-0153(01)00026-5.
47. Steffen JJ, Brehm BJ. The dimensions of obligatory exercise. Eat Disord. 1999;7(3):219–26. https://doi.org/10.1080/10640269908249287.
48. Szabo CP, Green K. Hospitalized anorexics and resistance training: impact on body composition and psychological well-being. A preliminary study. Eat Weight Disord. 2002;7(4):293–7. https://doi.org/10.1007/bf03324975.
49. Taranis L, Touyz S, Meyer C. Disordered eating and exercise: development and preliminary validation of the compulsive exercise test (CET). Eur Eat Disord Rev. 2011;19(3):256–68. https://doi.org/10.1002/erv.1108.
50. Tod D, Edwards C, Cranswick I. Muscle dysmorphia: current insights. Psychol Res Behav Manag. 2016;9:179–88. https://doi.org/10.2147/PRBM.S97404.
51. Trott M, Jackson SE, Firth J, Jacob L, Grabovac I, Mistry A, et al. A comparative meta-analysis of the prevalence of exercise addiction in adults with and without indicated eating disorders. Eat Weight Disord. 2020. https://doi.org/10.1007/s40519-019-00842-1.
52. Young S, Touyz S, Meyer C, Arcelus J, Rhodes P, Madden S, et al. Relationships between compulsive exercise, quality of life, psychological distress and motivation to change in adults with anorexia nervosa. J Eat Disord. 2018;6(1). https://doi.org/10.1186/s40337-018-0188-0.
53. Zunker C, Mitchell JE, Wonderlich SA. Exercise interventions for women with anorexia nervosa: a review of the literature. Int J Eat Disord. 2011;44(7):579–84. https://doi.org/10.1002/eat.20862.

12

Physical activity behaviors and attitudes among women with an eating disorder: a qualitative study

Jennifer Brunet[1,2,3*], Francis Del Duchetto[1,4] and Amanda Wurz[5]

Abstract

Background: Physical activity (PA) is an integral part of healthcare for the general population and individuals with psychiatric disorders. However, PA is significantly more complex for and related to both healthy (e.g., reduced anxiety and depressive symptoms) and unhealthy outcomes (e.g., intrusive, repetitive thoughts that lead to abnormally high levels of PA) among women with an eating disorder (ED). Consequently, many healthcare professionals recommend abstinence from PA during ED treatment. Despite this, women may remain engaged in PA during ED treatment or resume PA shortly thereafter. Little has been done to understand women's PA behaviors and attitudes and to explore how they integrate PA into their lives during and after ED treatment. Thus, this study sought to explore PA behaviors and attitudes among women with an ED.

Methods: Nine women who self-reported receiving an ED diagnosis participated in semi-structured interviews, which were transcribed and analysed thematically.

Results: Six interrelated themes were constructed to represent participants' PA experiences: *PA as a lifestyle, PA can be beneficial, How I feel when I can't do PA, Being cautious about PA, Reactions to healthcare professionals' practice of recommending abstinence from PA during ED treatment*, and *PA programming thoughts*.

Conclusions: Overcoming dysfunctional PA behaviors (e.g., engaging in abnormally high levels of PA) and attitudes (e.g., associating PA with caloric expenditure) can be a long and complicated journey for women with an ED. Nevertheless, women with an ED want PA to be integrated into their ED treatment protocol for two key reasons, namely to accrue the benefits associated with PA and to learn how to engage in PA in adaptive and healthy ways.

Keywords: Exercise, Women, Anorexia nervosa, Binge-eating disorder, Bulimia nervosa, Thematic analysis

Plain English Summary

Physical activity (PA) can be beneficial to the physical and mental health of women with an eating disorder (ED). However, little is known about women's PA behaviors and attitudes. Moreover, many healthcare professionals adopt the practice of recommending abstinence from PA during ED treatment. Despite this, women may remain engaged in PA during ED treatment or resume PA shortly thereafter. This study offers perspectives from nine women with an ED to better understand their PA behaviors and attitudes and to gain insight into how they integrated PA into their lives during and/or after ED treatment. Overall, the women's accounts reveal that overcoming dysfunctional PA behaviors (e.g., engaging in abnormally high levels of PA) and attitudes (e.g., associating PA with caloric expenditure) can be a long and complicated journey. At the same time, however, they

* Correspondence: jennifer.brunet@uottawa.ca
[1]School of Human Kinetics, University of Ottawa, 125 University Private, Montpetit Hall, Room 339, Ottawa, Ontario K1N 6N5, Canada
[2]Cancer Therapeutics Program, Ottawa Hospital Research Institute, 1053 Carling Avenue, Ottawa, Ontario K1Y 4E9, Canada
Full list of author information is available at the end of the article

suggest the benefits of PA warrant further consideration. In addition, the women expressed a desire for PA to be integrated into their ED treatment protocol when possible so they accrue benefits and learn how to engage in PA in adaptive and healthy ways.

Introduction

Eating disorders (EDs) are the most prevalent psychiatric disorder diagnosed in women [1]. The American Psychiatric Association [2] describes eight different feeding and EDs that share defining features, including obsessive preoccupations about food, body shape, and body weight: anorexia nervosa, bulimia nervosa, binge-eating disorder, pica, rumination disorder, avoidant/restrictive food intake disorder, other specified feeding or ED, and unspecified feeding or ED. There are also common behaviors associated with EDs, such as counting calories, frequent weighing/body checking, and hyperactivity [2]. EDs can have a negative impact on physical and psychosocial health. Indeed, physical complications arising from EDs can affect every organ system. Bradycardia, hypotension, anemia, hormonal imbalance, and low bone mass are just some of the negative physical effects commonly observed [3–7]. Also, EDs are associated with high rates of anxiety, depression, body image issues, and obsessive-compulsive disorders [8–10]. Whilst treatments such as pharmacological treatment, nutrition counselling, and cognitive behavioral therapy can help women manage their ED, many continue to experience compromised physical and psychosocial health, consequently re-accessing healthcare for years following their diagnosis [11, 12]. Identifying adjunct therapeutic approaches is necessary to improve both physical and psychosocial health in this population.

The physical and psychosocial health benefits of physical activity (PA), which is defined as any bodily movement that is produced by skeletal muscles that results in energy expenditure[1] and includes exercise [a subset of PA that is planned, structured and repetitive, with the objective of improving or maintaining physical fitness [13]], suggest it may be a potentially effective therapeutic adjunct to ED treatment to improve health. Literature reviews [14–19] and a meta-analysis [20] conclude that PA can be safe and beneficial for women with an ED, provided their nutritional needs are met. Furthermore, experimental studies report decreased compulsive PA, reduced drive for thinness and bulimic symptoms, improved body satisfaction, facilitated weight gain, enhanced muscular strength, and reversed cardiac abnormalities among women with an ED who engage in PA [21–23]. Additionally, PA can enhance mood, quality of life, and well-being among women with an ED [24, 25]. Last, PA can promote bone health [26], which is beneficial to women with anorexia nervosa because they often have decreased bone mass, impaired bone structure, and reduced bone strength [27].

Though the benefits of PA are notable, women with an ED may struggle to find a balanced approach to PA, with some being highly sedentary [e.g., many with binge eating disorder [28, 29]]. Others, however, engage in abnormally high levels of PA and feel anxious when unable to engage in PA [30, 31]. Some women with anorexia nervosa have described feeling addicted to PA such that their workouts remain unchanged despite social obligations or physical illness/injuries [32, 33]. Women with bulimia nervosa have also reported engaging in PA to compensate for energy surpluses due to binge eating in order to prevent weight gain and/or to regulate negative affect [30, 31, 34]. Anywhere from 30 to 80% of people with an ED engage in abnormally high levels of PA [35, 36], which is problematic because it has been associated with increased hospitalisation length, higher rates of inpatient dropout, compromised treatment efficacy, increased risk of relapse and chronicity, and increased psychological comorbidity [37–41]. Moreover, abnormally high levels of PA are associated with severe physical complications [e.g., absence of menstruation, reduced bone density, chronic energy deficit, reduced levels of growth hormone and insulin-like growth factor, increased levels of the stress hormone cortisol, changes to the microarchitectural skeletal structure, increased fracture risk, increased catecholamines and ghrelin, decreased leptin and thyroid hormones [42, 43]. Because PA is often a significant component of anorexia nervosa and other EDs, continuing to engage in PA before making significant progress during recovery could serve to maintain the obsessive-compulsive aspects of the ED. Consequently, many healthcare professionals may by wary of the risk-benefit ratio associated with PA, hesitate to formally address PA during the course of ED treatment, and understandably recommend abstinence from PA during ED treatment [44, 45]. Nevertheless, the practice of recommending abstinence from PA during ED treatment has been questioned [46] and many women remain engaged in PA during ED treatment or resume PA shortly thereafter to self-regulate, manage problematic feelings, and accrue the benefits associated with PA [33, 47]. Thus, it is important to help women establish a healthy relationship with PA at some point during ED treatment.

Whilst concerns about addressing PA during ED treatment continue to grow given that women with an ED can exhibit dysfunctional PA behaviors and hold different attitudes and motives for PA as compared to women without an ED [48, 49], little has been done to explore in-depth women's PA behaviors and attitudes and to understand how they integrate PA into their lives during

[1]Henceforth, the broader term of 'PA' will be used to describe all bodily movement, whether structured or unstructured.

and after ED treatment. An exception is Moola, Gairdner and Amara's [24] qualitative study in which they interviewed 11 women with anorexia nervosa about their PA experiences. Their findings revealed that women with anorexia nervosa have a complex relationship with PA over the course of their illness, with marked shifts in PA motives – ranging from intrinsically pleasurable pursuits (e.g., walking with friends) to instrumental outcomes (e.g., weight loss). Notwithstanding these contributions, there remains a lack of exploration of women's perspectives. In an attempt to extend Moola et al.'s [24] research, the aim of this study was to explore PA behaviors and attitudes among women who self-reported having been diagnosed with any type of ED. In turn, the information gained in this study could be used in practice to help women with an ED avoid engaging in abnormally high levels of PA, and instead engage in safe and appropriate amounts of PA once they have been cleared by their healthcare team.

Methods

A constructivist-interpretative research paradigm, as coined by Denzin and Lincoln [50], was adopted. This paradigm assumes a relativist ontology (i.e., multiple realities exist). Further, it assumes a subjective epistemology (i.e., knowledge is subjective and co-created). As such, a qualitative methodology using dialectical techniques for data collection and interpretation was used herein.

Participants

Purposeful sampling was used to identify and select information-rich cases who had firsthand experience with an ED. Accordingly, adult women who were willing to communicate their experiences were identified and selected based on the following criteria: (i) self-reported having been diagnosed with an ED by a healthcare professional, (ii) available to participate in this study, and (iii) able to read, understand, provide informed consent, and complete this study in English. Of note, no limit was imposed on type of ED and age to help ensure that the insights and experiences of women with varying ED diagnoses and ages could be captured. Moreover, the rationale behind recruiting women with varying ED diagnoses was to obtain a broad and comprehensive understanding of this phenomenon to lay a foundation for those wishing to continue this line of inquiry.

Sample size

Experts contend that there is no definitive numerical recommendation for determining sample size in qualitative research. Thus, the widely-used criterion of saturation was used. Specifically, Saunders et al.'s [51] notion of *data saturation* was used such that saturation was monitored continuously throughout recruitment and data collection, and sampling was discontinued when no additional information appeared to be forthcoming (i.e., no new information was heard or uncovered from the ongoing interviews). Following this criterion, potential participants were approached until data saturation was achieved; this was achieved after the seventh interview. However, two additional interviews were conducted with women who had expressed interest in this study before the seventh interview was conducted. Data from all interviewed women were analysed, yielding a total sample size of nine.

Procedures and data collection

Before recruitment began, ethics approval for this study was obtained from the University of Ottawa and administrative permission was obtained from the Hopewell Eating Disorder Support Centre – a community-based support centre for individuals diagnosed with an ED. A convenience sample of women with any type of ED was recruited by distributing information about this study through staff and placing posters at the Hopewell Eating Disorder Support Centre. Women were given information about this study and screened over the phone by FDD.

After providing written informed consent, participants completed a survey. The survey consisted of three sections. The first section served to collect self-reported personal information including age, ED diagnosis, height and weight (used to compute body mass index; BMI), and stage of treatment. The second section consisted of the Eating Attitudes Test-26 [EAT-26 [52]– a widely used self-report measure of symptoms and concerns characteristic of EDs. The third section consisted of the Exercise Dependence Scale-21 [EDS-21 [53]– a self-report measure widely used to determine risk for exercise dependence based on criteria presented in the Diagnostic and Statistical Manual of Mental Disorders. The data from all three sections were collected to describe the sample.

Once the survey was completed, participants took part in one face-to-face semi-structured interview. All interviews were arranged and conducted by FDD who had personal experience with women with an ED and had received training in qualitative methods (see below). FDD's knowledge, skills, and experience positioned him ideally to develop rapport with participants and exchange with them about their PA experiences within the context of an ED. During the interview, participants were asked a series of open-ended questions informed by the research aim [54]. After some introductory questions were asked to initiate conversation and establish rapport between FDD and participants, interview questions focused on participants' PA behaviors and attitudes. Participants were encouraged to deviate from the interview questions and discuss experiences that had significant meaning to them. Follow-up questions and probes were used to elicit more information, ask for further reflection, depth or context, and/or to clarify statements. All interviews ended with an opportunity for participants to make final comments and/or add additional pertinent information. The interviews lasted on average 80 min, were audio-recorded, and took place at the University of Ottawa in a private room. Participants received $25 CAD for participating in this study.

Prior to collecting data for this study, FDD tested the interview guide with three women who had a problematic relationship with food at some point in their lifetime, but fell short of meeting ED diagnostic criteria. The test interviews were conducted to determine if the questions were neutral, clear, facilitated open-ended responses, and flowed well. Additionally, the test interviews provided FDD an opportunity to practice developing follow-up questions and probes. Based on feedback obtained during the test interviews, some of the questions were revised, re-worded, and re-ordered prior to data collection.

Data analysis

Responses to the survey were analysed using descriptive statistics. For the EAT-26, total scores were computed and participants were classified as *positive* if they scored at or above 20 on the EAT-26, indicating a high level of concern about dieting, body weight, or problematic eating behaviors; otherwise, participants who scored less than 20 were classified as *negative*. For the EDS-21, total scores were computed and participants were classified into one of the three groups using the EDS-21 scoring manual that consists of flowchart decision rules, in which items or combinations of items determined if they should be classified in the dependent, symptomatic, or asymptomatic range on each of the seven Diagnostic and Statistical Manual of Mental Disorders criteria.

The interviews were transcribed verbatim and analysed inductively using thematic analysis [55]. First, JB and AW read each transcript thoroughly several times and took notes of initial thoughts. Next, they generated codes of salient features based on their judgement and relevance to the research aim. Third, they convened to discuss their findings and group similar codes into themes. Fourth, they labelled themes and prepared a table of themes in which subthemes were nested with supporting anonymised quotes to promote resonance. Fifth, they prepared descriptions for each theme.

Study rigor

Various strategies were followed to enhance the quality of this study [56, 57]. First, the interview guide comprised open-ended questions that allowed participants to enunciate what was important for them. Relatedly, the interview guide was decided upon by two experienced qualitative researchers from different disciplines (i.e., PA psychology and eating disorders) and by FDD allowing for triangulation between researchers. Third, JB and AW engaged in an exhaustive, systematic, and reflective analysis of the data. They also engaged in critical discussions while developing themes and subthemes, continuously reflecting upon and exploring multiple and alternative interpretations of the data. To this end, they listened to each other's interpretations of the data, offered each other critical feedback, and encouraged reflexivity by challenging each other's interpretations. Fourth, quotes are presented to give participants a voice, support the analysis, and allow readers to judge the authors' interpretations of the data. Fifth, participants shared the common experience of being diagnosed with an ED, and were able to communicate their experiences in an articulate, expressive, and reflective manner. Sixth, FDD received in-depth training to develop an understanding of the interview process, to practice his interviewing skills, and enhance his competence when speaking with women with an ED. To this end, he immersed himself in the literature, was given specific training by JB (a knowledgeable and experienced qualitative researcher), completed three test interviews wherein he received critical feedback, and transcribed each interview prior to subsequent interviews to gain insight into how to improve his interviewing skills. Finally, the authors acknowledged and reflected on their preconceptions, life experiences, and knowledge of the literature as they met with participants (FDD), read the transcripts and analysed the data (JB and AW), and interpreted the results (JB, FDD, AW) [see Additional file 1 for reflexivity statement].

Results

Participants

Nine women (M_{age} = 27.9; range = 19–56 years) participated in this study. The survey data (i.e., participants' age, ED diagnosis, stage of treatment, BMI, EAT-26 scores, and EDS-21 scores) are presented in Table 1. These data demonstrate that participants presented with varying symptoms and concerns that are characteristic of EDs (see Table 1, column 6 for EAT-26 scores), as well as with varying risks for exercise dependence (see Table 1, column 7 for EDS-21 scores).

Main results

The PA behaviors and attitudes collectively held by participants are presented in two sections. The first section, *PA behavior*, describes how active participants were when they were interviewed. The second section, *PA attitudes and experiences*, describes six overarching themes

Table 1 Participants' characteristics ($N = 9$)

Pseudonym	Age (years)	Self-reported ED diagnosis	Stage of treatment	BMI (kg/m^2)	EAT-26 scores / classification[a]	EDS-21 scores / classification[a]
Sarah	29	Anorexia nervosa	Recovery	19.42	5 / Negative	49 / Nondependent-symptomatic
Teresa	22	Anorexia nervosa	In-treatment	NR	32 / Positive	99 / At-risk for exercise dependence
Diane	56	Binge ED	Recovery	42.28	17 / Negative	40 / Nondependent-asymptomatic
Karen	25	Anorexia nervosa	Recovery	16.82	44 / Positive	58 / Nondependent-symptomatic
Julie	30	Bulimia nervosa	In-treatment	25.88	14 / Positive	44 / Nondependent-symptomatic
Donna	20	Anorexia nervosa	Recovery	19.73	53 / Positive	88 / At-risk for exercise dependence
Anna	30	Bulimia nervosa	Relapse / Seeking treatment	26.57	35 / Positive	60 / Nondependent-symptomatic
Isabelle	19	Other specified feeding or ED	Recovery	24.89	16 / Negative	48 / Nondependent-asymptomatic
Maude	20	Anorexia nervosa	Recovery	NR	7 / Negative	55 / Nondependent-symptomatic

Notes. BMI Body mass index, *ED* Eating disorder, *EAT-26* Eating Attitudes Test-26, *EDS-21* Exercise Dependence Scale-21, *NR* not reported

[a] See **Data analysis** section for classification details

and subthemes (indicated in italics in the text below) that resulted from the analysis of the interviews. This is followed by a third section, *PA programming thoughts*, which describes participants' thoughts about PA programming for women with an ED. Supporting, anonymised quotes for each section are presented in Tables 2, 3, 4, respectively. In the quotes, [...] signifies text that was removed for clarity.

Section 1: PA behavior

Participants were generally committed to PA regardless of their ED diagnosis and stage of treatment, though

Table 2 A snapshot of participants' PA behavior ($N = 9$)

Very Active	Sarah (anorexia nervosa): *"PA. So it's my way to get to work. I live about 10 km from where I work, and I usually bike or run to work so it's my main mode of transportation. And I also started competing again this year in road racing. So I deliberately exercise. Like my training is separate because [...] when I'm training, I have something that I need to accomplish like a defined goal at the end of it. And then when I'm commuting, it's PA to get to work."* Teresa (anorexia nervosa): *"I basically just do biking and that's usually like only 25 min. If I'm going to the gym, then I would do like 1 h of full-body weights workout and then if I'm not going to the gym but like going to a class, it tends to be like the group power class that focuses more on strength, but still has a cardio component. I do probably 5 days of PA ranging between 5 days of intentional PA where I'm at the gym and then the other days I would just probably try to get in some more walking. So it ranges from like 1 h to like 1 h and 45 min if I'm at the gym. Also, my goal is to go for a walk every day and the walk is about 40 min and I do 6 to 10 min of interval training every day and when I'm really feeling happy, I also do some Tai Chi and also do some muscle strengthening exercises for certain parts of my body."* Teresa (anorexia nervosa) Diane (binge ED): *"I go for a walk for about 160 min per week and then interval training is [...] 208 min total [per week]. I do a mix of PA and exercise. Exercise simply for exercise is about 50 min per week because it's the interval training. [...] Everything else I call PA but even my walking you know sometimes I walk with people who walk really fast and that's a cardiovascular workout."* Julie (bulimia nervosa): *"5 days a week at the moment. I do have a set routine. It's usually 30 to 45 min. Usually alternating between running or swimming. A lot of cardio. I try to incorporate weight lifting in a circuit training in once a week. And they [activities] are tied to social things so I have a swim class that I joined."* Donna (anorexia nervosa): *"Now I'm going towards 4 or 5 days a week for I think 1 h and a bit every time. So 5 to 6 h [per week]. [...] Usually it's just going to a gym, going on machines. Rowing or elliptical or treadmill to warm up and then just doing a bunch of weights. It depends what day it is. I do focus on groups. On one day, I just do shoulders, on another day, I do legs."*
Somewhat active	Karen (anorexia nervosa): *"I walk every day. I do yoga about every day and then again. I'm just up on my feet and active at work and that's about it. Usually 1 h of walking and then 20 or 30 min of yoga."* Anna (bulimia nervosa): *"1 h 6 days per week. Walking only."* Isabelle (other specified feeding or ED): *"Now, I guess I just go for a 30-min walk per day or maybe 1 h-long. [...] I haven't been really doing much in the past couple of weeks."*
Irregularly active	Maude (anorexia nervosa) *"If I want to exercise, I exercise. If I'm too tired or sick, I don't. [Now, I] do body [workout] and I do cardio."*

Note. ED Eating disorder, PA Physical activity

Table 3 *Quotes for themes related to participants' PA attitudes and experiences*

Themes	Subthemes	Quotes
PA as a lifestyle		Sarah (anorexia nervosa): *"It's probably like an 8 [out of 10]. It's a big part of everything. I think it's just a part of a way of being for me. It doesn't feel like I need to do anything extra. It just feels I need to do something that's just a part of my normal routine because it's just been ingrained for so long."* Donna (anorexia nervosa): *"I think it's important for your body to move around just so you're not doing nothing all day. You need to move around. That's what your body is meant to do. You can't just sit down and do nothing. I just think it's important to just workout and be healthy."* Teresa (anorexia nervosa): *"Exercise is one of the main focuses of my life. I grew up being very active playing sports and stuff. […] I guess [PA is] bringing some identity back to me because I feel like I was always the athletic one in school. It's important now that I can maybe start to reclaim some of that and be like 'Hey, you are still sporty and athletic and physically fit or whatever."* Karen (anorexia nervosa): *"There was just so much sports in my childhood. It was such a big part of my life. Growing up being that active, now I just want to be active because it's just part of my life, it's a part of me."* Diane (binge ED): *"As a kid and young adult I had not made it a priority. Nobody really ever helped me learn how to be physically active as a regular part of my life. But now, I need to make a priority. I'm proud of myself because it's all coming from me, nobody really ever helped me learn how to be physically active as regular part of my life."*
PA can be beneficial	Physical benefits	Diane (binge ED): *"I'm much healthier when I'm physically active. My body just feels good. I generally feel even if it's something that made me tired, I feel more energetic. I mean there are a lot of reasons. It means keeping my body able to move. It means cardiovascular health and it means to have enough strength to do what I want to do. It means flexibility and balance, everything that comes together that allows me to do the things that I want to do."* Maude (anorexia nervosa): *"I used to have asthma and doing exercise helped me to get rid of it and it keeps me strong and healthy and everything. I also want to live longer. I'm really interested in health in general. PA means taking care my body, my health."* Anna (bulimia nervosa): *"If I'm being completely honest, I would probably say I prefer exercising to lose weight because it makes me feel better about myself and makes me feel back in control."*
	Psychosocial benefits	Teresa (anorexia nervosa): *"Like reducing stress or if I'm upset about something then just going for a run is a really nice way to clear my mind. It's also been a really positive thing in a lot of times in my life. It has kept me, in a sense mentally, not sane* per se, *because I wouldn't say that I was ever like crazy or anything, but it just really eased a lot of my stress and anxiety around school or my body image."* Sarah (anorexia nervosa): *"I feel like I have a better time processing emotions if I'm exercising. I just feel calmer overall. I don't feel anxiety that much, and I don't feel stressed or worried as much as when I don't exercise."* Isabelle (other specified feeding or ED): *"I do think that I can feel a little bit better about myself when I do exercise. When I do exercise, I'm not a total waste of space. I feel like I have a little bit more control over my life. It helps my depression because of the serotonin."* Karen (anorexia nervosa): *"Like it has a good effect on my brain for sure. It releases endorphins and I feel good doing it. So when I'm active, I feel better. A healthy amount of exercise can be really really good for my mental health. It releases endorphins and I feel good about using my body."* Diane (binge ED): *"It's another factor that gives me a great sense of satisfaction and even joy, and as I say pride when I walk."* Julie (bulimia nervosa): *"I try to make it a social thing so it's not an isolating activity. I go for a run with a friend, go hiking with groups of friends."* Maude (anorexia nervosa): *"It has kind of opened up my social circle because I do Zumba in groups."*
	PA helps with ED management	Teresa (anorexia nervosa): *"Exercise plays such a central role in my ED and my ED kind of consumes my entire life. Exercise has really been like a helpful coping mechanism for me."* Diane (binge ED): *"My eating is more under control. I feel less necessity to binge and I'm more in touch with the real world. I found that I binge less*

Table 3 *Quotes for themes related to participants' PA attitudes and experiences (Continued)*

Themes	Subthemes	Quotes
		when I walk in particular. A huge part of the reason that I binge is that I'm feeling empty, lonely, bored, not a very useful person, all kind of negative sort of thoughts. And simply when I get lots of PA, I have far fewer of those thoughts. So it's a big influence on my kind of eating habits or ED." Julie (bulimia nervosa): *"It keeps my appetite regular. I'm less likely to binge and purge. [...] It's a component of the management of my ED. For me, it manages my appetite. I feel like I eat more normal meals at normal times and don't get as frequent an urge to binge. It manages my moods if I've had a rough day at work. Instead of going home and binging, I can go for a run and I feel a lot better afterwards. So it's been a helpful component of it."*
How I feel when I can't do PA	Physical effects	Diane (binge ED): *"If I don't get enough PA, first of all I get more pain. Secondly, I cannot then do the things I want. All of life becomes a chore if I'm not physically healthy."* Anna (bulimia nervosa): *"Kind of gross. It's a lot of like feeling like I'm losing that control I had and there's not much I can do about it. If it's for a while, then I can feel myself gaining the weight or losing the muscle. It just kind of feels like it's downhill from there. It's not really about not doing PA, it's more about losing the things that PA gives me. So like putting on a pair of jeans that are getting a little too tight because you're not doing what you're supposed to be doing and then kind of just feeling that if you're laying down on the couch and you're like 'I should not be doing this right now. I should be doing something else' and then it gets pretty stressful."*
	Psychosocial effects	Donna (anorexia nervosa): *"I feel really bad. If I have 1 day when I don't workout, I sometimes feel I didn't do anything even if I went to school or I went to work or something. [...] I saw some of my friends way less when I stopped going to the gym because that was something social too."* Sarah (anorexia nervosa): *"I just did not exercise for a week and I noticed a difference in term of like my attitude. It was like more negative and it felt like things were weighting on me heavier. So, it's difficult to be inactive."* Karen (anorexia nervosa): *"I'm not happy when I'm stagnant."* Teresa (anorexia nervosa): *"If I don't engage in PA and I'm 'that' size, then I feel shitty about it and feel like I should be smaller."*
	Effects on ED management	Teresa (anorexia nervosa): *"I get antsy when I am inactive. 1 or 2 days, then I think 'I am busy, I'm doing other things.' On day 3, I think 'I'm not taking care really. I should probably be getting back onto my routine.' By day 4, I think 'I'm having issues managing my ED.' I feel if I am not exercising, it is not a compulsion, but I can recognise that I have trouble managing my mood, trouble recognising my hunger cues. All these things that come up when I am not exercising regularly."* Sarah (anorexia nervosa): *"I know that the times where I know I'm going to be inactive, are times where I have to be vigilant of relapse."*
Being cautious about PA	Changing PA habits	Julie (bulimia nervosa): *"Although exercise helps, I don't want it to become something that I focus on to a point that it's detrimental. So, I am more conscious of the fact that if I am exercising for more than 30 or 45 min, it is being excessive. Also, I am conscious of trying to go to the gym 3 times a week."* Sarah (anorexia nervosa): *"I think it's just being really careful and honest with myself about where I'm at because sometimes I want to say like '10 more minutes but then I have to reel myself back in."* Teresa (anorexia nervosa): *"Now, it's definitely not as intense as it used to be. [...] I take rest days every week and I limit the amount of time I spend at the gym, I limit the intensity of my exercise. I don't force myself to go when I really don't want to go".* Maude (anorexia nervosa): *"I like doing it so I'll try to make time for it, but if I really don't have time or I'm tired or whatever, I'm like 'Okay, no you have to listen to your body' and I don't do it. My body knows best."* Donna (anorexia nervosa): *"I make sure that I don't go 2 days in a row. So, it's either every second day or you know. I still don't spend as much time as I used to go. I do different things. I'm not just on the cardio machines for 60 min at the highest."* Karen (anorexia nervosa): *"I loved running before the onset of my ED and at certain points in my recovery, but right now because I've only been out of the hospital for 3 months, I don't feel that I can run yet because I feel that if I run it will turn into a symptom. But I hope that one day I can run again and not feel it's for my ED and that I actually enjoy it."*

Table 3 *Quotes for themes related to participants' PA attitudes and experiences (Continued)*

Themes	Subthemes	*Quotes*
		Diane (binge ED): *"I'm not someone that goes overboard on PA. I don't really push myself. I'm not a marathon runner. I wouldn't go hiking for 8 h. I don't climb mountains. I don't do anything extreme."* Anna (bulimia nervosa): *"I don't feel that I'm overactive now because they say to get 1 h of activity per day. That's what I've heard. And I don't feel like I'm overdoing myself, like overworking myself. It doesn't feel excessive to me."*
	Re-thinking what PA means	Sarah (anorexia nervosa): *"I think when I was at the height of my ED, all I thought about was running or doing whatever burns the most amount of calories possible. [Now] I hit my steady weight. I'm aware of how many calories I'm burning while I'm running, but it's more to figure out what else I need to eat throughout the day."* Teresa (anorexia nervosa): *"There's still that mindset that I'm exercising to burn calories or I'm exercising to manipulate my body. [...] but [I try to find] things that are fun to do to take the focus off of burning calories."* Donna (anorexia nervosa): *"I still find I always switch to cardio machines so I can see how many calories I'm burning. For some reason, I have to know how many calories I'm burning. [...] And when I walk, I think of the calories I am burning, but I don't think of the actual number. I'm just thinking 'I'm burning calories'."* Karen (anorexia nervosa): *"I can very quickly think about it in terms of how much calories I am burning."*
Reactions to healthcare professionals' practice of recommending abstinence from PA during ED treatment		Julie (bulimia nervosa): *"Because of my ED, it [PA] has actually been recommended to me by my therapist as a means of managing my mood, anxiety."* Teresa (anorexia nervosa): *"I get where they are coming from. I understand that when you exercise, you are burning calories and when you want to gain weight because you are underweight, you probably shouldn't keep exercise because you're just going to prolong the process of gaining weight."* Anna (bulimia nervosa): *"It felt horrible. I was so upset. I was really, really upset and then actually a couple of days later, I was thankful. I was so thankful that she did that because I couldn't stop myself from doing it [PA]."* Maude (anorexia nervosa): *"It makes sense, but you're pissed when you're in that state and you're told not to do exercise. But in the long run, it's like you had such a pattern and a mindset around exercise that you kind of need to break to reframe and get back to it in a different mindset. So I don't 100% agree with it, but I'm not against it at all."* Karen (anorexia nervosa): *"I don't fully agree with the zero activity treatment. It's been proven over and over again that PA is good for people. So I don't understand why for people with EDs all of the sudden, it's not a good thing. I really struggled without it and I found it really annoying because I think it's going far in the other direction. I don't think the way of treating that is to eliminate exercise completely because the second you get out the hospital, you want to do it obsessively instead of reintroducing it in your life as something that can be a healthy part of it."* Donna (anorexia nervosa): *"It sucked that I couldn't be there and do those things that normal people do, that my friends do and everyone around me is doing."* Isabelle (other specified feeding or ED): *"I don't think I would suggest 'no PA at all'. I would suggest like 15 min walks or you know like half an hour of yoga or something like that. Something where you're not putting too much pressure on your body, but at the same time you still can do healthy things for you."*

Notes. ED Eating disorder, *PA* Physical activity

their behavior was highly variable. Participants were categorised inductively based on JB and AW's interpretations of their responses to questions asked during the interview into one of three overlapping categories (see Table 2). Sarah, Teresa, Diane, Julie, and Donna were categorised as *very active* given the extent of their involvement in PA, which included casual walking as well as more intense and targeted PA. They were consistently participating in high levels of structured PA throughout their week, and the activities they engaged in were mostly done with the intent of improving their cardiovascular endurance, muscular endurance, muscular strength, and flexibility. Karen, Anna, and Isabella were categorised as *somewhat active* as they described themselves as participating in weekly PA that usually consisted of walking (or other light-intensity PA). Though these three women sometimes engaged in PA to improve their cardiovascular endurance, muscular

Table 4 Quotes for theme related to PA programming thoughts

Theme	Quotes
PA programming thoughts	Julie (bulimia nervosa): *"Individuality, not necessarily in an ED but just in terms of people's preferences for the PA they do. People will always have things that they prefer."* Isabelle (other specified feeding or ED): *"I think that, in general, things that are personalised for people are always more helpful because it's based on you instead of based on the general demographic."* Sarah (anorexia nervosa): *"I would try to keep it looser. I guess it would be pretty similar to what I'm doing now just because that's where my goals are and that's where I'm able to maintain it."* Maude (anorexia nervosa): *"Everyone who has an ED is just so so different. So, what might be particularly helpful for someone is probably not going to be helpful for another person."* Teresa (anorexia nervosa): *"Everybody's intentions are different and you can't group all people with an ED into one basket and say 'Hey, this is your exercise program' because one person has an exercise compulsion and one hasn't, and one person is going to hate exercise no matter what and somebody is going to like it. So, it's got to be different. I think that there's going to be more commonalities between the ED subtypes, but I do still think an individual program is a lot more conducive to healing. [...] I think a big part of it is trying to change the mindset from doing PA because you feel like you have to to because you want to and you enjoy it so finding things that are fun to do. [...] More leisurely things focused more on actually enjoying it and having fun and finding pleasure out of it."* Teresa (anorexia nervosa): *"I would hate that. I would never want to be in an environment where I'm exercising with a bunch of other people who have EDs, especially in a class like setting. It would be quite the train wreck."* Sarah (anorexia nervosa): *"Every time you have a bunch of people with an ED in a room together it's already a little bit of tension. [...] There's competitiveness there because of the competitiveness and the comparisons."* Donna (anorexia nervosa): *"It would be pretty triggering to see people who are smaller than me or workout more than me. Just because you're always so competitive and you want to be the smallest one."* Julie (bulimia nervosa): *"I do like an environment where it's not a very competitive thing or where you're not comparing yourself against others. For me, that's something that's important."* Diane (binge ED): *"I would want it to be a group that is very inclusive that accepts that we all have different abilities and that were all different on a given day and all different from each other. If I was going to do it with other people, I would really want it to be inclusive and accepting essentially."*

Notes. ED Eating disorder, *PA* Physical activity

endurance, muscular strength, and flexibility, they mostly engaged in PA with the intent of staying mobile and feeling good. Finally, Maude was categorised as *irregularly active*. She commented that PA was not prioritised over other things in her life and engaged in minimal amounts of PA without a purpose.

Section 2: PA attitudes and experiences

PA as a lifestyle

This theme captures the enduring and important role of PA within participants' lives. Participants saw being active as essential to taking care of themselves. The positioning of PA as an important and central aspect of their lives was connected to their childhood experiences with PA and/or their ED. Participants described how their experiences with PA during their younger years and at the height of their ED impacted their attitudes toward PA now. However, for Diane, the importance attached to PA and the notion of PA as a lifestyle was new.

PA can be beneficial

Participants described how PA positively impacted their physical and psychosocial health, and explained that PA helped them manage their ED. In terms of the *physical benefits*, the favorable impact PA had on participants' health was clear, regardless of their ED diagnosis. In addition to maintaining their general health, participants described how PA helped them self-manage pre-existing medical conditions, and ultimately extend the length of their life. Additionally, they were acutely aware of how engaging in PA made them feel, and attributed periods of "feeling good" to their participation in PA. Weight loss, looking more toned, having better muscle definition, and improving appearance were also viewed as benefits of engaging in PA, which in turn allowed them to feel better.

In terms of the *psychosocial benefits*, participants described a range of psychological benefits associated with engaging in PA, including reduced stress, depression, and anxiety, adaptive emotional regulation, enhanced body image, as well as feeling a greater sense of control, accomplishment, self-acceptance, competence, confidence, and self-esteem. Participants offered that PA helped them manage stress and anxiety by providing them an opportunity to clear their minds. Some described that PA helped them feel better about themselves because it gave them a sense of control and helped them manage their depression. Moreover, participants discussed feeling accomplished and proud of themselves when they engaged in PA, and said they felt "much healthier and happier" when they engaged in PA. Social benefits of engaging in PA were also described. Although some participants enjoyed engaging in PA to have time to themselves, others saw engaging in PA as an opportunity to avoid isolation and connect with family and friends. For these participants, PA was seen as a way to forge new friendships, and they enjoyed their broader social network as a result of participating in group-based PA classes.

Participants were of the perspective that *PA helps with ED management*. The specific benefits reported, which differed from the aforementioned general benefits, related to coping with ED triggers (e.g., negative emotional states referring to feelings of anxiety, low mood, depression). For instance, participants explained that PA helped them manage some of the negative thoughts that contributed to their ED. Some said that PA was beneficial to them in managing their mood and hunger cues. As well, when discussing their thoughts about the role of PA in their ED, they explained that it helped them control and manage specific ED behaviors (e.g., binging, purging).

How I feel when I can't do PA

No matter their ED diagnosis, participants felt that being inactive negatively affected their physical and psychological health, and hindered their ability to manage their ED. In terms of the *physical effects*, they described how being inactive adversely impacted their body weight. In terms of the *psychosocial effects*, they explained that being inactive took a big toll on them, negatively impacting their general well-being. Indeed, they clearly articulated that their mood and body image were tied to their PA behavior. Participants also explained that being inactive made them feel agitated and antsy, which adversely affected their *ability to manage their ED*. Additionally, they feared relapsing during periods of inactivity and did not see their friends as much.

Being cautious about PA

Most participants discussed *changing PA habits*, which stemmed largely from their concern about being "overactive." For them, PA had dominated their life at the height of their ED. Now, they described seeking, or in some cases having found, a more balanced approach to PA. Overall, they felt their PA behavior was no longer dysfunctional; rather, it was now at a level they were content with. However, this only came as a result of hard work, self-monitoring, and self-imposed boundaries. Participants boundaries involved setting limits on the time spent at the gym, scaling back on intensity, avoiding certain types of PA, varying types of PA, and skipping PA at times of need (e.g., when they were tired or sick). Though most participants exerted a degree of vigilance over their PA, some did not feel this was necessary because PA was not associated with their ED and they did not obsess about PA or engage in abnormally high levels of PA.

For participants for whom PA had dominated their life at the height of their ED, insights were offered into how they were *re-thinking what PA means*. They explained that their proneness to obsess about PA and engage in abnormally high levels of PA in the past was influenced by a dominant discourse of PA in the media – PA burns calories. As a result, they were cognisant of calories burnt by PA and saw caloric expenditure as a key reason for taking part in PA in the past, especially at the height of their ED. Yet, some had managed to distance themselves from this thinking, and others who were still hung up on the idea that PA burns calories were actively trying to move away from that thinking. They noted that the shift in thinking was facilitated by instead taking part in fun, enjoyable low-intensity PA, and using PA to connect with nature and other people.

Reactions to healthcare professionals' practice of recommending abstinence from PA during ED treatment

Participants recounted that their healthcare provider recommended they abstain from PA during treatment, with the exception of Julie who was diagnosed with bulimia nervosa and was encouraged to engage in PA to help her manage her mood. Participants generally understood the rationale behind the practice of recommending PA abstinence during ED treatment. Some even appreciated being told to abstain from PA at the height of their ED once their initial reaction of being upset dissipated. This said, Karen and Donna maintained stronger, opposing feelings against the practice of recommending PA abstinence.

Regardless of the feelings participant had, they commented that having to abstain from PA during ED treatment and not receiving support to address their dysfunctional PA behaviors and attitudes from their healthcare team made it difficult for them to initiate or maintain healthy PA patterns. Participants explained how support to manage and integrate PA into their lives would be useful during ED treatment. They also felt that being encouraged to engage in less intensive and shorter bouts of PA when it would be safe would be more helpful to learn how to safely engage in PA than receiving recommendation to abstain from PA altogether.

Section 3: PA programming thoughts

When asked to describe their thoughts about PA programming for women with an ED, participants highlighted the necessity of customised, individually tailored PA programs based on personal preferences, abilities, and goals. Beyond this, participants stressed the importance of tailoring programs based on each women's ED symptoms and that PA programs should be focused on showing women with an ED that PA can be a fun, relaxing, mood-modulating, and overall healthy activity.

Though participants recognised that PA can provide social opportunities and facilitate engagement with family and friends, they expressed hesitation and worry about participating in PA with other women with an ED.

Participants explained that they would dislike an ED-specific group-based PA program, explaining that being around other women with an ED would likely heighten their natural desire to compare themselves to others, and thus foster a judgmental, competitive environment. Rather, they proposed that if PA programs are to be offered to women with an ED in a group setting, care would be needed to stop women from comparing themselves to others and learn to appreciate others.

Discussion

The aim of this qualitative study was to explore PA behaviors and attitudes among women with any type of ED. The results revealed that there are important risks associated with PA (e.g., engaging in abnormally high levels), and that overcoming dysfunctional PA behaviors and attitudes can be a long and complicated journey for women with an ED. At the same time, the general assertion that PA confers physical and psychosocial benefits was confirmed. As well, the results suggest that PA may help women with an ED cope with ED triggers (e.g., negative emotional states), manage ED behaviors (e.g., binging, purging), and reduce the risk of relapse. Accordingly, healthcare professionals should remain open to women's desire for PA support during ED treatment and help them learn to engage in PA in adaptive and healthy ways so as to allow them to reap benefits and better manage their ED. In doing so, it will be critical to address the dysfunctional PA behaviors and attitudes women with an ED hold that can lead them to engage in abnormally high levels of PA, and to investigate the specific benefits of PA for women with different ED diagnoses. Moreover, given that some issues raised with respect to PA behaviors and attitudes during the interviews may be linked with specific EDs and/or stage of treatment, potential variations in women's experiences via subgroup analyses according to ED diagnosis and/or stage of treatment warrants further investigation.

Participants admitted to engaging in abnormally high levels of PA in the past. They used terms such as "compulsive exercise,"[2] "unhealthy exercise," "over-exercise," "overactivity," and "exercise dependence" when describing their PA behavior at the onset and/or height of their ED. This aligns with reports that suggest the prevalence of dysfunctional PA behavior varies between 30 and 80% [35, 36], and that it is higher among adults with anorexia nervosa than in healthy controls [see [58] for a review]. Collectively, these findings highlight the need to address women's dysfunctional PA behaviors and attitudes to help them establish healthy PA levels and cope effectively with periods of inactivity. There is promising evidence that adding structured PA consisting of varied, low-intensity activities to treatment, offering cognitive behavior therapy, and/or providing physical therapy that follows guidelines [14] may reduce dysfunctional PA behaviors and attitudes in women with an ED [59–61].

Although participants were only interviewed once, they described that their PA behaviors and attitudes changed over time and became less dysfunctional. They explained that they participated in various, less intensive activities, and engaged in PA less often and for shorter bouts. Their accounts show that changing PA behaviors and attitudes was a complex and taxing endeavor, which in some cases was still ongoing, but that adopting new motives for PA (e.g., to socialize, regulate emotions, enjoyment, improve health and quality of life, manage ED triggers and behaviors) and avoiding activities that trigger dysfunctional PA was helpful. The finding that participants' attitudes, not just their behaviors, changed is important given the recently reported paradox observed in people with bulimia nervosa and binge eating disorder [62], which demonstrates that people may score high on compulsive PA instruments alongside low levels of PA because they maintain obsessive beliefs of PA. In contrast, women in this study seemed to lower both their levels and their obsessive beliefs of PA. As this coincided with them adopting PA motives that align with intrinsic origins, encouraging women with an ED to engage in PA for intrinsic reasons (i.e., fun, enjoyment) may help to address dysfunctional PA attitudes, as well as actual PA behavior.

Whilst society in general is bombarded with messages that PA is health-enhancing, such messaging can mask the ways in which PA may contribute to the development and/or maintenance of an ED, and that in some cases PA can be associated with adverse consequences [e.g., lowered BMI, maintained obsessive-compulsive aspect of ED [30, 63]. Anywhere from 30 to 80% of people with an ED engage in abnormally high levels of PA [35, 36], which can have dangerous and possibly life-threatening consequences (e.g., physical damage to the heart and muscles, electrolytic imbalances, demyelination of the nerves, increased risk of fracture, fatal heart fibrillation). For these reasons, healthcare professionals understandably may adopt the practice of recommending abstinence from PA during ED treatment, especially if they see signs of dysfunctional PA. Participants in this study generally understood that abstinence from PA at certain stages of their treatment was prudent (especially in light of ED-induced medical complications), though a minority maintained that the practice of recommending abstinence from PA during ED treatment ignores the notion that PA is good for health. This likely

[2]The use of the word "exercise" has not been replaced by PA when quoting participants.

harks back to the pervasive messaging that people need to engage in PA to be healthy. Indeed, alongside their expression of discontent, they argued that PA is a healthy pursuit and that refraining from PA during ED treatment would equate to becoming unhealthy. As such, it may be important to clarify the rationale for PA abstinence and to help women discover new adaptive coping mechanisms to manage their physical and psychosocial health – underscoring that living a healthy and long life can be realised through many avenues – not just PA.

On the other hand, it is imperative for women to develop a healthy relationship with PA at some point in their life, and thus it is important to formally address PA during the course of ED treatment. Results from this study suggest that recommending abstinence from PA was viewed as failing to provide women with the help they need to engage in PA safely and avoid engaging in abnormally high levels of PA. So while abstinence from PA may be necessary at certain stages of treatment (especially during weight restoration), closely monitored, nutritionally supported therapeutic PA can be safely introduced and confer numerous benefits for women during or after ED treatment [20]. This said, more research is needed to understand how best to help women break the rigid attitudes they may have towards PA, and help them truly enjoy PA as a fun, relaxing, mood-modulating, and overall healthy activity.

Practical implications

Some women in this study admitted to engaging in abnormally high levels of PA in the past, and two seemed to ignore the potential adverse effects of continuing to engage in PA and/or did not consider their PA behavior a problem warranting treatment; rather, they maintained the belief that PA is always good. Thus, healthcare professionals should remain attuned to dysfunctional PA behaviors and attitudes, and formally address these during ED treatment. Whilst there is little evidence on how to address dysfunctional PA behaviors and attitudes, cognitive behavioral therapy and behavioral strategies (e.g., contingency management, rewarding PA abstinence or low levels of PA) have been recommended [64]. As well, strategies to promote intuitive movement (i.e., movement performed with attention, purpose, self-compassion, acceptance, awareness, and joy, and that focuses on becoming more connected, healthier, and stronger) are emerging as promising, though they require further investigation.

Related to the previous point, careful attention should be paid to women who use PA to control and manage their ED symptoms and behaviors. Although participants in this study shared that engaging in PA helped them regulate their ED symptoms and behaviors, there is the risk that they could fall back into their previous dysfunctional PA behaviors and engage in abnormally high levels of PA but justify it as 'harmless' in comparison to other ED behaviors (e.g., binging, purging) or perhaps brush it aside as 'mild' compared to their previous PA behavior. Accordingly, ensuring women participate in PA for non-ED related reasons (e.g., to socialize, regulate emotions, improve health and quality of life) and addressing the underlying issues associated with women's ED will be necessary to treat dysfunctional PA behaviors and attitudes, and promote optimal healing, recovery, and relapse prevention. To this end, it might be valuable to offer post-PA debriefing sessions where women can discuss their experiences during PA and confirm that sessions were fun, enjoyable, relaxing, mood-modulating, and overall deemed healthy.

In addition, even if the practice of recommending abstinence from PA is understandable given the risks, the results from this study suggest that the benefits of PA may warrant its integration during ED treatment, contingent upon treatment compliance and when weight requirements and/or weight gain goals are met. When integrating PA, individually tailored approaches that include a graded PA program beginning with short bouts of low-intensity PA are suggested [65]. Furthermore, bearing in mind that women with an ED are sensitive to what others around them are doing and seem motivated to do more than others, it is not advised to have them engage in PA with others with whom they can compare themselves with.

Moreover, when inquiring about women's PA history, understanding their preferences and abilities is important to facilitate the development of programs that favor enjoyment and that could potentially yield more positive experiences. Beyond this, ensuring PA programs and opportunities educate women and equip them to self-manage their PA behavior, while mitigating competition, may also encourage healthy PA integration. Accordingly, those offering PA opportunities to women with an ED should remove means of tracking progress (e.g., equipment that provide caloric expenditure data), incorporate activities that necessitate teamwork, and seek to foster an inclusive environment. Finally, there is a need to train PA professionals using guidance such as the Safe Exercise at Every Stage Guidelines. These guidelines can help PA professionals make informed decisions on how to help women safely (re)engage in PA during ED treatment and may even be used by healthcare professionals when having discussions about PA with their patients.

Study limitations

The limitations of this study should be kept in mind when interpreting the findings. First, participants may have been reluctant to disclose certain experiences because they were interviewed by a male. Second, participants self-reported their PA behavior, ED diagnosis, and stage of treatment, and no contact was made with healthcare providers to confirm ED diagnoses. Consequently, there may be errors due to the self-reported nature of these data. Indeed, methods of self-report have been criticised with ED patients because they are known to hide/underestimate their symptoms [66]. Third, the depth of the information gathered on PA behavior varied in richness across participants, which made it difficult to categorise some participants based on both quantitative (i.e., intensity, frequency, duration, and type of PA) and qualitative (i.e., motives for PA) elements. Relatedly, participants were categorised into one of three categories based on JB and AW's interpretations of their responses to some of the questions asked during the interview. To eliminate the possibility of misclassification and to allow for more precise classification in future studies, additional questions that require participants to report full PA behavior details should be asked. Fourth, this study was conducted in a Western, economically developed country with women who self-reported being employed and had a postsecondary education. Fifth, most participants were between 19 and 30 years of age, making it necessary to further explore women's experiences across the lifespan as additional perspectives might have emerged if more middle-aged and older women had participated. Accordingly, recruitment strategies may need to be tailored to different age groups to ensure middle-age and older women with an ED are recruited into PA studies as they have the potential to generate data that can be translated into more effective ED management. To this end, exploring strategies to recruit middle-age and older women with an ED into PA studies is crucial to advancing this area of research. Sixth, though questions asked about change over time, participants were only interviewed once. Last, although data saturation was achieved, it is possible that continuing to interview additional women may have further contributed to the understanding of one or more themes.

Conclusions

Based on the current study, as well as previous literature [14–19], PA is associated with numerous benefits for women with an ED. However, PA behaviors and attitudes are highly complex for this population. As such, findings suggest that treating women with any type ED and supporting them in their recovery will require holistic approaches that include education alongside opportunities to discover varied, intrinsically motivated low-intensity PA options. This said, it is clear that more work is needed to understand how healthcare and PA professionals can work together to empower and support women with an ED and to delineate if and how these findings differ amongst samples comprised of women with specific EDs, who are at specific stages of treatment and recovery, and who are younger or older. A next logical step would be to explore experiences among subsets of the ED population and to engage stakeholders (e.g., women with an ED, healthcare professionals, PA professionals) to review the current findings and co-develop programs to offer women with an ED support for PA.

What is already known on this subject?

Among women with an eating disorder (ED), physical activity (PA) is related to both healthy and unhealthy outcomes. Consequently, PA is typically restricted during treatment. Yet, women may remain engaged in PA during treatment or resume PA shortly thereafter. There is a critical need to understand women's PA behaviors and attitudes and to explore how they integrate PA into their lives during and after ED treatment.

What your study adds?

The exploration of PA behaviors and attitudes among women with an ED revealed that overcoming dysfunctional PA behaviors (e.g., engaging in abnormally high levels) and attitudes (e.g., associating PA with caloric expenditure) can be a long and complicated journey, but that the benefits of PA warrant further consideration. It also revealed that helping women engage in PA in adaptive and healthy ways when possible during ED treatment may be beneficial.

Abbreviations

BMI: Body mass index; EAT-26: Eating Attitudes Test-26; ED: Eating disorder; EDS-21: Exercise Dependence Scale-21; PA: Physical activity

Acknowledgements

The authors would like to thank the women who were involved in this study for their willingness to share their experiences and time. The authors would also like to thank the staff at the Hopewell Eating Disorder Support Centre who assisted with recruitment and Dr. Georgio Tasca from the University of Ottawa for his assistance developing and refining the interview guide.

Authors' contributions

JB conceptualised the work, analysed and interpreted the data, drafted the manuscript. FDD conceptualised the work, and led the data collection. AW analysed and interpreted the data, and revised the work critically. All authors provided final approval of the version to be published.

Competing interests

The authors declare that they have no conflicts of interest.

Author details

[1]School of Human Kinetics, University of Ottawa, 125 University Private, Montpetit Hall, Room 339, Ottawa, Ontario K1N 6N5, Canada. [2]Cancer Therapeutics Program, Ottawa Hospital Research Institute, 1053 Carling Avenue, Ottawa, Ontario K1Y 4E9, Canada. [3]Institut du savoir Montfort,

Hôpital Montfort, 713 Montreal Road, Ottawa, Ontario K1K 0T2, Canada. [4]Present address: Université du Québec à Trois-Rivières, 3351 Boulevard des Forges, Trois-Rivières, Québec G8Z 4M3, Canada. [5]Faculty of Kinesiology, University of Calgary, 2500 University Drive, Calgary, Alberta T2N 1N4, Canada.

References

1. Pritts SD, Susman J. Diagnosis of eating disorders in primary care. Am Fam Physician. 2003;67(2):297–304.
2. American Psychiatric Association. Diagnostic and statistical manual of mental disorders: DSM-5. 5th ed. Arlington: American Psychiatric Association; 2013.
3. Kaplan AS, Noble S. Medical complications of eating disorders. In: Wonderlich S, Mitchell J, de Zwaan M, editors. Annual review of eating disorders. London: CRC Press; 2007.
4. Forney KJ, Buchman-Schmitt JM, Keel PK, Frank GK. The medical complications associated with purging. Int J Eat Disord. 2016;49(3):249–59. https://doi.org/10.1002/eat.22504.
5. Mitchell JE. Medical comorbidity and medical complications associated with binge-eating disorder. Int J Eat Disord. 2016;49(3):319–23. https://doi.org/10.1002/eat.22452.
6. Sachs KV, Harnke B, Mehler PS, Krantz MJ. Cardiovascular complications of anorexia nervosa: a systematic review. Int J Eat Disord. 2016;49(3):238–48. https://doi.org/10.1002/eat.22481.
7. Westmoreland P, Krantz MJ, Mehler PS. Medical complications of anorexia nervosa and bulimia. Am J Med. 2016;129(1):30–7. https://doi.org/10.1016/j.amjmed.2015.06.031.
8. Jenkins PE, Hoste RR, Meyer C, Blissett JM. Eating disorders and quality of life: a review of the literature. Clin Psychol Rev. 2011;31(1):113–21. 0.1016/j.cpr.2010.08.003.
9. Swinbourne JM, Touyz SW. The co-morbidity of eating disorders and anxiety disorders: a review. Eur Eat Disord Rev. 2007;15(4):253–74. https://doi.org/10.1002/erv.784.
10. Altman SE, Shankman SA. What is the association between obsessive-compulsive disorder and eating disorders? Clin Psychol Rev. 2009;29(7):638 46. https://doi.org/10.1016/j.cpr.2009.08.001.
11. Wonderlich S, Mitchell JE, Crosby RD, Myers TC, Kadlec K, Lahaise K, et al. Minimizing and treating chronicity in the eating disorders: a clinical overview. Int J Eat Disord. 2012;45(4):467–75. https://doi.org/10.1002/eat.20978.
12. Mitchell JE, Myers T, Crosby R, O'Neill G, Carlisle J, Gerlach S. Health care utilization in patients with eating disorders. Int J Eat Disord. 2009;42(6):571 4. https://doi.org/10.1002/eat.20651.
13. Caspersen CJ, Powell KE, Christenson GM. Physical activity, exercise, and physical fitness: definitions and distinctions for health-related research. Public Health Rep. 1985;100(2):126–31.
14. Cook BJ, Wonderlich SA, Mitchell JE, Thompson R, Sherman R, McCallum K. Exercise in eating disorders treatment: systematic review and proposal of guidelines. Med Sci Sports Exerc. 2016;48(7):1408–14. https://doi.org/10.1249/MSS.0000000000000912.
15. Hoie LH, Myking E, Reine EC, Bruusgaard D. Diet and exercise in addition to psychotherapy, in the treatment of patients suffering from eating disorders with obesity. Eat Weight Disord. 1997;2(4):207–10. https://doi.org/10.1007/BF03339977.
16. Zunker C, Mitchell JE, Wonderlich SA. Exercise interventions for women with anorexia nervosa: a review of the literature. Int J Eat Disord. 2011;44(7):579–84. https://doi.org/10.1002/eat.20862.
17. Hausenblas HA, Cook BJ, Chittester NI. Can exercise treat eating disorders? Exerc Sport Sci Rev. 2008;36(1):43–7. https://doi.org/10.1097/jes.0b013e31815e4040.
18. Moola FJ, Gairdner S, Amara C. Exercise in the care of patients with anorexia nervosa: a systematic review of the literature. Ment Health Phys Act. 2013; 6(2):59–68.
19. Vancampfort D, Vanderlinden J, De Hert M, Soundy A, Adamkova M, Skjaerven LH, et al. A systematic review of physical therapy interventions for patients with anorexia and bulemia nervosa. Disabil Rehabil. 2014;36(8):628–34. https://doi.org/10.3109/09638288.2013.808271
20. Ng LWC, Ng DP, Wong WP. Is supervised exercise training safe in patients with anorexia nervosa? A meta analysis. Physiotherapy. 2013;99:1–11. https://doi.org/10.1016/j.physio.2012.05.006.
21. Carei TR, Fyfe-Johnson AL, Breuner CC, Brown MA. Randomized controlled clinical trial of yoga in the treatment of eating disorders. J Adolesc Health. 2010;46(4):346–51. https://doi.org/10.1016/j.jadohealth.2009.08.007.
22. Chantler I, Szabo CP, Green K. Muscular strength changes in hospitalized anorexic patients after an eight week resistance training program. Int J Sports Med. 2006;27(8):660–5. https://doi.org/10.1055/s-2005-865812.
23. Szabo CP, Green K. Hospitalized anorexics and resistance training: impact on body composition and psychological well-being. A preliminary study. Eat Weight Disord. 2002;7(4):293–7. https://doi.org/10.1007/BF03324975.
24. Moola FJ, Gairdner S, Amara C. Speaking on behalf of the body and activity: investigating the activity experiences of Canadian women living with anorexia nervosa. Ment Health Phys Act. 2015;8:44–55. https://doi.org/10.1016/j.mhpa.2015.02.002.
25. Hall A, Ofei-Tenkorang NA, Machan JT, Gordon CM. Use of yoga in outpatient eating disorder treatment: a pilot study. J Eat Disord. 2016;4:38. https://doi.org/10.1186/s40337-016-0130-2.
26. Santos L, Elliott-Sale KJ, Sale C. Exercise and bone health across the lifespan. Biogerontology. 2017;18(6):931–46. https://doi.org/10.1007/s10522-017-9732-6.
27. Misra M, Klibanski A. Anorexia nervosa and bone. J Endocrinol. 2014;221(3): R163–76. https://doi.org/10.1530/JOE-14-0039.
28. Hrabosky JI, White MA, Masheb RM, Grilo CM. Physical activity and its correlates in treatment-seeking obese patients with binge eating disorder. Int J Eat Disord. 2007;40(1):72–6. https://doi.org/10.1002/eat.20323.
29. Vancampfort D, De Herdt A, Vanderlinden J, Lannoo M, Adriaens A, De Hert M, et al. The functional exercise capacity and its correlates in obese treatment-seeking people with binge eating disorder: an exploratory study. Disabil Rehabil. 2015;37(9):777–82. https://doi.org/10.3109/09638288.2014.942000.
30. Meyer C, Taranis L, Goodwin H, Haycraft E. Compulsive exercise and eating disorders. Eur Eat Disord Rev. 2011;19(3):174–89.
31. Meyer C, Taranis L. Exercise in the eating disorders: terms and definitions. Eur Eat Disord Rev. 2011;19(3):169–73. https://doi.org/10.1002/erv.1122.
32. Godier LR, Park RJ. Does compulsive behavior in anorexia nervosa resemble an addiction? A qualitative investigation. Front Psychol. 2015;6:1608. https://doi.org/10.3389/fpsyg.2015.01608.
33. Kolnes L-J. 'Feelings stronger than reason': conflicting experiences of exercise in women with anorexia nervosa. J Eat Disord. 2016;4:6. https://doi.org/10.1186/s40337-016-0100-8.
34. Tobin DL, Johnson CL, Dennis AB. Divergent forms of purging behavior in bulimia nervosa patients. Int J Eat Disord. 1996;11(1):17–24.
35. Davis C, Katzman DK, Kaptein S, Kirsh C, Brewer H, Kalmbach K, et al. The prevalence of high-level exercise in the eating disorders: etiological implications. Compr Psychiatry. 1997;38(6):321–6. https://doi.org/10.1016/s0010-440x(97)90927-5.
36. Dalle Grave R, Calugi S, Marchesini G. Compulsive exercise to control shape or weight in eating disorders: prevalence, associated features, and treatment outcome. Compr Psychiatry. 2008;49(4):346–52. https://doi.org/10.1016/j.comppsych.2007.12.007.
37. Stiles-Shields C, Bamford B, Lock J, Le Grange D. The effect of driven exercise on treatment outcomes for adolescents with anorexia and bulimia nervosa. Int J Eat Disord. 2015;48(4):392–6. https://doi.org/10.1002/eat.22281.
38. Strober M, Freeman R, Morrell W. The long-term course of severe anorexia nervosa in adolescents: survival analysis of recovery, relapse, and outcome predictors over 10-15 years in a prospective study. Int J Eat Disord. 1997; 22(4):339–60.
39. El Ghoch M, Calugi S, Pellegrini M, Milanese C, Busacchi M, Battistini NC, et al. Measured physical activity in anorexia nervosa: features and treatment outcome. Int J Eat Disord. 2013;46(7):709–12. https://doi.org/10.1002/eat.22140.
40. Young S, Touyz S, Meyer C, Arcelus J, Rhodes P, Madden S, et al. Relationships between compulsive exercise, quality of life, psychological distress and motivation to change in adults with anorexia nervosa. J Eat Disord. 2018;6:2. https://doi.org/10.1186/s40337-018-0188-0.
41. Beumont PJ, Touyz SW. What kind of illness is anorexia nervosa? Eur Child Adolesc Psychiatry. 2003;12(Suppl 1):I20–4. https://doi.org/10.1007/s00787-003-1103-y.
42. Fuqua JS, Rogol AD. Neuroendocrine alterations in the exercising human: implications for energy homeostasis. Metabolism. 2013;62(7):911–21. https://doi.org/10.1016/j.metabol.2013.01.016

43. Allaway HCM, Southmayd EA, De Souza MJ. The physiology of functional hypothalamic amenorrhea associated with energy deficiency in exercising women and in women with anorexia nervosa. Horm Mol Biol Clin Investig. 2016;25(2):1868–91.
44. Davies R. The treatment of compulsive physical activity in anorexia nervosa lacks a conceptual base. Adv Eat Disord. 2015;3(1):103–12. https://doi.org/10.1080/21662630.2014.892835.
45. Hechler T, Beaumont P, Marks P, Touyz S. How do clinical specialists understand the role of physical activity in eating disorders? Eur Eat Disord Rev. 2005;13(2):125–32. https://doi.org/10.1002/erv.630.
46. Quesnel DA, Libben M, Oelke ND, Clark MI, Willis-Stewart S, Caperchione CM. Is abstinence really the best option? Exploring the role of exercise in the treatment and management of eating disorders. Eat Disord. 2018;26(3): 290–310. https://doi.org/10.1080/10640266.2017.1397421.
47. Bratland-Sanda S, Martinsen EW, Rosenvinge JH, Ro O, Hoffart A, Sundgot-Borgen J. Exercise dependence score in patients with longstanding eating disorders and controls: the importance of affect regulation and physical activity intensity. Eur Eat Disord Rev. 2011;19(3):249–55. https://doi.org/10.1002/erv.971.
48. Schlegl S, Dittmer N, Hoffmann S, Voderholzer U. Self-reported quantity, compulsiveness and motives of exercise in patients with eating disorders and healthy controls: differences and similarities. J Eat Disord. 2018;6:17. https://doi.org/10.1186/s40337-018-0202-6.
49. Bardone-Cone AM, Higgins MK, St George SM, Rosenzweig I, Schaefer LM, Fitzsimmons-Craft EE, et al. Behavioral and psychological aspects of exercise across stages of eating disorder recovery. Eat Disord. 2016;24(5):424–39. https://doi.org/10.1080/10640266.2016.1207452.
50. Denzin ND, Lincoln YS. Introduction: the discipline and practice of qualitative research. In: Denzin ND, Lincoln YS, editors. The sage handbook of qualitative research. Thousand Oaks: Sage Publications; 2005.
51. Saunders B, Sim J, Kingstone T, Baker S, Waterfield J, Bartlam B, et al. Saturation in qualitative research: exploring its conceptualization and operationalization. Qual Quant. 2018;52(4):1893–907. https://doi.org/10.1007/s11135-017-0574-8.
52. Garner DM, Olmsted MP, Bohr Y, Garfinkel PE. The eating attitudes test: psychometric features and clinical correlates. Psychol Med. 1982;12(4):871–8. https://doi.org/10.1017/s0033291700049163.
53. Hausenblas HA, Symons Downs D. How much is too much? The development and validation of the exercise dependence scale. Psychol Health. 2000:17. https://doi.org/10.1080/08870440220000004894.
54. Kvale S. Interviews: an introduction to qualitative research interviewing. USA: Sage; 1996.
55. Braun V, Clarke V, Weate P. Using thematic analysis in sport and exercise research. In: Smith B, Sparkes AC, editors. Routledge handbook of qualitative research in sport and exercise. London: Routledge; 2016. p. 191–205.
56. Smith B, McGannon KR. Developing rigor in qualitative research: problems and opportunities within sport and exercise psychology. Int Rev Sport Exerc Psych. 2018;11(1):101–21. https://doi.org/10.1080/1750984X.2017.1317357.
57. Yardley L. Dilemmas in qualitative health research. Psychol Health. 2000; 15(2):215–28. https://doi.org/10.1080/08870440008400302.
58. Rizk M, Mattar L, Kern L, Berthoz S, Duclos J, Viltart O, et al. Physical activity in eating disorders: a systematic review. Nutrients. 2020;12(1). https://doi.org/10.3390/nu12010183.
59. Mathisen TF, Bratland-Sanda S, Rosenvinge JH, Friborg O, Pettersen G, Vrabel KA, et al. Treatment effects on compulsive exercise and physical activity in eating disorders. J Eat Disord. 2018;6:43. https://doi.org/10.1186/s40337-018-0215-1.
60. Dittmer N, Voderholzer U, Monch C, Cuntz U, Jacobi C, Schlegl S. Efficacy of a specialized group intervention for compulsive exercise in inpatients with anorexia nervosa: a randomized controlled trial. Psychother Psychosom. 2020;89(3):161–73. https://doi.org/10.1159/000504583.
61. Calogero RM, Pedrotty KN. The practice and process of healthy exercise: an investigation of the treatment of exercise abuse in women with eating disorders. Eat Disord. 2004;12(4):273–91. https://doi.org/10.1080/10640260490521352.
62. Bratland-Sanda S, Mathisen TF, Sundgot-Borgen J, Harald RJ. Defining compulsive exercise in eating disorders: acknowledging the exercise paradox and exercise obsessions. J Eat Disord. 2019;7(8):1–3.
63. Shroff H, Reba L, Thornton LM, Tozzi F, Klump KL, Berrettini WH, et al. Features associated with excessive exercise in women with eating disorders. Int J Eat Disord. 2006;39(6):454–61. https://doi.org/10.1002/eat.20247
64. Adams J. Understanding exercise addiction. J Contemp Psychother. 2009;39: 231–40.
65. Danielsen M, Ro O, Bjornelv S. How to integrate physical activity and exercise approaches into inpatient treatment for eating disorders: fifteen years of clinical experience and research. J Eat Disord. 2018;6:34. https://doi.org/10.1186/s40337-018-0203-5.
66. Bezzina L, Touyz S, Young S, Foroughi N, Clemes S, Meyer C, et al. Accuracy of self-reported physical activity in patients with anorexia nervosa: links with clinical features. J Eat Disord. 2019;7:28. https://doi.org/10.1186/s40337-019-0258-y.

13

Interventional sialendoscopy in parotidomegaly related to eating disorders

Giuseppe Colella[1], Giorgio Lo Giudice[2*], Roberto De Luca[2], Antonio Troiano[2], Carmelo Lo Faro[2], Vincenzo Santillo[1] and Gianpaolo Tartaro[1]

Abstract

Background: To evaluate the viability and efficacy of sialendoscopy for the management of parotidomegaly related to eating disorders, 6 patients suffering from eating disorders and recurring symptoms of glandular swelling were followed up at the Multidisciplinary Department of Medical-Surgical and Dental Specialties, Oral and Maxillofacial Surgery Unit, AOU University of Campania "Luigi Vanvitelli". After the detection of the impaired gland through clinical and radiographical analysis, the diagnostic unit was introduced into the duct and was advanced in, reaching the ductal system. Plaques were washed out, any strictures were dilated both by hydrostatic pressure application and steroid solution injection directly in the fibrotic area.

Results: Both glands resulted affected in 83% of patients. 11 parotid glands were explored and treated. Strictures were found in 2 glands (33%), sialectasis in 3 glands (50%), strictures and sialectasis together in 1 glands (17%). In 3 parotid glands (50%) Stenon's duct was affected, in two (33%) only secondary ducts, in 1 (17%) both. We reached symptomatic improvement in 5 patients (83%), reporting the spherical volume of the parotid region and pain reduction.

Conclusions: Our results demonstrate that sialendoscopy is a safe and effective therapeutic method to treat EDs salivary symptoms. Treating the underlining psychiatric pathology should be the primary goal in patient care to lower the possible recurrence rate and increase the successful outcome of this technique.

Keywords: Sialendoscopy, Sialoendoscopy, Parotidomegaly, Sialadenosis, Sialoadenosis, Sialadenitis, Sialoadenitis, Eating disorders, Anorexia, Bulimia

Plain English summary

Patients affected by Eating Disorders such as Anorexia Nervosa and Bulimia Nervosa often follow compensatory behaviors to control their weight. Among all behaviors, if self-induced vomiting is protracted over time, oral health can be affected on both anatomical and biochemical level. Salivary gland swelling is a pathological alteration that these patients can manifest. The glands can become visible and sometimes painful, changing the facial profile. Sialendoscopy is a technique that offers a minimally invasive approach to non-neoplastic diseases, allowing the endoscopic visualization of the salivary glands and their ducts, offering a tool to treat ductal system pathologies. The aim of this research was then to assess the validity of this non-invasive technique to treat salivary symptoms related to Eating Disorders. The results showed a reduction of salivary gland volume and symptom relief in most patients, opening a new path to treat the consequences of such conditions.

Background

Eating disorders (EDs) are psychological conditions based on self-misperception of body shape and weight,

* Correspondence: Giorgio.logiudice@gmail.com
[2]Department of Neurosciences, Reproductive and Odontostomatological Sciences, Maxillofacial Surgery Unit, University of Naples "Federico II", 80138 Naples, Italy
Full list of author information is available at the end of the article

often leading to severe systemic conditions that require medical treatment. DSM-V lists different behavioral syndromes in the Feeding and Eating Disorders chapter: Pica, Rumination Disorder, Avoidant/Restrictive Food Intake Disorder, Anorexia Nervosa (AN), Bulimia Nervosa (BN), Binge-Eating Disorder and Unspecified Feeding or Eating Disorder [1]. AN clinical characteristics lead to two subtypes: Anorexia Nervosa Restricting type (AN-R) and Anorexia Nervosa Binge-eating/Purging type (AN-BP) whereas BN is distinguished by compensatory actions after binge eating. Patients may follow inappropriate compensatory behaviors in order to avoid guilt perceived after eating or weight gain, such as chewing and spitting, self-induced vomiting, fasting or intake restriction after food consumption, drug intake such as laxatives or diuretics, inappropriate use of enemas, and over-exercising. The self-induced vomiting behaviour exhibited by some patients sabotages the oral health status, affecting both hard and soft tissues. Clinically, the patients may show enamel erosion, tooth decay, periodontal diseases, mucositis, and glossitis. The salivary profile is also affected both biochemically and anatomically showing altered salivary flow, increased amylase levels, decreased pH and bicarbonate salivary levels, salivary gland swelling (mostly affecting the parotid gland), sialadenosis, and facial swelling coming from parotidomegaly [2]. Although the mechanisms underlining salivary gland swelling are still up to debate, this condition must be treated by the physician: the impact on the patients' body image is significant, furthermore magnified by the social pressure to pursuit a symmetric, imperfection-free face, possibly worsening their dysmorphic disorder. Nahlieli and Baruchin introduced rigid salivary gland endoscopy in 1994 [3]. Since that time, sialendoscopy has been used for diagnostic and therapeutic purposes [4]. Sialendoscopy offers a minimally invasive approach to non-neoplastic diseases, allowing endoscopic intraluminal visualization and offering a tool to treat ductal system pathologies, reducing or eliminating the need for sialadenectomy thus avoiding the related surgical risks [5–8]. This paper aims to evaluate the reliability of sialendoscopy in the management of parotidomegaly related to eating disorders.

Materials and methods

Six patients were referred to the Multidisciplinary Department of Medical-Surgical and Dental Specialties, Oral and Maxillofacial Surgery Unit, AOU University of Campania "Luigi Vanvitelli" and were recruited for this prospective study from November 2012 to December 2016. The inclusion criteria were: diagnosis of EDs, recurring symptoms of glandular swelling either with or without pain, enlarged volume of the parotid region. Exclusion criteria were: any previous sialendoscopic treatment and/or botulinum toxin treatment of the parotid, previous facial surgery.

Patients were diagnosed with EDs by our center according to DSM-V. ED related parotidomegaly and sialadenosis was diagnosed after clinical and radiological examination, and exclusion of drinking history, parotid gland infective diseases, sialolithiasis or tumors.. Morphological analysis was performed through ultrasound and MRI scans. The spherical volume of the parotid region was measured according to Metzger at baseline (T0) and 6 months follow-up (T1) as "$V = 4/3 \times \pi \times (r1 \times r2 \times r3)$" where r1, r2, and r3 are the semidiameters for gland height, width, and depth [9]. Signs and symptoms improvement were considered as the primary endpoint of this study and it was evaluated assessing salivary swelling and pain reduction compared to baseline.

After the detection of the impaired gland, local anesthesia with lidocaine 2% was achieved on the orifice region. Gradual dilatation of the duct orifice was then performed, using salivary probes of increased diameter from 0000 to 0 size and with a 0.5 mm lacrimal probe, reaching 1.3 mm diameter, matching the outer diameter of the sialendoscope diagnostic unit (Marchal Sialendoscope - Karl Storz). The larger scopes (1.6 mm diameter) were introduced as needed and a 5 mm papillotomy was performed in order to prevent false roads creation. The diagnostic unit was introduced into the duct and was advanced, until reaching the ductal system while carrying out continuous lavage with isotonic saline solution. Care is taken to avoid puncturing or lacerating the duct. The plaques were washed out; any strictures were dilated both by hydrostatic pressure application and steroid solution injection directly in the fibrotic area; mucous plugs and debris were removed with irrigation or forceps. At the end of the procedure, the ductal system was irrigated with a betamethasone solution (Bentelan 4 mg/2 ml – Alfasigma S.p.a., Milano, Italy) under direct vision while withdrawing the scope, in order to treat the inflammation of the ductal epithelium (sialodochitis) and to promote the dilatation of ductal strictures.

Sialendoscopy was considered successful when the entire ductal lumen and its branches were clear of any disease. An antibiotic prophylaxis treatment was performed with twice a day doses of Amoxicillin 875 mg and Clavulanic acid 125 mg on post-operative phase for one week. The patients were followed-up at 3 months, 6 months (T1), and 1 year.

Results

Our cohort included 6 female patients with a mean age of 22 years. 4 patients came to our attention with a diagnosis of AN-BP, 2 with a diagnosis of BN. In patients 1, 3 and 4, eating disorders familiarity was discovered during anamnesis. In patients 2 and 4, Generalized Anxiety

Table 1 Patients' demographics. (AN-BP - *Anorexia Nervosa Binge eating/Purging type; BN - Bulimia Nervosa)*

Patient	Sex	Age	Symptoms Onset (months)	Eating Disorder	Eds Familiarity	Comorbidities	Ultrasound Findings
1	F	18	12	BN	yes	None	Hypoechogenic areas and punctate calcifications
2	F	23	6	AN-BP	no	Generalized Anxiety Disorder and Major Depression	Hypoechogenic areas
3	F	25	6	BN	yes	None	Hypoechogenic areas and reactive lymph nodes
4	F	27	18	AN-BP	yes	Generalized Anxiety Disorder and Major Depression	Hypoechogenic areas and punctate calcifications
5	F	17	4	AN-BP	no	Autoimmune Thyroiditis	Hypoechogenic areas
6	F	20	3	AN-BP	no	DM1, Fibromialgia	Hypoechogenic areas

Disorder and Major Depression treated with benzodiazepines were associated. Symptoms onset average from our medical examination was 12.6 months (Table 1, Fig. 1).

Before performing this technique, all patients carried out analgesic and antibiotic drug therapy without any relief. All patients performed ultrasonography and MRI scans: in 3 patients the preoperative imaging evidenced hypoechogenic areas, in 2 patients hypoechogenic areas and punctate calcifications, in 1 patient hypoechogenic areas and reactive lymph nodes (Table 1, Fig. 2).

Both glands resulted affected in 5 out of 6 patients (83%). 11 parotid glands were explored and treated; in 5 patients the procedure was completed with no complications. However, in 1 case the procedure was discontinued at the initial stage due to pain intolerance and anxiety. The procedure was then performed again after 1 week (Table 2).

Strictures were found in 2 glands (33%), sialectasis in 3 glands (50%), strictures and sialectasis together in 1 gland (17%). In 3 parotid glands (50%) Stenon's duct was affected, in 2 glands (33%) only secondary ducts, in 1 (17%) both (Fig. 3).

No diagnosis of sialolithiasis was made in our patients. No major complications such as nerve damage, hemorrhage, airway impairment, ductal perforation or kinks were observed. Symptomatic improvement was reached in 5 patients at T1 (83%). The patients showed spherical volume reduction of the parotid region and pain reduction at T1 (Table 2, Fig. 4).

One patient (patient 6) with bilateral parotidomegaly did not reach symptom relief nor spherical volume reduction after performing 4 sialendoscopies in succession at a time interval of 6 months. In this case, we observed an endoscopic pattern of sialectasis bilaterally. One patient (patient 5) did not show immediate improvement and they underwent a further sialendoscopy within a 3–5 months interval from their first treatment, obtaining success.

Discussion

Studies found in literature describe non-inflammatory swelling of the salivary glands as a symptom underlining eating disorders [10, 11]. The enlarged area of the anatomical region of the parotid gland and, occasionally, of the submandibular gland, are described in patients with AN and BN, while other glands may not show any macroscopic alterations [12, 13]. Parotid swelling incidence has been estimated from 10 to 50% and may be either uni- or bilateral [14–17]. Some studies presume the etiology of this condition to be a combination of an abnormally low body mass index (BMI), nutritional deficiency, functional hypertrophy, and neurovegetative/hormonal dysregulation. Binge eating and purging behaviour by vomiting seems to be directly connected to

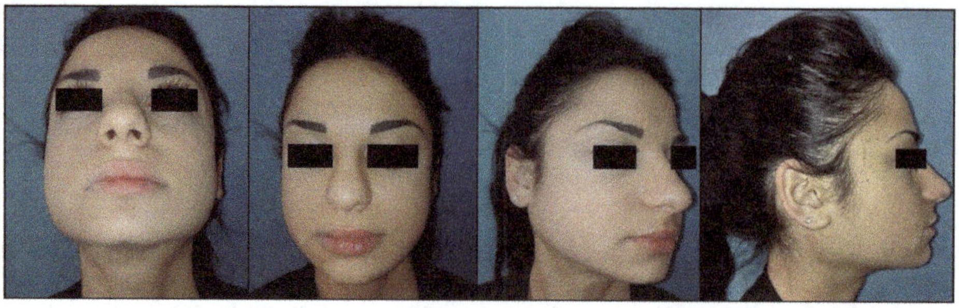

Fig. 1 T0 external view examination

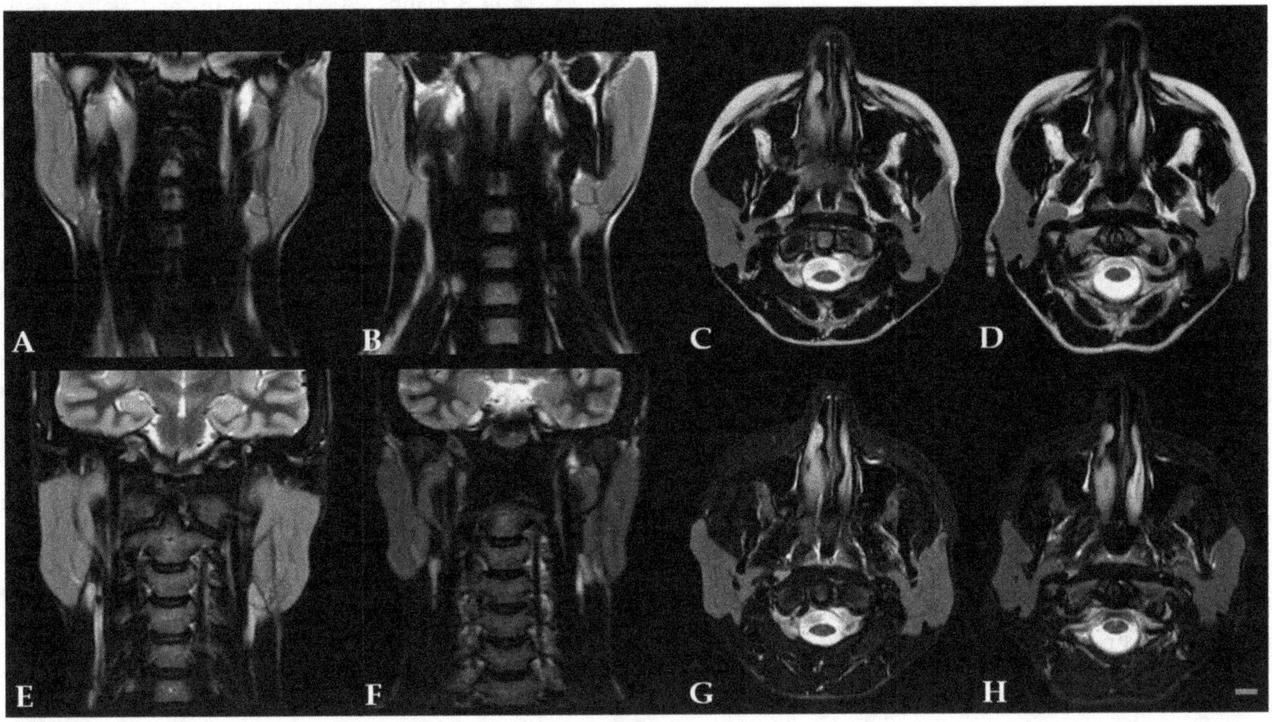

Fig. 2 MRI assessment shows reduction of the parotid gland volume bilaterally. Coronal T2w at T0 (**a**) and T1 (**b**); axial T2w at T0 (**c**) and T1 (**d**); coronal STIR at T0 (**e**) and T1 (**f**); axial STIR at T0 (**g**) and T1 (H). BAR: 1 cm

Table 2 Sialendoscopic features and outcomes. (*StD - Stenon's duct; SeD - Secondary ducts*)

Patient	Gland	Findings	Intervention	Complications	Parotid region spherical volume (T0)	Parotid region spherical volume (T1)
1	L Parotid R Parotid	Sialectasis StD	Dilatation and removal	None	5 cm L 4,8 cm R	4.5 cm L 3.2 cm R
2	R Parotid	Stricture StD Stricture SeD	Dilatation and removal	None	4.5 cm	2 cm
3	L Parotid R Parotid	Stricture SeD	Dilatation and removal	None	2.9 cm L 4 cm R	1.2 cm L 3 cm R
4	L Parotid R Parotid	Stricture SeD Sialectasis SeD	Dilatation and removal	None	3.7 cm L 4.4 cm R	2.1 cm L 3.2 cm R
5	L Parotid R Parotid	Sialectasis StD	Dilatation and removal	None	6.2 cm L 6.5 cm R	2.5 cm L 1.8 cm R
6	L Parotid R Parotid	Sialectasis StD	Dilatation and removal	Failed 4 endoscopies	6.3 cm L 4.5 cm R	6.2 cm L 4.5 cm R

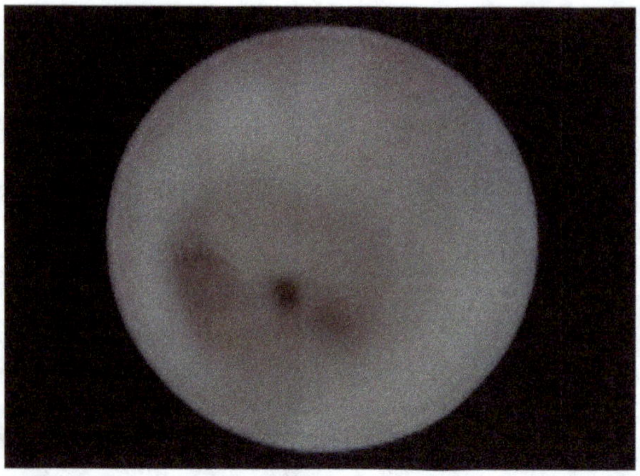

Fig. 3 Sialendoscopic photogram of right parotid primary duct stricture

the onset of the swelling, usually beginning 2–6 days after the trigger episode. This sign tends to fade in early stages if the behaviour is not protracted in time and is generally painless [18]. Histological examinations show changes within the parenchyma of the parotids, including hypertrophy of the cells and increased storage of adipose tissue [10, 14–16]. Hyposalivation is another typical feature reported in patients affected by both AN subtypes and BN, thus possibly concurring to the persistence of the glands inflammatory state. The genesis of this phenomenon could come from vomiting, starvation and antidepressant medications that have antisialagogue side effects. The appetite suppressant may also play a role in this pathological sign [2, 19]. Since this plethora of signs tend to subside after ED treatment and resolution, due to the inflammatory trigger removal, a step-by-step treatment approach should be followed: intensive pharmacological, sialendoscopic and then surgical approaches should be kept for refractory cases in long-history ED patients. Reports of effective sialogogue drug use such as pilocarpine, can be found in literature and could be used as primary treatment in such patients [20, 21].

While performing sialoendoscopy, phlogistic findings were detected. Strictures were founded in 2 glands (33%), sialectasis in 3 glands (50%), strictures and sialectasis together in 1 gland (17%). Each of these features, typical of chronic sialoadenitis, is widely described in literature and successfully treated with sialendoscopy [21, 22].

Sialendoscopy is a technique able to offer a minimally invasive and gland-preserving approach to non-neoplastic salivary glands diseases. In our work, we obtained encouraging results that justify the possibility of treating EDs salivary symptoms with a conservative procedure reaching symptomatic improvement in most of the patients treated. The morphological analysis showed spherical volume reduction of the parotid region, less incidence of salivary swelling and pain reduction (Table 2). Only 1 patient with bilateral parotidomegaly reached neither symptoms relief nor spherical volume reduction after performing 4 sialendoscopies in succession at a time interval of 6 months. Botulinum toxin injection of the salivary glands is used to treat sialorrhea, salivary fistulae, first bite syndrome, Frey syndrome and sialoadenitis [23]. Cosmetic off-label use has been reported in literature due to its parenchymal atrophy effects in order to reduce gland volume thus performing facial recontouring [24]. This treatment, reported to be possible in both percutaneous and intraductal infusion, could be used to treat those parotidomegaly cases refractory to the sialendoscopic therapy [25]. The surgical treatment (superficial or total parotidectomy) should be carefully pondered by the surgeon and used as a last resort, considering that a slight significant percentage of symptomatic pain is usually referred, the young mean age of the patients in question, and the related risks of such surgical procedures.

Conclusions

Sialendoscopy is a versatile procedure, worthwhile to treat EDs salivary symptoms refractory to common therapy. Despite the small cohort of patients considered, our results are promising and should push the researchers to widen its application fields. Treating the underlining psychiatric pathology should be the primary goal in patient care, in order to lower the possible recurrence rate and increase the successful outcomes of this technique.

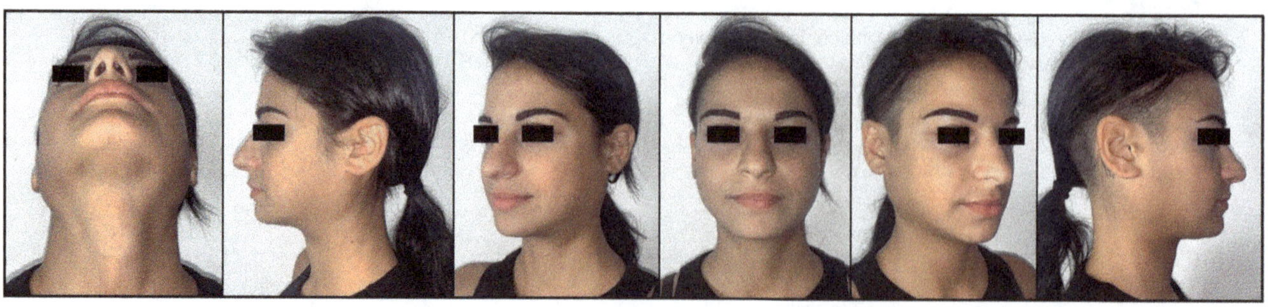

Fig. 4 T1 external view examination

Abbreviations

AN: Anorexia Nervosa; AN-BP: Anorexia Nervosa Binge eating/Purging type; AN-R: Anorexia Nervosa Restricting type; BN: Bulimia Nervosa; DSM-V: Diagnostic and statistical manual of mental disorders - 5th edition; ED: Eating disorder; MRI: Magnetic Resonance Imaging

Authors' contributions

Data curation, A.T; formal analysis, C.L.F.; investigation, V.S.; project administration, G.C.; supervision, G.T.; writing—original draft, R.D.L.; writing—review and editing, G.L.G. All authors read and approved the final manuscript.

Competing interests

The authors declare that they have no competing interests.

Author details

[1]Multidisciplinary Department of Medical-Surgical and Dental Specialties, Oral and Maxillofacial Surgery Unit, University of Campania "Luigi Vanvitelli", 80138 Naples, Italy. [2]Department of Neurosciences, Reproductive and Odontostomatological Sciences, Maxillofacial Surgery Unit, University of Naples "Federico II", 80138 Naples, Italy.

References

1. American Psychiatric Association. Diagnostic and statistical manual of mental disorders. 5th ed. Arlington, VA: American Psychiatric Association; 2013. p. 2013.
2. Frydrych AM, Davies GR, McDermott BM. Eating disorders and oral health: a review of the literature. Aust Dent J. 2005;50(1):6–15 quiz 56.
3. Nahlieli O, Baruchin AM. Sialoendoscopy: three years' experience as a diagnostic and treatment modality. J Oral Maxillofac Surg. 1997;55(9):912–8 discussion 9–20.
4. Capaccio P, Torretta S, Ottavian F, Sambataro G, Pignataro L. Modern management of obstructive salivary diseases. Acta Otorhinolaryngol Ital. 2007;27(4):161–72.
5. Strychowsky JE, Sommer DD, Gupta MK, Cohen N, Nahlieli O. Sialendoscopy for the management of obstructive salivary gland disease: a systematic review and meta-analysis. Arch Otolaryngol Head Neck Surg. 2012;138(6): 541–7.
6. Shacham R, Puterman MB, Ohana N, Nahlieli O. Endoscopic treatment of salivary glands affected by autoimmune diseases. J Oral Maxillofac Surg. 2011;69(2):476–81.
7. Marchal F, Dulguerov P, Becker M, Barki G, Disant F, Lehmann W. Specificity of parotid sialendoscopy. Laryngoscope. 2001;111(2):264–71.
8. De Luca R, Trodella M, Vicidomini A, Colella G, Tartaro G. Endoscopic management of salivary gland obstructive diseases in patients with Sjogren's syndrome. J Craniomaxillofac Surg. 2015;43(8):1643–9.
9. Metzger ED, Levine JM, McArdle CR, Wolfe BE, Jimerson DC. Salivary gland enlargement and elevated serum amylase in bulimia nervosa. Biol Psychiatry. 1999;45(11):1520–2.
10. Bozzato A, Burger P, Zenk J, Uter W, Iro H. Salivary gland biometry in female patients with eating disorders. Eur Arch Otorhinolaryngol. 2008;265(9):1095–102.
11. Walsh BT, Croft CB, Katz JL. Anorexia nervosa and salivary gland enlargement. Int J Psychiatry Med. 1981;11(3):255–61.
12. Buchanan JA, Fortune F. Bilateral parotid enlargement as a presenting feature of bulimia nervosa in a post-adolescent male. Postgrad Med J. 1994; 70(819):27–30.
13. Het S, Vocks S, Wolf JM, Hammelstein P, Herpertz S, Wolf OT. Blunted neuroendocrine stress reactivity in young women with eating disorders. J Psychosom Res. 2015;78(3):260–7.
14. Coleman H, Altini M, Nayler S, Richards A. Sialadenosis: a presenting sign in bulimia. Head Neck. 1998;20(8):758–62.
15. Du Plessis DJ. Parotid enlargement in malnutrition. S Afr Med J. 1956;30(30): 700–3.
16. Vavrina J, Muller W, Gebbers JO. Enlargement of salivary glands in bulimia. J Laryngol Otol. 1994;108(6):516–8.
17. Mandel L, Kaynar A. Bulimia and parotid swelling: a review and case report. J Oral Maxillofac Surg. 1992;50(10):1122–5.
18. Brown S, Bonifazi DZ. An overview of anorexia and bulimia nervosa, and the impact of eating disorders on the oral cavity. Compendium. 1993;14(12): 1594 6-602, 604-8; quiz 608.
19. Tschoppe P, Wolgin M, Pischon N, et al. Etiologic factors of hyposalivation and consequences for oral health. Quintessence Int. 2010;41(4):321–33.
20. Mehler PS, Wallace JA. Sialadenosis in bulimia. A new treatment. Arch Otolaryngol Head Neck Surg. 1993;119(7):787–8.
21. Mignogna MD, Fedele S, Lo RL. Anorexia/bulimia-related sialadenosis of palatal minor salivary glands. J Oral Pathol Med. 2004;33(7):441–2.
22. Ziegler CM, Steveling H, Seubert M, Muhling J. Endoscopy: a minimally invasive procedure for diagnosis and treatment of diseases of the salivary glands. Six years of practical experience. Br J Oral Maxillofac Surg. 2004; 42(1):1–7.
23. Gillespie MB, Intaphan J, Nguyen SA. Endoscopic-assisted management of chronic sialadenitis. Head Neck. 2011;33(9):1346–51.
24. Jung GS, Cho IK, Sung HM. Submandibular gland reduction using Botulinum toxin type a for a smooth jawline. Plast Reconstr Surg Glob Open. 2019;7(4):e2192.
25. Schwalje AT, Hoffman HT. Intraductal salivary gland infusion with Botulinum toxin. Laryngoscope Investig Otolaryngol. 2019;4(5):520–5.

14

The abrupt transition from face-to-face to online treatment for eating disorders: a pilot examination of patients' perspectives during the COVID-19 lockdown

Yael Doreen Lewis[1,2*], Roni Elran-Barak[3], Rinat Grundman-Shem Tov[1,2] and Eynat Zubery[1,2]

Abstract

Background: Studies investigating patients' perspectives towards an abrupt transition from face-to-face to online treatment in eating disorders (EDs) are scarce. The current study aimed to (1) conduct a preliminary assessment of patients' perspectives regarding this transition, and (2) explore potential demographic, clinical, and treatment-related factors associated with these perspectives.

Methods: Sixty-three patients with EDs whose treatment was moved to an online format, were surveyed during the COVID-19 lockdown (April–May 2020). A 6-item measure was developed to examine their perspectives toward this transition. Exploratory factor analyses (EFAs) were conducted to confirm the rational-theoretical structure of the measure (Eigenvalue = 3.745, explaining 62.4% of variance). The Cronbach's alpha value was excellent ($\alpha = 0.878$). Validated questionnaires were used to measure ED symptoms, general psychopathology, therapeutic alliance, and pandemic anxiety, and their associations with our transition-focused scale and telemedicine satisfaction were examined.

Results: Mixed views were found regarding the transition, with the majority (68%) stating that they would not choose to continue online therapy given the option. Longer duration of treatment ($r = 0.291$, $p = 0.022$), stronger therapeutic alliance ($r = 0.293$, $p = 0.028$), and higher COVID-19 anxiety ($r = 0.276$, $p = 0.029$) were linked with more positive views towards the transition.

Conclusions: Analyses suggest that patients' perspectives towards the transition can be measured using a Likert-type 6-item scale. Findings highlight the various responses to online treatment and indicate a need to identify patients who may face difficulties in the transition to this newly ubiquitous treatment mode. Clinicians should be cognizant of these potential difficulties and consider appropriate modes of treatment in the ongoing pandemic situation.

Keywords: Eating disorders, COVID-19, Coronavirus, Lockdown, Telemedicine, Telehealth, eHealth, Metal health

* Correspondence: yael.d.lewis@gmail.com
[1]Hadarim Eating Disorders Treatment Center, Shalvata Mental Health Center, Hod Hasharon, Israel
[2]Sackler Faculty of Medicine, Tel Aviv University, Tel Aviv, Israel
Full list of author information is available at the end of the article

Plain English summary

The topic of forced and abrupt changes of setting in psychological treatment was, until the COVID-19 pandemic struck, scarcely ever addressed. Despite the obligatory massive shift to online treatment because of worldwide lockdowns, little was previously known about patients' attitudes towards such a transition and/or possible outcomes. The aim of the current study was to conduct a preliminary assessment of patients' perspectives regarding the transition to online therapy during the first COVID-19 lockdown, and explore potential factors associated with these perspectives. We found that longer duration of pre-lockdown treatment, stronger therapeutic alliance, and high COVID-19 anxiety were associated with a more positive perspective toward the transition. These findings could inform further research on similar transitions, as well as drawing clinicians' attention to the various implications of such transitions.

Background

The subject of obligatory changes in the setting of psychological treatment has received little attention in the scientific literature. Efforts to control the spread of the novel severe acute respiratory syndrome coronavirus 2 (SARS-CoV-2) have led to quarantining and social distancing, across the globe, accompanied by considerable psychological implications [1, 2]. In this context, ambulatory mental health services shifted from conventional face-to-face treatment to remote online treatment. Although some preliminary reports have emerged regarding therapists' attitudes [3], patients' experiences of this abrupt transition have received little attention [4].

Online mental health treatment, including psychological and psychiatric services, has been found to be effective in both the assessment and delivery of care across diagnoses [5, 6], including eating disorders (EDs) [7], although more research is warranted to understand benefits and possible adverse effects. During the coronavirus disease (COVID-19) lockdown, patients with EDs experienced altered access to services [8]. A rapid shift from the previous limited scale of tele-mental health care, to its wide usage, was thus urged worldwide [9–11], including in the area of EDs [12]. Taking into account predictions for an increase in ED risks and symptoms during the COVID-19 crisis via several pathways related to disrupted food access and routines, movement and exercise constraints, heightened stress and anxiety, decreased support and, in some cases, the increased possibility of violence [13, 14], the provision of continuous therapy remained a principal goal. However, this unprecedented and abrupt transition was forced upon patients as well as on therapists, with no prior warning or preparation. For guidance, and due to the lack of studies describing patients' perspectives, therapists were suddenly in a position of having to rely on the limited literature [15], on in-house institutional professional peer support [16], and on an international exchange of viewpoints and expertise [17].

In the absence of existing knowledge about the patient experience concerning such an abrupt change, we wished to conduct a pilot study investigating how patients in ambulatory treatment for EDs perceived the transition from traditional face-to-face treatment to remote online treatment. We sought to study a unique "real-world setting" situation created by the imposition of the first lockdown, in contrast to previous studies of telehealth in EDs in which participants had a choice of treatment. Therefore, our aims were to (1) assess patients' perspectives regarding this transition, and (2) explore potential demographic, clinical, and treatment-related factors associated with these perspectives. Specifically, we chose to consider the factors of depression and anxiety symptoms, which are significant comorbidities and have been suggested to be linked with EDs [18], as well as COVID-19 anxiety. With respect to therapy-related factors, it seemed crucial to investigate the therapeutic alliance, which has been shown to be related to patients' perceptions of their therapy outcome [19]. Patient satisfaction with online treatment was also measured in order to draw a clear distinction between patients' perceptions towards the transition to online treatment and their satisfaction with it.

Considering that the initial phase of therapy is a critical period for the formation of the therapeutic alliance, necessary for the building of trust and collaborative work [20], and in light of the unexpected challenge of building an alliance remotely [21], we hypothesized that patients with established therapeutic relationships (i.e., those who had been in face-to-face therapy for a longer time before the outbreak and had a stronger working alliance), would perceive the transition more favorably and experience it as less harmful than those in the initial stages of treatment. We further hypothesized that greater concerns relating to the virus and potential contagion [22] would cause patients to adhere to confinement measures and would therefore be associated with a more positive attitude toward online treatment.

The new measure developed in the current study could be used in future research about obligatory transitions from traditional to online treatment. In addition, identification of the potential factors influencing patient perspectives could guide further research regarding this process of transition and inform our knowledge regarding any future such changes resulting from the ongoing COVID-19 pandemic or other disruptive events.

Methods

Participants

Participants included 63 patients recruited from the patient population of the Hadarim Eating Disorders Treatment Center (EDTC) in Kfar Saba, Israel, a part of the Shavata Mental Health Center. Twenty-four (38%) of these patients were diagnosed with anorexia nervosa (AN) (AN: $n = 17$, atypical AN: $n = 7$), 20 (32%) with bulimia nervosa (BN), 16 (25%) with binge eating disorder (BED), and 3 (5%) with other EDs (purging disorder: $n = 1$, avoidant restrictive food intake disorder: $n = 2$). As presented in Table 1, most participants were female ($n = 57$, 91%), their mean age was 27 (SD = 11.47, 27% under the age of 18), and their mean time in treatment was almost one year (M = 317 days, SD = 195). In order to obtain a broad understanding of patients' perspectives, all patients who had commenced treatment prior to the lockdown were eligible for participation. As the study did not include any intervention, no further inclusion or exclusion criteria were applied.

Table 1 Demographic and clinical characteristics ($N = 63$)

Demographic characteristics	
Age, years: M (SD), range	27.25 (11.47), 12–56
Gender: n (%)	
Female	57 (90.50)
Male	6 (9.50)
Marital Status: n (%)	
Single	38 (60.32)
Married/living with partner	23 (36.51)
Divorced	2 (3.17)
Other	
Level of Education: n (%)	
Student	17 (27.0)
High school graduate	15 (23.80)
University student	8 (12.70)
University/college graduate	23 (36.50)
Clinical characteristics	
Diagnosis: n (%)	
Anorexia nervosa	24 (38.10)
Bulimia nervosa	20 (31.75)
Binge eating disorder	16 (25.40)
Other ED	3 (4.75)
Age of ED onset: M (SD), range	15.39 (4.99), 12–56
BMI (last measured), kg/m^2: M (SD), range	24.82 (7.40), 16.36–52.61
Duration of treatment, days: M (SD), range	317 (195), 42–909
Past ED hospitalization: n (%), range	14 (22.22)

Abbreviations: M mean, *SD* standard deviation, *BMI* body mass index, *ED* eating disorder

Procedure

The institutional review board (IRB) of the Shalvata Mental Health Center approved the study in a special meeting convened to discuss COVID-19 related studies. In terms of social distancing concerns, the IRB required that when informed consent could not be signed in the clinic, it would be obtained via email. In the case of minors, parents signed the informed consent, in addition to which the under-18 participants also signed an assent form. Eating disorder diagnoses were decided in accordance with the DSM-5 and in clinic discussions held among a trained psychiatrist (YDL) with 5 years of experience in the field, a qualified dietician (RGS) with 20 years of experience, and the head of the center (EZ), with over 30 years of experience in the field. Demographic and ED-related information were collected in the survey, and the last measured body mass index (BMI) was collected from the patient files. Approximately 95% of patients in the clinic were invited to participate in the study. Those who were not approached were those for whom there were certain clinical indicators suggesting that participation would have a negative impact, or those who could not be reached during the lockdown. Fifty-one adult patients were contacted of whom 46 completed the survey. Thirty minor patients and their parents were contacted, and 17 of them participated in the study, with about half of the refusals being due to a parental decision. Overall, consent for participation was approximately 80%, with a higher rate in the adult patients.

Data were collected between mid-April and mid-May 2020, following the March–April lockdown in Israel, which was gradually lifted during the month of May. As of the second week of March, all non-urgent services in the Hadarim clinic (including psychotherapy, and dietetic and psychiatric consultations) were switched to online platforms.

Measures

The Telemedicine Satisfaction Questionnaire (TSQ [23]) was used to evaluate reactions to remote treatment. This validated tool includes 15 items rated on a 1–5 Likert-type scale and comprises three factors including quality of care, similarity of remote meetings to face-to-face meetings, and perception of the interaction. It has been previously used in studies of videoconferencing-psychotherapy [24, 25]. The internal consistency of the TSQ in this study was $\alpha = 0.67$ for the total score, with $\alpha = 0.50$ for the similarity to face-to-face encounter subscale and $\alpha = 0.63$ for the quality of care subscale.

The Eating Disorder Examination Questionnaire (EDE-Q [26]) was used to assess ED symptoms. The EDE-Q has been used extensively in the study of EDs [27], and the Hebrew version has demonstrated good convergent validity [28]. The internal consistency of the EDE-Q in the present study was α = 0.93 for the global score, and α = 0.63, α =0.79 α = 0.75 α = 0.74 for the restraint, eating concerns, shape concerns, and weight concerns subscales, respectively.

The Depression Anxiety and Stress Scales – Version 21 was used to examine general psychopathology (DASS-21 [29]). This instrument has shown high internal consistency and concurrent validity scores [30]. The internal consistency of the DASS-21 in the present study was α = 0.95, with α = 0.92, α =0.84 and α = 0.90 for depression, anxiety, and stress scores, respectively, similar to reliability scores reported in previous studies of the Hebrew version [31].

Working alliance was assessed using the short version of the Working Alliance Inventory (WAI-S [32]), a widely used instrument, the Hebrew version of which has also been used extensively in studies [33]. The internal consistency in the present study was α = 0.82.

Fears and worries related to the COVID-19 pandemic were assessed with an instrument recently and purposively developed: the fear of COVID-19 scale (FCV-19S [34]). The Hebrew version of the questionnaire was found to have good psychometric properties [22]. The internal consistency in the present study was α = 0.84.

Perspectives toward the transition to online treatment were measured using the six items that we developed for this study. As detailed above, we utilized the TSQ [23] to evaluate reactions and technical aspects of remote treatment. However, the TSQ does not address the obligatory change in mode of therapy that was at the heart of our study. As such, we used previous studies to identify central themes related to patients' perceptions toward telehealth services, including quality of professional care, preference of telehealth vs. traditional face-to-face treatment, possible future use, and promotion of service to others [35, 36]. Based on these emerging themes we composed six statements, focusing on the transition, to be rated on a 1–5 Likert-type scale. The first and second authors generated the items, which were then reviewed in discussions regarding content by all authors – a psychiatrist, two social workers, and a dietician – all of whom have worked clinically with patients with EDs for many years. The items were also reviewed by several patients with EDs.

Statements 1–4 addressed the perception of the care given as either beneficial or adverse. Statement 5 addressed the preference for online vs. face-to-face treatment, and Statement 6 related to the promotion of this mode of therapy to others. A higher score indicated a more favorable attitude towards online treatment, except for items 1 and 2, which were reversed.

1. I feel the transition to online treatment adversely affected the quality of care I receive at the clinic.
2. I feel the transition to online treatment adversely affected the effectiveness of the treatment I receive at the clinic.
3. I feel the transition to online treatment contributed to the quality of care I receive at the clinic.
4. I feel the transition to online treatment contributed to the effectiveness of the treatment I receive at the clinic.
5. If it were possible to continue using online treatment after the COVID-19 pandemic, I would prefer it rather than going back to conventional face-to-face treatment.
6. I would recommend moving to online treatment to my family members and friends.

These six items are not disorder-specific and may be used among a diverse psychiatric patient population (e.g., patients with depression/anxiety). That said, in the current study we utilized this measure only among patients with EDs. The measure is designed to be answered either with paper and pencil or online. Internal consistency of the six items was excellent: Cronbach's α = 0.878 (internal consistency above 0.7 is considered acceptable for new instruments [37]). For each of the six items, we assessed Cronbach's α if the item were deleted, and the results ranged from α = 0.866 (Items 1,5) to α = 0.846 (Item 4).

Data analysis

Data were analyzed using IBM SPSS-25. Results of the exploratory factor analysis (EFA) verified that all six of the items we developed to measure perceptions toward the transition to online treatment belonged to one single factor: Eigenvalue = 3.745 (explaining 62.4% of variance), Kaiser-Meyer-Olkin (KMO) = 0.794 (a value above 0.6 is considered preferred [37]), Bartlett's Test of Sphericity chi-square (df = 15) = 208.3, $p < 0.001$. Table 2 demonstrates that component loading for each item ranged from 0.848 (Item 4) to 0.735 (Item 1), meaning that no item had to be removed. T-tests and Pearson's correlations were computed to examine univariate associations of participants' characteristics with the 6-item measure and the TSQ scales.

Results

Sample clinical and therapy-related characteristics

Demographic and clinical characteristics are detailed in Table 1. The mean score of the EDE-Q global score was 3.51 (SD = 1.30), comparable with clinical ED samples [38, 39] and above 95% of the general population [40]. Mean scores in the EDE-Q subscales – that is, restraint (M = 3.45, SD = 1.66), eating concerns (M = 2.72, SD = 1.53), shape concerns (M = 4.18, SD = 1.76), and weight

Table 2 Means and SDs, factor loadings and item total correlations of the 6 items measuring patients' perspectives towards the transition to online treatment

	Loading	Mean	SD	Item correlation
1. I feel the transition to online treatment adversely affected the quality of care I receive at the clinic.[a]	.735	2.94	1.17	.630
2. I feel the transition to online treatment adversely affected the effectiveness of the treatment I receive at the clinic.[a]	.802	2.97	1.22	.708
3. I feel the transition to online treatment contributed to the quality of care I receive at the clinic.	.805	2.57	1.09	.692
4. I feel the transition to online treatment contributed to the effectiveness of the treatment I receive at the clinic.[a]	.848	2.63	1.08	.753
5. If it were possible to continue using online treatment after the COVID-19 pandemic, I would prefer it rather than going back to conventional face-to-face treatment.	.741	1.95	1.13	.629
6. I would recommend moving to online treatment to my family members and friends.	.803	2.17	1.17	.700

[a] Items are reversed. *Abbreviations: SD* standard deviation

concerns (M = 3.69, SD = 1.59) – were also above 95% general population [41].

The DASS-21 depression score was found to be moderate (M = 15.14, SD = 11.27), whereas the anxiety score was mild (M = 8.79, SD = 8.79), similar to the stress score (M = 17.55, SD = 10.60).

Pandemic-related anxiety as measured by the FCV-19S (M = 13.16, SD = 4.89) was slightly lower than what was measured in a larger non-clinical sample in Israel [22].

The therapeutic alliance total score was found to indicate a relatively strong alliance, in the range of previous ED studies (M = 5.32, SD = 1.24 [42, 43];) with similar results in the subscales of task (M = 5.16 (SD-1.51), bond (M = 5.59, SD = 1.24), and goal (M = 5.19, SD = 1.34).

Perception of online treatment

Figure 1 illustrates participants' responses to the six Likert-type scale statements on the transition to

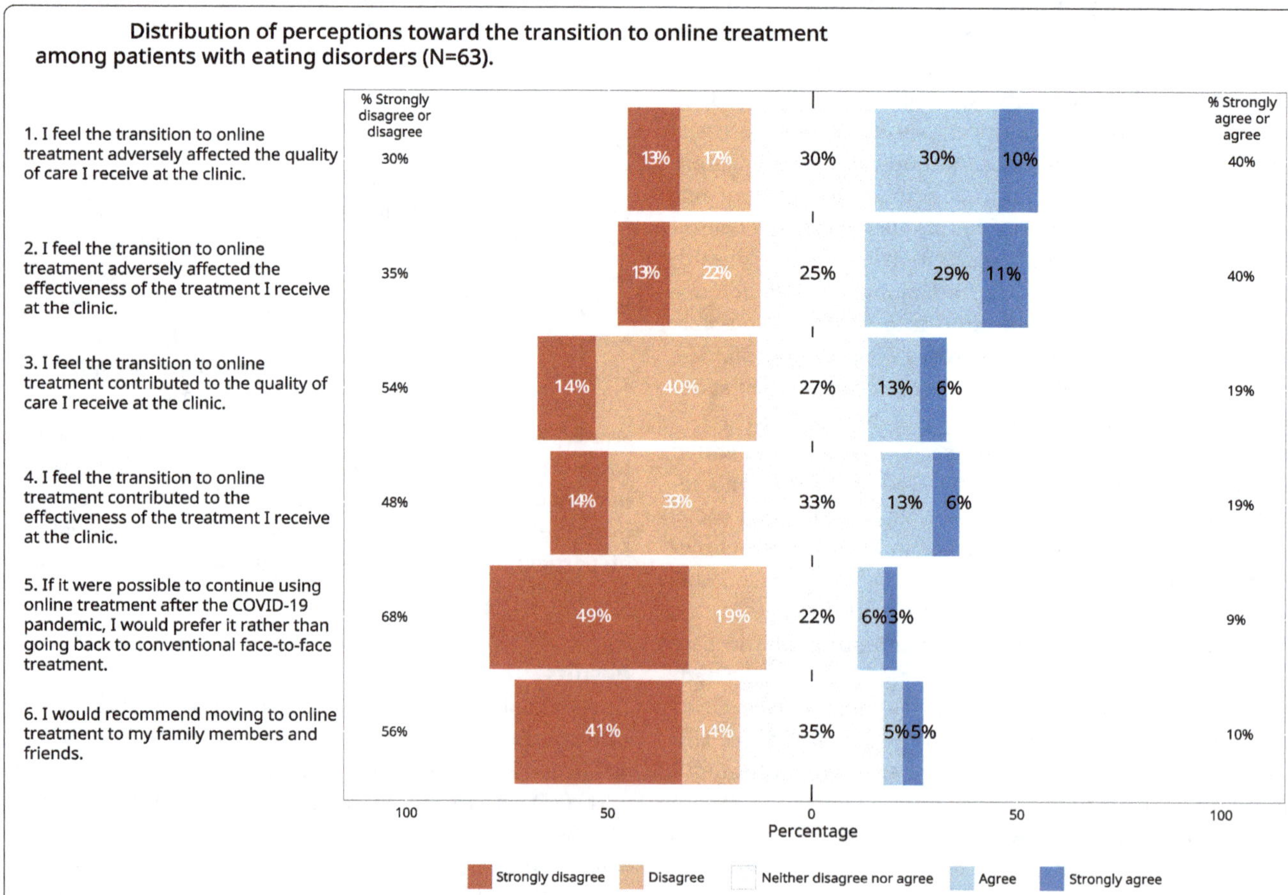

Fig. 1 Distribution of perceptions toward the transition to online treatment among patients with eating disorders (*N* = 63)

online treatment. Twenty-five (40%) of the participants agreed that the transition to online treatment adversely affected the effectiveness/quality of their treatment at the clinic, while 22 (34%) disagreed that the effectiveness had been negatively influenced and 19 (30%) disagreed the quality had worsened, leaving the remaining 16 (25%) neutral about the effectiveness and the remaining 19 (30%) neutral about the quality. Twelve (19%) of the participants agreed that the transition to online treatment contributed to the effectiveness/quality of their treatment at the clinic, while 30 (48%) disagreed that the effectiveness had been enhanced and 34 (54%) disagreed that the quality of treatment improved, leaving and the remaining 21 (33%) neutral about the effectiveness and 17 (27%) neutral about the quality.

Most participants ($n = 43$, 68%) stated that they would not prefer continuing online therapy given the choice, with only six participants (9%) opting to continue. Thirty-four participants (54%) stated that they would not recommend online treatment to friends and family members, with 22 (34%) remaining neutral, and only six participants (9%) endorsing it.

The mean score of the TSQ was 3.08 (SD = 0.69), which is lower relative to a mean of around 4.7 in prior reports [24, 25], with subscale means of 3.11 (SD = 0.73) for similarity of online to face-to-face encounter, 3.06 (SD = 0.90) for quality of care provided, and 3.02 (SD = 1.17) for perception of the interaction.

Univariate associations between demographic, clinical, and treatment-related factors and perceptions of online treatment

Table 3 shows the associations between the Likert-type scale statements and demographic and illness-related characteristics of the participants. Longer duration in treatment was significantly correlated with more positive perceptions towards the transition to online treatment ($r = 0.291$, $p = 0.022$). Other demographic and clinical characteristics (including BMI and ED diagnosis) were not found to have any significant correlations with the views toward the transition to online therapy.

Table 4 shows the associations between the perceptions and clinical and treatment-related factors. Strength of therapeutic alliance (as measured by the WAI-S total score) was significantly correlated with more favorable perspectives towards the transition to online treatment ($r = 0.293$, $p = 0.028$). Goal and task scores also correlated with favorable perspectives towards the transition ($r = 0.295$, $p = 0.027$; $r = 0.346$, $p = 0.00$, respectively). Fear of COVID-19 significantly correlated with favorable perspectives towards the transition ($r = 0.276$, $p = 0.029$).

The TSQ was found to be correlated only with the therapeutic alliance bond score (similarity: $r = 0.291$, $p = 0.030$), and goal score (quality: $r = 0.268$, $p = 0.045$). We also examined whether patients with different ED diagnoses (AN, BN, BED) had different perspectives toward the transition and/or different TSQ scores, and we found no significant results.

Table 3 The univariate associations of demographic and clinical characteristics with TSQ and the 6-item measure of patients' perspectives towards the transition to online treatment ($N = 63$)

		TSQ similarity	TSQ quality	Perspectives towards the transition to online treatment
Demographic characteristics				
Age	r =	.182	−.047	.036
	p =	.154	.717	.777
Gender	r =	.067	.146	.006
	p =	.604	.254	.964
Education	r =	.093	−.017	.092
	p =	.469	.893	.471
Clinical characteristics				
BMI (last measured), Kg/m^2	r =	.221	−.011	.226
	p =	.085	.931	.077
Duration of treatment, days	r =	.124	−.144	**.291**
	p =	.338	.263	**.022**
Past ED hospitalization	t =	.149	.061	.152
	p =	.242	.634	.235

Note: Perspectives towards the transition to online treatment were measured using the six items developed for the current study. A higher score represents more positive attitude towards the transition. Bold font indicates statistically significant results (p-value< 0.05). *Abbreviations*: *TSQ* Telemedicine Satisfaction Questionnaire, *BMI* body mass index, *ED* eating disorder

Table 4 The univariate associations of eating disorder (ED) psychopathology, general psychopathology, therapeutic alliance, COVID-19 anxiety with TSQ and the 6-item measure of patients' perspectives towards the transition to online treatment ($N = 63$)

		TSQ similarity	TSQ quality	Perspectives towards the transition to online treatment
ED psychopathology (EDE-Q)				
Dietary restraints	*r* =	−.096	.101	−.121
	p =	.454	.432	.347
Eating concerns	*r* =	.045	.041	−.094
	p =	.726	.751	.466
Shape concerns	*r* =	−.070	−.100	−.168
	p =	.587	.435	.187
Weight concerns	*r* =	−.038	−.053	−.155
	p =	.767	.678	.224
General psychopathology (DASS-21)				
Depression	*r* =	−.121	.094	−.162
	p =	.344	.466	.205
Stress	*r* =	−.037	.094	−.158
	p =	.772	.461	.215
Anxiety	*r* =	−.114	.026	−.080
	p =	.376	.840	.531
COVID-19 anxiety (FCV-19S)				
	r =	−.193	−.143	**.276**
	p =	.129	.263	**.029**
Therapeutic alliance (WAI-S)				
Total	*r* =	.196	.173	**.293**
	p =	.147	.203	**.028**
Task	*r* =	.033	.086	**.346**
	p =	.806	.530	**.009**
Bond	*r* =	**.291**	.119	.140
	p =	**.030**	.384	.302
Goal	*r* =	.204	**.268**	**.295**
	p =	.131	**.045**	**.027**

Note: Perspectives towards the transition to online treatment were measured using the six items developed for the current study. A higher score represents a more positive attitude towards the transition. Bold font indicates statistically significant results (p-value< 0.05). *Abbreviations*: *ED* eating disorder, *EDE-Q* Eating Disorder Examination Questionnaire, *DASS-21* Depression, Anxiety and Stress Scale – Version 21, *WAI-S* Working Alliance Inventory – short version, *COVID-19* coronavirus disease 2019, *FCV-19S* Fear of COVID-19 Scale (FCV-19S), *TSQ* Telemedicine Satisfaction Questionnaire

Discussion

The aim of the current study was to conduct a pilot investigation into the perspectives of ambulatory patients with EDs toward the transition from conventional face-to-face treatment to online treatment during the COVID-19 lockdown and to provide a measure for their assessment. Analyses demonstrated three main findings. First, preliminary analyses suggested that these views can be measured using a Likert-type 6-item scale. Second, a mixed distribution of views was observed in our sample with regard to the transition to online treatment. Third, the key factors that were linked with a more favorable attitude toward the transition were longer duration of treatment, stronger therapeutic alliance and stronger COVID-19 anxiety. These findings highlight the need to identify patients who may face difficulties with transitioning to online therapy as well as offering them appropriate support or a service package to meet their needs.

Our preliminary analyses revealed that the six items we developed could provide an accurate measure evaluating patients' perspectives toward the transition to online treatment. The results of the exploratory factor analysis (EFA) revealed a unidimensional factor structure which explained 62.4% of the variance. Cronbach's alpha for the unidimensional model was excellent (α =0.878). An examination of the construct validity indicated that the scale was not related to telemedicine satisfaction (as measured by the TSQ), suggesting that the construct measuring patients' perspectives toward the transition to online treatment should be studied in parallel with the construct measuring patients' satisfaction with online treatment. Of note is that a prior study analyzing the impact of the lockdown on patients with EDs and obesity did not distinguish between these two constucts [4].

A roughly normal distribution of perspectives was found toward the positive contribution or adverse effect of the transition: an expression of varied perspectives on the transition. Interestingly, although most participants did not report an adverse effect of their online care (Items 1,2), as many as two thirds stated that they would not choose to continue with online treatment (Item 5), and more than half were sure that they would not recommend online treatment to family members and friends (Item 6). This finding suggests that patients understand remote online treatment to be a situation-specific necessity rather than a choice, a finding further supported by the association we found between the goal component of the therapeutic alliance and satisfaction with the quality of telemedicine. Indeed, this transition was previously described by patients with AN as being accompanied by feelings of great uncertainty and a lack of preparedness [44]. Along the same lines, we found lower satisfaction scores across quality, similarity, and perception of encounter measures, compared with previous studies that used the same tool to investigate satisfaction of online treatment for mental health issues in unrelated circumstances [24, 25]. Online treatment in our study was closely connected with the COVID-19 pandemic, an overall negative and anxiety-provoking experience for patients with EDs [45], implicated in the worsening of ED symptoms for many patients [8, 46, 47], and prompting the strong wish to "go back to normal." Our results contrast with those from a recent report by Fernández-Aranda et al. where a newly developed comprehensive tool to assess the impact of confinement on ED symptoms and acceptance of telemedicine described telemedicine as well accepted [4]. However, the novelty of the tool used in that study precludes comparison to other studies, and the data were collected retrospectively. Our finding that most participants would not willingly choose online treatment is important, as recent publications have called on the professional world to "seize the opportunity" and embrace online therapy, not as a requirement but as an indicated and preferred treatment [48]. Patients may be reluctant to make this transition, and it is important that their views be considered.

With respect to potential contributing factors, no demographic characteristics, including age, were found to be correlated with views on the transition. As hypothesized, longer pre-lockdown duration and a stronger therapeutic alliance were found to be associated with a more positive view of the transition. A meta-analysis comparing videoconferencing-psychotherapy (VCP) to in-person therapy found the working alliance to be good in VCP, but inferior in relation to face-to-face therapy, although symptom reduction was comparable in both groups [49]. Given the challenge of establishing an early alliance remotely [7], it could be that participants who did not have a chance to develop a strong therapeutic alliance before the lockdown (e.g., due to short treatment duration or preexisting tensions with the therapist) had difficulties strengthening their alliance during the lockdown in the context of VCP usage. This lack of alliance may have thus contributed to their negative perception of online treatment. These findings stress the importance of the therapeutic alliance as a central component of therapy [50], which in this context likely facilitated (or impeded, where there was no such alliance) the transition from the patient's perspective. Our findings mirror the recent experience as described by clinicians; namely, previous face-to-face engagement with a therapist was found to allow for a smoother transition to distant ED protocol-based treatment during the pandemic, whereas initiating the program distantly was greeted by difficulty in building a collaborative relationship [51].

Clinical factors including severity of ED symptoms, depression, or general anxiety showed no overall effect on perceptions toward the transition. Patients with different ED diagnoses (AN, BN, or BED) did not vary in their satisfaction with online treatment or in their perceptions towards the transition, a finding that may be attributed to the transdiagnostic view of EDs [52], which focuses on the common features, rather on the dissimilarities, of ED diagnoses [53]. This finding differs from that described by Fernández-Aranda et al. who found lower acceptance of online therapy among AN patient. Future studies using larger samples with more patients in each diagnostic group would be helpful in clarifying these conflicting results.

As predicted, fear of the novel coronavirus and the disease that it causes was associated with positive views toward online treatment. Concerns among people with EDs regarding the impact of COVID-19 on their health and mental health have been found to be common [45]. For health-anxious patients, online therapy was advantageous for two reasons. First, their fear would have prevented them from leaving home and arriving at clinics for therapy anyway; as such, remote treatment enabled them to continue care. Second, as fears of COVID-19 have indeed been found to predict mental health symptoms [54] (e.g. depression, anxiety), therapy could potentially provide a containing environment to ease these fears and alleviate their possible harmful results.

The strengths of our study include the use of validated questionnaires as well as a dedicated measure, developed specifically for this study, and conducting a rapid real-world data collection among a clinical sample during the lockdown period, thus capturing patients' perceptions during this unique and unprecedented time. Some important limitations should be noted. Our sample size was limited by the size of our center and the short time in which the study was conducted. In our study we grouped together patients with different ED diagnoses, an approach which is supported by the ED transdiagnostic model [53]. Future studies using a larger sample size may uncover differences among the main ED diagnoses. Such studies could also expose variance between attitudes of patients undergoing different models of therapy, for example enhanced cognitive behavioral therapy (CBT-E) against insight-directed therapy. Given the exploratory nature of our study, alpha correction for multiple comparisons was not used in the analyses. Future studies may verify our results using a larger sample size which would allow alpha correction. The design of the study was cross-sectional, and therefore causal relations cannot be deduced from our findings. Last, it could be that our clinic has specific characteristics (e.g., a large portion of chronic patients with a relatively long treatment duration) that may have impacted results, thus limiting the generalizability of our findings to other clinical ED populations.

Conclusions

Our pilot study demonstrates that the views of ED outpatients can be assessed using a short 6-item Likert-type scale. Our main preliminary conclusions are that a longer pre-lockdown treatment duration, stronger therapeutic alliance, and more severe COVID-19 anxiety are associated with a positive attitude toward online treatment. These findings require further investigation in larger samples, potentially via the utilization of our transition-focused measure. Amidst the ongoing pandemic situation and confinement measures that may be instituted on a not infrequent basis, initial clinical implications drawn from our findings are that special consideration may be needed in newly-begun treatments, and that attentiveness and a flexible approach should be taken towards those prone to health anxieties. Future studies might wish to utilize a prospective longitudinal design in order to determine how views on the transition are related to long-term treatment outcomes.

Abbreviations

AN: Anorexia Nervosa; BED: Binge Eating Disorder; BMI: body mass index; BN: Bulimia Nervosa; CBT-E: Enhanced Cognitive Behavioral Therapy; COVID-19: Coronavirus disease of 2019; DASS-21: Depression Anxiety and Stress Scales; ED: Eating disorder; EDE-Q: Eating Disorder Examination Questionnaire; EFA: Exploratory Factor Analysis; FCV-19S: Fear of COVID-19 Scale; IRB: Institutional Review Board; KMO: Kaiser-Meyer-Olkin; SARS-CoV-2: Severe Acute Respiratory Syndrome Coronavirus 2; TSQ: Telemedicine Satisfaction Questionnaire; VCP: Video-Conferencing Psychotherapy; WAI-S: Working Alliance Inventory

Authors' contributions

YDL and REB initiated the study, and all authors developed the protocol. YDL, RGS and EZ recruited participants. REB analyzed the data, and all authors interpreted it. YDL wrote the initial manuscript and all authors critically reviewed and approved the final manuscript.

Competing interests

The authors have no conflict of interests to declare.

Author details

[1]Hadarim Eating Disorders Treatment Center, Shalvata Mental Health Center, Hod Hasharon, Israel. [2]Sackler Faculty of Medicine, Tel Aviv University, Tel Aviv, Israel. [3]School of Public Health, University of Haifa, Haifa, Israel.

References

1. Brooks SK, Webster RK, Smith LE, Woodland L, Wessely S, Greenberg N, et al. The psychological impact of quarantine and how to reduce it: rapid review of the evidence. Lancet. 2020;395:912–20. https://doi.org/10.1016/S0140-6736(20)30460-8.
2. Elran-Barak R, Mozeikov M. One month into the reinforcement of social distancing due to the COVID-19 outbreak: subjective health, health behaviors, and loneliness among people with chronic medical conditions. Int J Environ Res Public Health. 2020;17(15):5403. https://doi.org/10.3390/ijerph17155403.
3. Békés V, van Doorn KA. Psychotherapists' attitudes toward online therapy during the COVID-19 pandemic. J Psychother Integr. 2020;30(2):238–47. https://doi.org/10.1037/int0000214.
4. Fernández-Aranda F, Munguía L, Mestre-Bach G, Steward T, Etxandi M, Baenas I, et al. COVID isolation eating scale (CIES): analysis of the impact of confinement in eating disorders and obesity—a collaborative international study. Eur Eat Disord Rev. 2020;28(6):871–83. https://doi.org/10.1002/erv.2784.
5. Lamb T, Pachana NA, Dissanayaka N. Update of recent literature on remotely delivered psychotherapy interventions for anxiety and depression. Telemed e-Health. 2019;25(8):671–7. https://doi.org/10.1089/tmj.2018.0079.
6. Hilty DM, Ferrer DC, Parish MB, Johnston B, Callahan EJ, Yellowlees PM. The effectiveness of telemental health: a 2013 review. Telemed e-Health. 2013;19(6):444–54. https://doi.org/10.1089/tmj.2013.0075.
7. Sproch LE, Anderson KP. Clinician-delivered Teletherapy for eating disorders. Psychiatr Clin North Am. 2019;42(2):243–52. https://doi.org/10.1016/j.psc.2019.01.008.
8. Fernández-Aranda F, Casas M, Claes L, Clark Bryan D, Favaro A, Granero R, et al. COVID-19 and implications for eating disorders. Eur Eat Disord Rev. 2020;28(3):239–45. https://doi.org/10.1002/erv.2738.
9. Liu S, Yang L, Zhang C, Xiang Y-T, Liu Z, Hu S, et al. Online mental health services in China during the COVID-19 outbreak. Lancet Psychiatry. 2020;7(4):e17–8. https://doi.org/10.1016/S2215-0366(20)30077-8.
10. Torous J, Jän Myrick K, Rauseo-Ricupero N, Firth J. Digital mental health and COVID-19: using technology today to accelerate the curve on access and quality tomorrow. JMIR Ment Heal. 2020;7(3):e18848. https://doi.org/10.2196/18848.
11. Kahnna R, Forbes M. Telepsychiatry as a public health imperative: slowing COVID-19. Aust New Zeal J Psychiatry. 2020;54(7):758–61. https://doi.org/10.1177/0004867420924480.
12. Shah M, Sachdeva M, Johnston H. Eating disorders in the age of COVID-19. Psychiatry Res. 2020;290:113122. https://doi.org/10.1016/j.psychres.2020.113122.
13. Cooper M, Reilly EE, Siegel JA, Coniglio K, Sadeh-Sharvit S, Pizetsky EM, et al. Eating disorders during the COVID-19 pandemic: an overview of risks and recommendations for treatment and early intervention. Eat Disord. 2020;00(00):1–23. https://doi.org/10.1080/10640266.2020.1790271.

14. Rodgers RF, Lombardo C, Cerolini S, Franko DL, Omori M, Fuller-Tyszkiewicz M, et al. The impact of the COVID-19 pandemic on eating disorder risk and symptoms. Int J Eat Disord. 2020;(May):1166–70. https://doi.org/10.1002/eat.23318.
15. Weissman RS, Bauer S, Thomas JJ. Access to evidence-based care for eating disorders during the COVID-19 crisis. Int J Eat Disord. 2020;53(5):369–76. https://doi.org/10.1002/eat.23279.
16. Davis C, Ng KC, Oh JY, Baeg A, Rajasegaran K, Chew CSE. Caring for children and adolescents with eating disorders in the current coronavirus 19 pandemic: a Singapore perspective. J Adolesc Heal. 2020;67(1):131–4. https://doi.org/10.1016/j.jadohealth.2020.03.037.
17. Waller G, Pugh M, Mulkens S, Moore E, Mountford VA, Carter J, Wicksteed A, Maharaj A, Wade TD, Wisniewski L, Farrell NR. Cognitive-behavioral therapy in the time of coronavirus: clinician tips for working with eating disorders via telehealth when face-to-face meetings are not possible. Int J Eat Disord. 2020;53(7):1132–41.
18. Treasure J, Claudino AM, Zucker N. Eating disorders. Lancet. 2010;375(9714): 583–93. https://doi.org/10.1016/S0140-6736(09)61748-7.
19. Horvath AO, Symonds D. Relation between alliance and outcome in psychotherapy: a metaanalysis. J Couns Psychol. 1991;38(2):139–49. https://doi.org/10.1037/0022-0167.38.2.139.
20. Horvath AO, Luborsky L. The role of the therapeutic alliance in psychotherapy. J Consult Clin Psychol. 1993;61(4):561–73.
21. Aafjes-van Doorn K, Békés V, Prout TA. Grappling with our therapeutic relationship and professional self-doubt during COVID-19: will we use video therapy again? Couns Psychol Q. 2020;00(00):1–12. https://doi.org/10.1080/09515070.2020.1773404.
22. Tzur Bitan D, Grossman-Giron A, Bloch Y, Mayer Y, Shiffman N, Mendlovic S. Fear of COVID-19 scale: psychometric characteristics, reliability and validity in the Israeli population. Psychiatry Res. 2020;289(May):113100. https://doi.org/10.1016/j.psychres.2020.113100.
23. Yip MP, Chang AM, Chan J, Mackenzie AE. Development of the telemedicine satisfaction questionnaire to evaluate patient satisfaction with telemedicine: a preliminary study. J Telemed Telecare. 2003;9(1):46–50. https://doi.org/10.1258/135763303321159693.
24. Stubbings DR, Rees CS, Roberts LD, Kane RT. Comparing in-person to videoconference-based cognitive behavioral therapy for mood and anxiety disorders : randomized controlled trial. J Med Internet Res. 2013;15(11)): e258. https://doi.org/10.2196/jmir.2564.
25. Yang R, Vigod SN, Hensel JM. Optional web-based videoconferencing added to office-based Care for Women Receiving Psychotherapy during the postpartum period : pilot randomized controlled trial. J Med. 2019;21(6): e13172. https://doi.org/10.2196/13172.
26. Fairburn CG, Beglin SJ. Assessment of eating disorders: interview or self-report questionnaire? Int J Eat Disord. 1994;16(4):363–70 Available from: https://doi.org/10.1002/1098-108X(199412)16:4%3C363::AID-EAT2260160405%3E3.0.CO;2-%23.
27. Berg KC, Peterson CB, Frazier P, Crow SJ. Psychometric evaluation of the eating disorder examination and eating disorder examination-questionnaire: A systematic review of the literature. Int J Eat Disord. 2012. https://doi.org/10.1002/eat.20931.
28. Zohar AH, Lev-Ari L, Bachner-Melman R. The EDE-Q in Hebrew: structural and convergent/divergent validity in a population sample. Isr J Psychiatry. 2017;54(3):15–21.
29. Lovibond SH, Lovibond PF. Manual for the Depression Anxiety Stress Scales. Sydney: Psychology Foundation of Australia; 1995.
30. Antony MM, Bieling PJ, Enns MW, Swinson RP. Psychometric properties of the 42-item and the 21-item version of the DASS in clinical groups and a community sample. Psychol Assess. 1998;10(2):176–81 Available from: https://psycnet.apa.org/doi/10.1037/1040-3590.10.2.176.
31. Anghel E. Longitudinal invariance and information of the depression, anxiety, and stress scales. J Clin Psychol. 2020;76(10):1923–37. https://doi.org/10.1002/jclp.22968.
32. Tracey TJ, Kokotovic AM. Factor structure of the working Alliance inventory. Psychol Assess A J Consult Clin Psychol. 1989;1(3):207–10.
33. Nakash O, Nagar M, Kanat-Maymon Y. "What should we talk about?" the association between the information exchanged during the mental health intake and the quality of the working alliance. J Couns Psychol. 2015;62(3): 514–20 Available from: https://doi.apa.org/doi/10.1037/cou0000074.
34. Ahorsu DK, Lin C-Y, Imani V, Saffari M, Griffiths MD, Pakpour AH. The Fear of COVID-19 Scale: Development and Initial Validation. Int J Ment Health Addict. 2020:1–9 Available from: http://www.ncbi.nlm.nih.gov/pubmed/32226353%0A; http://www.pubmedcentral.nih.gov/articlerender.fcgi?artid=PMC7100496.
35. Constanzo F, Aracena-Sherck P, Hidalgo JP, Muñoz M, Vergara G, Alvarado C. Validation of a patient satisfaction survey of the Teleneurology program in Chile. BMC Res Notes. 2019;12(1):1–7. https://doi.org/10.1186/s13104-019-4358-1.
36. Fitzsimmons DA, Thompson J, Bentley CL, Mountain GA. Comparison of patient perceptions of Telehealth-supported and specialist nursing interventions for early stage COPD: a qualitative study. BMC Health Serv Res. 2016;16(1):1–12. https://doi.org/10.1186/s12913-016-1623-z.
37. Vogt WP, Johnson B. Dictionary of statistics & methodology: a nontechnical guide for the social sciences. Thousand Oaks: Sage; 2011.
38. Dahlgren CL, Stedal K, Rø Ø. Eating disorder examination questionnaire (EDE-Q) and clinical impairment assessment (CIA): clinical norms and functional impairment in male and female adults with eating disorders. Nord J Psychiatry. 2017;71(4):256–61. https://doi.org/10.1080/08039488.2016.1271452.
39. Calugi S, Milanese C, Sartirana M, El Ghoch M, Sartori F, Geccherle E, et al. The eating disorder examination questionnaire: reliability and validity of the Italian version. Eat Weight Disord. 2017;22(3):509–14. https://doi.org/10.1007/s40519-016-0276-6.
40. Aardoom JJ, Dingemans AE, Slof Op't Landt MCT, Van Furth EF. Norms and discriminative validity of the eating disorder examination questionnaire (EDE-Q). Eat Behav. 2012;13(4):305–9. https://doi.org/10.1016/j.eatbeh.2012.09.002.
41. Hilbert A, de Zwaan M, Braehler E. How frequent are eating disturbances in the population? Norms of the eating disorder examination-questionnaire. PLoS One. 2012;7(1). https://doi.org/10.1371/journal.pone.0029125.
42. Sly R, Morgan JF, Mountford VA, Lacey JH. Predicting premature termination of hospitalised treatment for anorexia nervosa: the roles of therapeutic alliance, motivation, and behaviour change. Eat Behav. 2013;14(2):119–23. https://doi.org/10.1016/j.eatbeh.2013.01.007.
43. Waller G, Tatham M, Turner H, Mountford VA, Bennetts A, Bramwell K, et al. A 10-session cognitive-behavioral therapy (CBT-T) for eating disorders: outcomes from a case series of nonunderweight adult patients. Int J Eat Disord. 2018;51(3):262–9. https://doi.org/10.1002/eat.22837.
44. Clark Bryan D, Macdonald P, Ambwani S, Cardi V, Rowlands K, Willmott D, et al. Exploring the ways in which COVID-19 and lockdown has affected the lives of adult patients with anorexia nervosa and their carers. Eur Eat Disord Rev. 2020;(June):1–10 Available from: http://www.ncbi.nlm.nih.gov/pubmed/32643844.
45. Termorshuizen JD, Watson HJ, Thornton LM, Borg S, Flatt RE, MacDermod CM, et al. Early Impact of COVID-19 on Individuals with Eating Disorders: A survey of ~1000 Individuals in the United States and the Netherlands. Int J Eat Disord. 2020;(June):1–11 Available from: http://www.ncbi.nlm.nih.gov/pubmed/32511555%0A; http://www.pubmedcentral.nih.gov/articlerender.fcgi?artid=PMC7274236.
46. Schlegl S, Meule A, Voderholzer U. Bulimia nervosa in times of the COVID-19 pandemic — results from an online survey of former inpatients. Eur Eat Disord Rev. 2020;28(6):847–54. https://doi.org/10.1002/erv.2773.
47. Schlegl S, Maier J, Voderholzer U. Eating disorders in times of the COVID-19 pandemic — results from an online survey of patients with anorexia nervosa. Int J Eat Disord. 2020;53(11):1791–800. https://doi.org/10.1002/eat.23374.
48. Taylor CB, Fitzsimmons-craft EE, Graham AK. Digital technology can revolutionize mental health services delivery : the COVID-19 crisis as a catalyst for change. Int J Eat Disord. 2020;53(7):1155–7. https://doi.org/10.1002/eat.23300.
49. Norwood C, Moghaddam NG, Malins S, Sabin-Farrell R. Working alliance and outcome effectiveness in videoconferencing psychotherapy: a systematic review and noninferiority meta-analysis. Clin Psychol Psychother. 2018;25(6): 797–808. https://doi.org/10.1002/cpp.2315.
50. Zilcha-Mano S. Is the alliance really therapeutic? Revisiting this question in light of recent methodological advances. Am Psychol. 2017;74(4):311–25. https://doi.org/10.1037/a0040435.
51. Murphy R, Calugi S, Cooper Z, Dalle GR. Challenges and opportunities for enhanced cognitive behaviour therapy (CBT-E) in light of COVID-19. Cogn Behav Ther. 2020;13:e14. https://doi.org/10.1017/S1754470X20000161.
52. Elran-Barak R, Sztainer M, Goldschmidt AB, Crow SJ, Peterson CB, Hill LL, et al. Dietary restriction behaviors and binge eating in anorexia nervosa, bulimia nervosa and binge eating disorder: trans-diagnostic examination of

the restraint model. Eat Behav. 2015;18:192–6. https://doi.org/10.1016/j.eatbeh.2015.05.012.

53. Fairburn CG, Cooper Z, Shafran R, Wilson GT. Eating disorders: a transdiagnostic protocol; 2008.

54. Liu CH, Zhang E, Wong GTF, Hyun S, Chris HH. Factors associated with depression, anxiety, and PTSD symptomatology during the COVID-19 pandemic: Clinical implications for U.S. young adult mental health. Psychiatry Res. 2020;290(June). https://doi.org/10.1016/j.psychres.2020.113172.

15

Economic burden of eating disorders in South Korea

Sang Min Lee[1], Minha Hong[2], Saengryeol Park[3], Won Sub Kang[1] and In-Hwan Oh[4*]

Abstract

Background: Few studies have investigated the epidemiology of eating disorders using national representative data. In this study, we investigated the treatment prevalence and economic burden of eating disorders in South Korea.

Methods: The aim of this study was to estimate the treatment prevalence and the medical expenditure of diagnosed eating disorders (ICD F50.x) in South Korea between 2010 and 2015. We also examined the economic costs of eating disorders, including the direct medical cost, direct non-medical costs, and indirect costs, in order to calculate the economic burden of such disorders.

Results: The total treatment prevalence of eating disorders in South Korea was 12.02 people (per 100,000) in 2010, and 13.28 in 2015. The cost of medical expenditures due to eating disorders increased from USD 1229724 in 2010 to USD 1843706 in 2015. The total economic cost of eating disorders was USD 5455626 in 2015. In 2015, the economic cost and prevalence of eating disorders was the highest in the 20–29 age group.

Conclusions: The results showed the eating disorders are insufficiently managed in the medical insurance system. Further research is therefore warranted to better understand the economic burdens of each type of eating disorder.

Keywords: Eating disorder, Prevalence, Burden of disease, Bulimia nervosa, Anorexia nervosa

Plain English summary

This article is the result of estimating the overall medical expenditures due to eating disorders in South Korea, a country that has introduced the National Health Insurance system, the prevalence rate based on this, and further the economic burden. It is a data that can grasp the status and actual condition of medical expenses due to eating disorders, and can be the basis for appropriate distribution of medical expenses and policy-making process in the future.

Background

There is evidence that eating disorders are increasing worldwide, and that they affect approximately 2% of the world's population [1, 2]. Eating disorders may occur at a relatively young age, often beginning between 10 and 20 years of age [3], and may be chronic, lifelong conditions that are associated with various physical and psychiatric components [4, 5]. They are also one of the most common adolescent chronic disorders [6, 7], and friends and family often become informal long-term caregivers [8]. Among mental illnesses, eating disorders have the highest lifetime mortality rate (up to 20%); the mortality rate among women with eating disorders is twelve times higher than it is for unaffected women [9, 10]. When compared with the general population, people with eating disorders have nearly double the mortality rate of those who are unaffected [11].

A study of patients with eating disorders in the United States found that the majority of patients did not seek treatment for the eating disorder itself [5]. It was similar phenomenon in Asia that the proportion of patients

* Correspondence: parenchyme@gmail.com
[4]Department of Preventive Medicine, Kyung Hee University School of Medicine, 1 Hoegi-Dong, Dongdaemug-Gu, Seoul 130-701, South Korea
Full list of author information is available at the end of the article

within the healthcare setting is low [12, 13]. Even when eating disorders are treated, medication has limited efficacy and, in general, more than half the patients with anorexia and bulimia nervosa do not recover fully [1, 6]. One in four people with anorexia nervosa develops long-term impairment in social functioning and employment, to the extent that they cannot be gainfully employed. The quality of life for patients with eating disorders deteriorates more than it does for patients with symptomatic coronary heart disease or major depression, and the duration of illness tends to be longer [14].

Treatment guidelines recommend the active involvement of family members in the treatment of eating disorders [15]. Patients with severe and long-lasting anorexia nervosa are highly dependent on their families, creating a subsequently high caregiving burden [16]. The socio-economic burden and costs of anorexia nervosa and bulimia nervosa are similar to those of anxiety disorders and depression [6], as quantified by the Global Burden of Disease Study conducted in 2013 [17].

Studies have been conducted in Europe to estimate the size and cost of eating disorders, but most have included only anorexia nervosa and bulimia nervosa; this led to a gross underestimation of the problem, because binge eating and unspecified eating disorders are in fact the most commonly occurring disorders [18]. Those studies also did not include key resource items: the cost of lost productivity for the entire family, and indirect costs due to reduced length of life and health [6, 18].

Only some recently published studies presented a partial aspect of epidemiology of eating disorders in Asia [12, 13, 19]. There have been very few studies of epidemiology of eating disorders completed in South Korea. Lee et al. published a psychiatric epidemiology of major disorders using DSM-III criteria [20, 21]. Cho et al. reported that the lifetime prevalence of eating disorders using DSM-IV criteria in Korea was 0.2% [22].

Globally, several studies have systematically reviewed the disease burden of eating disorders. Extant studies of eating disorders tend to have poor data representation due to the lack of large-scale population based studies and the inconsistencies of studies [17]. This study analyzed the healthcare costs of anorexia nervosa, bulimia nervosa, and other eating disorders, such as binge eating disorder and eating disorders not otherwise specified, over a six-year period. Using representative health statistics and health insurance data from 2010 to 2015, we attempted to estimate the national burden and economic costs of eating disorders on medical care utilization and to explore the characteristics of this burden with respect to gender and age groups.

Methods

Data sources

This study utilized two government data sources for its analysis. The prevalence rates and medical expenditure of eating disorders were calculated using data from the Health Insurance Review & Assessment Service (HIRA). The database provided records of patient numbers and specified outpatient, inpatient, and hospitalization days by gender. The economic cost of eating disorders was derived from the data of the National Health Insurance Services (NHIS), which is the single insurer in South Korea [23]. The NHIS provides medical costs based on the medical utilization records from the National Health Information Database (NHID). Data from January 1, 2020 to December 31, 2015 were collected from both HIRA and NHIS. Population statistics were adopted from the Korean Statistical Information Service (KOSIS). Average currency rates per year were adopted from the Bank of Korea (http://ecos.bok.or.kr) to convert the Korean Won to US dollars (USD). The data supporting this study's findings are available on request from the corresponding author, but are not publicly available due to privacy or ethical restrictions.

Case definition

Eating disorders (F50) were defined using the International Classification of Diseases, Tenth Revision (ICD-10) [24]. For estimation of the economic burden, eating disorders were as: anorexia nervosa (F50.0); bulimia nervosa (F50.2); and other eating disorders (OED) (F50.1–F50.9). OED included atypical anorexia nervosa (F50.1); atypical bulimia nervosa (F50.3); overeating associated with other psychological disturbances (F50.4); vomiting associated with other psychological disturbances (F50.5); other eating disorders (F50.8); and unspecified eating disorder (F50.9).

Treatment prevalence rates of eating disorders

The treatment prevalence rates of eating disorders from 2010 to 2015 were estimated using the number of cases from HIRA Service. The number of cases was divided by the total population and then multiplied by 100,000.

Estimation of the economic burden of eating disorders

The present study estimated the medical expenditure and economic cost of eating disorders (anorexia nervosa, bulimia nervosa, OED) using data from HIRA and NHIS. Medical expenditure was determined by the HIRA data regarding expenditures from both the national insurance service and patients. Economic cost, both direct and indirect, was estimated using a prevalence-based approach from NHIS data.

Direct costs included the total costs associated with medical treatment, transportation, and caregivers.

Medical costs included non-covered care costs, insured and non-insured costs, and drug costs. Direct non-medical costs included transportation costs and caregiver costs. Transportation costs associated with eating disorders were defined as the products of the number of outpatient visits and hospitalizations with the average roundtrip transportation costs. The average roundtrip transportation costs were 4.34 USD per outpatient visit and 46.70 USD per hospitalization according to Korean Health Panel data. The time spent for an outpatient visit was estimated as one-third of the cost for an inpatient visit for determination of outpatient caregiver costs. Also, caregiver costs were calculated using data from the Korea Patient Helper Society.

Indirect costs-2 was estimated to explain productivity loss caused by the absence from work for hospital admissions or outpatient visits. Indirect costs-2 was included in the total costs. For sensitivity purposes, indirect costs-1 was estimated by considering lost productivity. Productivity lost was defined as the loss of ones' time due to medical care. To estimate the productivity lost we used time spent traveling to hospital and waiting for treatment and multiplied the average time spent by the average daily wage. For example, when a patient took the day off due to hospitalization, it was considered as the loss of one day's income. In case of an outpatient visit, it was considered as the loss of one-third of daily income. Data were not available for those under 20 years old as they are too young to work. Indirect costs-1 was not included in the total costs. Total economic cost was taken as the sum of direct and indirect costs.

All analyses were performed using SAS (ver. 9.4; SAS institute, Cary, NC, USA).

Ethics statement

Ethical review was obtained by a University review board (IRB No. KHSIRB-19-354 (EA)). Informed consent was exempted due to the public nature of the NHIS data. The information is gathered by ID number, it is not identifiable.

Results

The current study investigated the treatment prevalence rates of eating disorders and patients' use of medical care between 2010 and 2015, in addition to evaluating the economic burden of eating disorders in Korea in 2015.

The results of this study showed that the treatment prevalence rates of eating disorders tended to increase from 2010 to 2013 and then decreased slightly from 2014 to 2015 (Table 1 and Fig. 1). The medical expenditure of eating disorders consistently increased from USD 1229724 in 2010 to USD 1843706 in 2015. Cases of bulimia nervosa increased from 2010 to 2015. In addition, a gender differential was observed in the economic burden of eating disorders from 2010 to 2015; the discrepancy was higher in female patients than in to male patients.

Table 2 shows the medical care use of eating disorders, including anorexia nervosa, bulimia nervosa, and OED, from 2010 to 2015. There was an inconsistent increase in the number of outpatient visits of patients afflicted with different types of eating disorders. The number of

Table 1 Treatment Prevalence of eating disorders in Korea from 2010 to 2015 by gender (per 100,000)

	Eating disorders Number of patients Prevalence			**Anorexia nervosa Number of patients Prevalence**			**Bulimia nervosa Number of patients Prevalence**			**Other eating disorders Number of patients Prevalence**			**Medical expenditure of eating disorders**		
Year	Sub total	Male	Female	Sub total	Male	Female	Sub total	Male	Female	Sub total	Male	Female	Male	Female	Total cost
2010	6074	1010	5064	1511	376	1135	1399	72	1327	3366	572	2794	131,770	1,097,954	1,229,724
	12.02	3.99	20.09	2.99	1.49	4.50	2.77	0.28	5.26	6.66	2.26	11.08			
2011	6694	1070	5624	1570	405	1165	1440	74	1366	3888	607	3281	135,824	1,298,591	1,434,415
	13.19	4.21	22.21	3.09	1.59	4.60	2.84	0.29	5.39	7.66	2.39	12.95			
2012	7052	1187	5865	1534	369	1165	1600	92	1508	4151	754	3397	155,809	1,314,500	1,470,310
	13.84	4.65	23.05	3.01	1.45	4.58	3.14	0.36	5.93	8.15	2.96	13.35			
2013	7388	1301	6087	1905	478	1427	1597	111	1486	4099	727	3372	123,037	1,506,356	1,629,394
	14.45	5.08	23.82	3.72	1.87	5.58	3.12	0.43	5.82	8.02	2.84	13.20			
2014	7364	1204	6160	1793	457	1336	1681	93	1588	4110	680	3430	175,329	1,631,515	1,806,843
	14.35	4.69	24.01	3.49	1.78	5.21	3.28	0.36	6.19	8.01	2.65	13.37			
2015	6845	1129	5716	1604	397	1207	1832	123	1709	3614	630	2984	138,939	1,704,767	1,843,706
	13.28	4.38	22.18	3.11	1.54	4.68	3.56	0.48	6.63	7.01	2.45	11.58			

Note. Data sources from Healthcare Bigdata Hub (https://opendata.hira.or.kr/) and Korean Statistical Information Service (KOSIS); size of population = 50,515,666 (female 25,205,281; 2010); 50,734,284 (female 25,327,350; 2011); 50,948,272 (female 25,444,212; 2012); 51,141,463 (female 25,553,127; 2013); 51,327,916 (female 25,658,620; 2014); 51,529,338 (female 25,771,152; 2015); Exchange rate US dollar: 1 Korean won = 1132 US dollar (2015); 1053 (2014); 1095 (2013); 1127 (2012); 1108 (2011); 1156 (2010); from the Bank of Korea (http://ecos.bok.or.kr/)

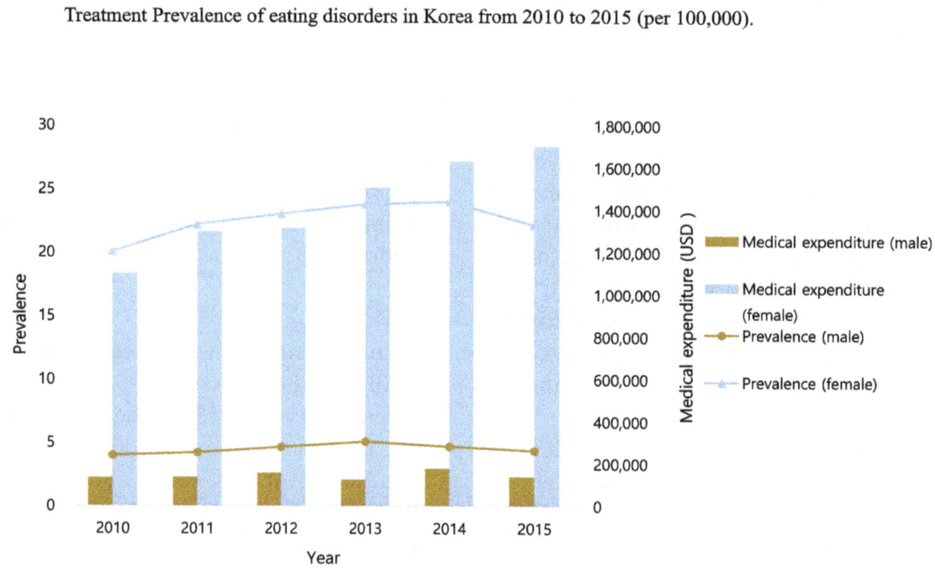

Fig. 1 Treatment Prevalence of eating disorders in Korea from 2010 to 2015 (per 100,000)

inpatient admissions decreased for patients with bulimia nervosa but increased in the cases with anorexia nervosa and OED. Hospitalization days per patient inconsistently decreased in anorexia nervosa and bulimia nervosa, but increased in OED.

Table 3 shows the economic burden of eating disorders including anorexia nervosa, bulimia nervosa, and OED by gender in 2015. The economic cost of eating disorders was 5,455,626 USD. Total costs were approximately 6 times higher in female patients than male patients. Direct costs were higher than indirect costs-2 in all types of eating disorders. OED were the highest contributor to the economic burden among anorexia nervosa, bulimia nervosa, and OED.

Table 4 shows the results of the sensitivity analysis for the economic burden of eating disorders in 2015. OED were the highest contributor to the economic burden and females were a higher contributor to the economic burden than males in indirect costs-1.

Table 5 and Figs. 2 and 3 show the economic burden of eating disorders in Korea in 2015 by age and gender. The economic burden of eating disorders was higher in patients aged between 20 years and 29 years than other age ranges. Anorexia nervosa was higher in patients aged between 10 years and 19 years than other age ranges. Bulimia nervosa was higher in patients aged between 20 years and 29 years than other age ranges. OED were higher in patients aged 50 years and 59 years than other age ranges. In general, female patients showed higher economic burden than male patients. In addition, younger generations showed a higher economic burden than older generations, except for in the case of OED.

Discussion

Population-representative epidemiological research studies on eating disorders are rare. Despite the knowledge that eating disorders have an early onset, few studies have been conducted on eating disorders among children and young people under the age of 18 [25]. The current study is meaningful, in that its use of a nationwide database means that it represents all of South Korea, including patients of all ages. It included eating disorder with ICD F50.x in its entirety and was not limited to anorexia nervosa and bulimia nervosa alone.

The recent systematic review reported that the estimated lifetime prevalence of eating disorder was 1.01% (95% CI, 0.54–1.89) [26]. It is noteworthy that the lifetime prevalence reported from studies conducted in Western countries (1.29%) was 6.1-fold greater than that reported in a single study from South Korea (0.21%) [26]. The current study found that the prevalence of eating disorders in South Korea was between 12.02 (0.012%) in 2010 and 13.28 (0.013%)in 2015. This implies that it can update the prevalence of eating disorders in South Korea, even though our study method and case definition varied from that of Cho et al. [22]. The estimated total economic cost of eating disorders in the current study was USD 5455626, which is equivalent to 0.0039% of Korean GDP in 2015. Those with OED, including binge eating disorder, accounted for 42% of the economic burden; anorexia nervosa, 34.7%; and bulimia nervosa, 22.3%. Our results are underestimated because the study did not take into account the negative impact of eating disorders on individual health,

Table 2 Patient's medical care use for eating disorders from 2010 to 2015

Year	Eating disorders			Anorexia nervosa			Bulimia nervosa			Other eating disorders		
	Number of outpatient visits (per patient)	Number of inpatient admissions (per patient)	Hospitalization days (per patient)	Number of outpatient visits (per patient)	Number of inpatient admissions (per patient)	Hospitalization days (per patient)	Number of outpatient visits (per patient)	Number of inpatient admissions (per patient)	Hospitalization days (per patient)	Number of outpatient visits (per patient)	Number of inpatient admissions (per patient)	Hospitalization days (per patient)
2010	3.27	1.72	31.16	2.43	1.51	28.32	4.03	1.67	37.62	3.19	1.33	17.76
2011	3.07	1.80	30.40	2.30	1.93	34.26	4.20	1.77	32.95	2.92	1.13	14.65
2012	3.54	1.79	30.48	2.73	1.97	35.17	4.57	1.63	29.07	3.25	1.24	17.58
2013	3.49	1.82	29.83	2.49	1.90	35.11	4.44	1.78	22.76	3.42	1.40	17.97
2014	3.51	1.71	28.69	2.71	1.65	29.42	4.16	1.66	25.78	3.15	1.34	17.14
2015	3.86	1.65	27.01	2.86	1.62	27.26	4.52	1.63	28.25	3.40	1.47	22.05

Note. Data source from Healthcare Bigdata Hub (https://opendata.hira.or.kr/)

Table 3 Economic cost of eating disorders in 2015

Classification	Eating disorders			Anorexia nervosa			Bulimia nervosa			Other eating disorders		
	Male	Female	Sub total	Male	Female	Sub total	Male	Female	Sub total	Male	Female	Sub total
Direct costs												
Direct medical costs	246,792	2,572,075	2,818,867	91,585	1,037,569	1129 154	31,420	737,817	769,237	123,786	796,690	920,476
Direct non-medical costs												
Transportation cost for hospital visits	11,492	84,283	95,776	4402	20,806	25,208	1275	27,047	28,322	5815	36,430	42,245
Caregiver cost	79,798	405,167	484,965	44,865	213,194	258,059	5964	67,603	73,568	28,969	124,370	153,339
Total direct costs	338,082	3,061,526	3,399,608	140,852	1,271,569	1,412,421	38,660	832,467	871,127	158,570	957,490	1,116,060
Indirect costs-2	453,177	1,602,841	2,056,018	132,185	353,510	485,694	18,772	328,218	346,991	302,220	921,113	1,223,333
Total costs	791,259	4,664,367	5,455,626	273,037	1,625,078	1,898,115	57,432	1,160,686	1,218,118	460,790	1,878,602	2,339,393

Note. Exchange rate US dollar: 1 Korean won = 1132 US dollar from the Bank of Korea (http://ecos.bok.or.kr/); For indirect costs-2, productivity loss from the absence from work due to hospital admission and outpatient visits were included

or socio-economic well-being. Given this, the actual economic costs can be expected to be much higher. In terms of gender, the treatment prevalence of eating disorders among females was high (4.68–5.27 times) in our study, and the medical expenditure for females was more than twice as high (8.33–12.26 times), compared to the treatment prevalence. In addition, in the proportion of economic burden, the ratio of direct medical cost is significantly higher for women compared to men (55% vs 31%). This is thought to be, in part, due to general gender differences in seeking diagnostic evaluation or healthcare treatment, and receiving more prescription drugs [27–29]. As shown by previous studies, the current study found that the disease burden of eating disorders was high in adolescent and early adult ages. This implies that disease burden is likely underestimated, because it is a condition that can be chronic and progressive [30].

A few limitations in the present study must be noted. First, the data was collected from a secondary database, the NHIS claims database, and not from medical records. It considers only the burden of disease based on patients who sought treatment. Also, we did not consider either psychiatric or physical comorbid disorders. Therefore, questions about the validity of the diagnosis and comorbidity information across hospitals may be raised. In addition, we used the number of hospitalizations and frequency of outpatient visits to ensure accuracy. Another limitation is that binge eating disorder, which has of clinical importance was added to the DSM-5 in 2013, and was not reflected in the ICD diagnostic system during the study period; therefore in our study, it is included under unspecified eating disorders. Although, we used the nationally representative database (i.e. HIRA), the treatment prevalence rates may not represent patients with eating disorders of South Korea, due to the nature of the database using medical records. Thus, future research may replicate this study by assessing another database to calculate the prevalence rates of South Korea.

Conclusion

Despite these limitations, this study is meaningful in that it has calculated the treatment prevalence and economic burden of eating disorders using national representative data. Eating disorders create severe and disabling conditions for the afflicted individual, their families, and society at large, but are often overlooked. In particular, this study is unique in its inclusion of other eating disorder groups, including binge eating disorder; most previous studies examined only bulimia nervosa and anorexia nervosa. The findings from the current study contribute to the evidence base from which suggestions for improvements in health service can be made, and to make policy- and service-planning more effective.

Table 4 Sensitivity analysis of indirect costs for economic cost of eating disorders in 2015

Classification	Eating disorders			Anorexia nervosa			Bulimia nervosa			Other eating disorders		
	Male	Female	Sub total	Male	Female	Sub total	Male	Female	Sub total	Male	Female	Sub total
Indirect costs-1	920,012	3,064,617	3,984,629	157,353	638,689	796,043	24,599	552,534	577,132	738,060	1,873,394	2,611,454

Note. Indirect costs-1 is different from indirect costs-2. Indirect costs-1 was estimated for the purpose of sensitivity analysis without the employment-to-population ratio (i.e., proportion of the population employed). Indirect costs-1 was not included in the total costs

Table 5 Economic cost of disease due to eating disorders in Korea in 2015 by age group

	Eating disorders						Anorexia nervosa						Bulimia nervosa						Other eating disorders					
	Direct cost			Indirect cost			Direct cost			Indirect cost			Direct cost			Indirect cost			Direct cost			Indirect cost		
Age range	Male	Female	Sub total	Male	Female	Sub total	Male	Female	Sub total	Male	Female	Sub total	Male	Female	Sub total	Male	Female	Sub total	Male	Female	Sub total	Male	Female	Sub total
0–9	29,659	41,561	71,220	–	–	–	16,507	20,429	36,936	–	–	–	–	1253	1253	–	–	–	13,152	19,879	33,031	–	–	–
10–19	58,076	766,065	824,141	–	–	–	29,904	507,441	537,345	–	–	–	15,145	130,128	145,273	–	–	–	13,027	128,496	141,523	–	–	–
20–29	59,903	913,172	973,075	22,652	390,672	413,324	12,388	274,955	287,343	5134	126,763	131,897	13,288	388,018	401,306	5231	152,803	158,034	34,227	250,199	284,427	12,287	111,105	123,392
30–39	42,248	688,260	730,507	126,348	427,966	554,314	26,783	237,700	264,483	105,300	166,309	271,609	6174	198,800	204,974	8619	106,144	114,763	9290	251,760	261,050	12,429	155,513	167,941
40–49	16,621	293,279	309,900	30,714	200,841	231,555	4100	118,678	122,778	7081	42,819	49,901	2130	75,690	77,820	3705	56,011	59,716	10,391	98,911	109,302	19,927	102,011	121,938
50–59	16,330	89,894	106,224	23,474	574,452	597,925	7170	25,813	32,984	10,143	13,574	23,717	286	25,356	25,641	1014	12,263	13,277	8874	38,725	47,599	12,317	548,614	560,931
60–69	27,404	34,994	62,398	240,666	4301	244,967	5041	10,934	15,975	1894	1321	3215	19	8126	8145	27	892	919	22,344	15,934	38,278	238,745	2088	240,833
70–79	47,007	98,324	145,331	4483	3213	7697	24,946	45,507	70,453	2544	1555	4099	1618	4200	5818	176	103	279	20,444	48,617	69,061	1764	1555	3319
80–89	40,834	135,978	176,812	4840	1395	6236	14,013	30,113	44,125	88	1167	1255	–	897	897	–	1	1	26,821	104,968	131,790	4752	227	4979
Total	338,082	3,061,526	3,399,608	453,177	1,602,841	2,056,018	140,852	1,271,569	1,412,421	132,185	353,510	485,694	38,660	832,467	871,127	18,772	328,218	346,991	158,570	957,490	1,116,060	302,220	921,113	1,223,333

Note. Exchange rate US dollar: 1 Korean won = 1132 US dollar from the Bank of Korea (http://ecos.bok.or.kr/)

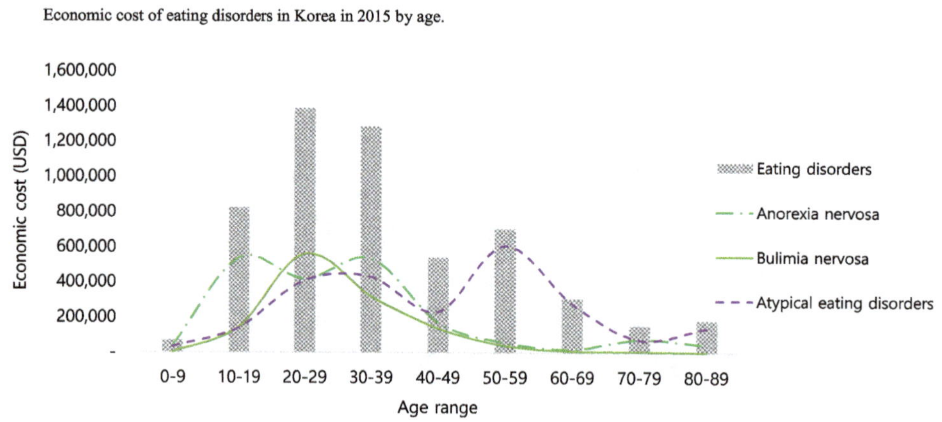

Fig. 2 Economic burden of eating disorders in Korea in 2015 by age

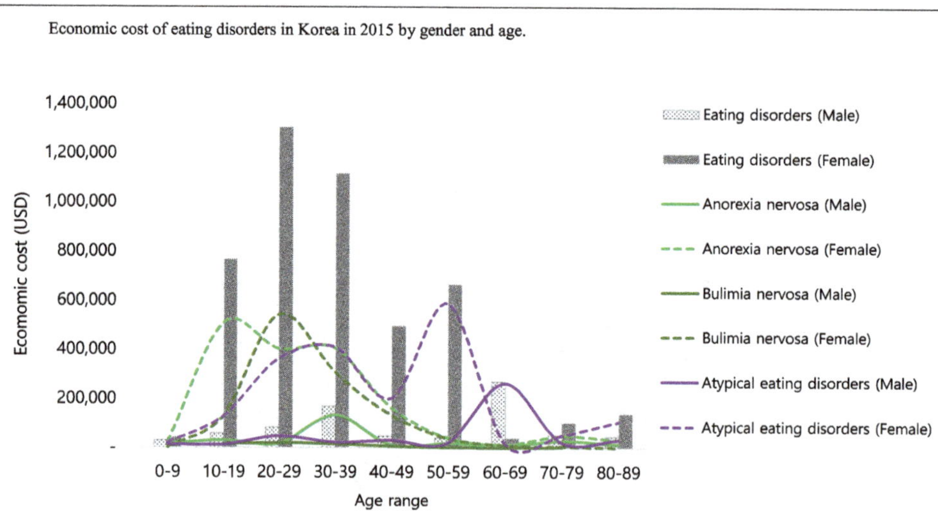

Fig. 3 Economic burden of eating disorders in Korea in 2015 by gender and age

Abbreviations

DSM: Diagnostic and Statistical Manual; HIRA: Health Insurance Review & Assessment Service; NHIS: National Health Insurance Services; NHID: National Health Information Database; KOSIS: Korean Statistical Information Service; ICD: International Classification of Diseases; OED: other eating disorders

Acknowledgements

A part of this study was presented at WPA 2019 as an oral presentation.

Authors' contributions

S.M.L and I.H.O conceptualized the study and were major contributors to writing the manuscript. S. P and M. H analyzed the data and contributed to organizing data collection. W.S.K assisted in manuscript revision and interpretation. All authors read and approved of the final manuscript.

Competing interests

The authors declare that they have no competing interests.

Author details

[1]Department of Psychiatry, Kyung Hee University Hospital, Kyung Hee University College of Medicine, 1 Hoegi-Dong, Dongdaemug-Gu, Seoul 130-701, South Korea. [2]Department of Psychiatry, Myongji Hospital, Hanyang University College of Medicine, 55 Hwasu-ro 14 beon-gil, Deogyang-gu, Goyang 10475, South Korea. [3]Department of Physical Education, College of Education, Chonnam National University, 77 Yongbong-ro, Buk-gu, Gwangju 61186, South Korea. [4]Department of Preventive Medicine, Kyung Hee University School of Medicine, 1 Hoegi-Dong, Dongdaemug-Gu, Seoul 130-701, South Korea.

References

1. Kessler RC, et al. The prevalence and correlates of binge eating disorder in the World Health Organization world mental health surveys. Biol Psychiatry. 2013;73(9):904–14.
2. Micali N, et al. The incidence of eating disorders in the UK in 2000–2009: findings from the General Practice Research Database. BMJ Open. 2013;3: e002646. https://doi.org/10.1136/bmjopen-2013-002646.
3. Smink FR, van Hoeken D, Hoek HW. Epidemiology, course, and outcome of eating disorders. Curr Opin Psychiatry. 2013;26(6):543–8.
4. Jacobi F, et al. Prevalence, co-morbidity and correlates of mental disorders in the general population: results from the German health interview and examination survey (GHS). Psychol Med. 2004;34(4):597–611.
5. Hudson JI, et al. The prevalence and correlates of eating disorders in the National Comorbidity Survey Replication. Biol Psychiatry. 2007;61(3):348–58.
6. Schmidt U, et al. Eating disorders: the big issue. Lancet Psychiatry. 2016;3(4): 313–5.
7. Lewinsohn PM, Striegel-Moore RH, Seeley JR. Epidemiology and natural course of eating disorders in young women from adolescence to young adulthood. J Am Acad Child Adolesc Psychiatry. 2000;39(10):1284–92.
8. Coomber K, King RM. A longitudinal examination of burden and psychological distress in carers of people with an eating disorder. Soc Psychiatry Psychiatr Epidemiol. 2013;48(1):163–71.
9. Steinhausen HC. The outcome of anorexia nervosa in the 20th century. Am J Psychiatry. 2002;159(8):1284–93.
10. Sullivan PF. Mortality in anorexia nervosa. Am J Psychiatry. 1995;152(7):1073–4.
11. Zipfel S, et al. Anorexia nervosa: aetiology, assessment, and treatment. Lancet Psychiatry. 2015;2(12):1099–111.
12. Tseng MM, et al. Rates and trends in healthcare-detected incidence of anorexia nervosa and bulimia nervosa: a national health insurance claim data study in Taiwan, 2002-2013. Int J Eat Disord. 2020;53(3):331–8.
13. Chua SN, et al. Estimated prevalence of eating disorders in Singapore. Int J Eat Disord. 2021;54(1):7–18.
14. Treasure J, et al. Anorexia nervosa. Nat Rev Dis Primers. 2015;1:15074.
15. National Collaborating Centre for Mental Health (UK). Eating disorders: core interventions in the treatment and management of anorexia nervosa, bulimia nervosa and related eating disorders. Leicester: British Psychological Society (UK); 2004.
16. Zabala MJ, Macdonald P, Treasure J. Appraisal of caregiving burden, expressed emotion and psychological distress in families of people with eating disorders: a systematic review. Eur Eat Disord Rev. 2009;17(5):338–49.
17. Erskine HE, Whiteford HA, Pike KM. The global burden of eating disorders. Curr Opin Psychiatry. 2016;29(6):346–53.
18. Gustavsson A, et al. Cost of disorders of the brain in Europe 2010. Eur Neuropsychopharmacol. 2011;21(10):718–79.
19. Yao S, et al. Screen-detected disordered eating and related traits in a large population sample of females in mainland China: China health and nutrition survey. Int J Eat Disord. 2021;54(1):24–35.
20. Lee CK, et al. Psychiatric epidemiology in Korea. Part I: gender and age differences in Seoul. J Nerv Ment Dis. 1990;178(4):242–6.
21. Lee CK, et al. Psychiatric epidemiology in Korea. Part II: urban and rural differences. J Nerv Ment Dis. 1990;178(4):247–52.
22. Cho MJ, et al. Lifetime and 12-month prevalence of DSM-IV psychiatric disorders among Korean adults. J Nerv Ment Dis. 2007;195(3):203–10.
23. Cheol Seong S, et al. Data resource profile: the national health information database of the National Health Insurance Service in South Korea. Int J Epidemiol. 2017;46(3):799–800.
24. World Health Organization. The ICD-10 classification of mental and behavioural disorders: clinical descriptions and diagnostic guidelines. Geneva: World Health Organization; 1992.
25. Erskine HE, et al. The global coverage of prevalence data for mental disorders in children and adolescents. Epidemiol Psychiatr Sci. 2017;26(4): 395–402.
26. Qian J, et al. Prevalence of eating disorders in the general population: a systematic review. Shanghai Arch Psychiatry. 2013;25(4):212–23.
27. Anthony M, et al. Gender and age differences in medications dispensed from a national chain drugstore. J Women's Health (Larchmt). 2008;17(5): 735–43.
28. Owens GM. Gender differences in health care expenditures, resource utilization, and quality of care. J Manag Care Pharm. 2008;14(3 Suppl):2–6.
29. Schappert SM, Burt CW. Ambulatory care visits to physician offices, hospital outpatient departments, and emergency departments: United States, 2001–02. Vital Health Stat. 2006;13(159):1–66.
30. Franko DL, et al. A longitudinal investigation of mortality in anorexia nervosa and bulimia nervosa. Am J Psychiatry. 2013;170(8):917–25.

16

Examination of eating disorder risk among university marching band artists

Nancy A. Uriegas[1], Dawn M. Emerson[2], Allison B. Smith[1], Melani R. Kelly[2] and Toni M. Torres-McGehee[1*]

Abstract

Background: Marching band artists are a physically active population, composed of approximately 27,000 people in the United States. University marching band artists face many of the same physically active demands and mental stressors as student athletes, potentially predisposing them to injury, illness, and risk for eating disorders (EDs). The purpose of this study was to examine ED risk across sex in university marching band artists, and to determine the type of risk based on the Eating Disorder Inventory-3 (EDI-3) and Eating Disorder Inventory-3 Symptom Check List (EDI-3 SC). A secondary aim examined marching band artists and pathogenic weight control behavior use across sex.

Methods: This was a cross-sectional study. A total of 150 marching band artists (female: $n = 84$, male: $n = 66$, age = 19.9 ± 1.1 years) from three National Collegiate Athletic Association Division I university marching bands participated in the study. We screened for ED risk using the EDI-3, and the EDI-3 SC.

Results: Overall, marching band artists were at risk for EDs, using only the EDI-3, 45.3% ($n = 68$) were at risk, with females at significant higher risk than males [$\chi^2 = 5.228$, $p = .022$]; using only the EDI-3 SC, 54% ($n = 81$) were at risk and no significant differences were found across sex. Overall, 48% of all participants reported dieting and 20.7% engaged in excessive exercise to control weight. Significant differences were found between sex and purging to control weight [$\chi^2 = 3.94$, $p = .047$] and laxative use [$\chi^2 = 4.064$, $p = .044$], with females engaging in behavior more than males.

Conclusions: Eating disorder risk was prevalent for both female and male marching band artists, with females displaying higher risk for EDs than males. Furthermore, marching band artists are engaging in pathogenic behaviors to control their weight. Healthcare providers (e.g., physicians, athletic trainers, physical therapist, dietitians, etc.) working in this setting should be aware of the risk factors displayed in marching band artists, and be able to provide education, prevention, and clinical interventions to this population. Additionally, marching band administrators should be aware of all medical risk factors and the benefit of having a healthcare provider (e.g., athletic trainer) to oversee the healthcare and wellness of marching band artists.

Keywords: Disordered eating behaviors, Behavioral health, Marching arts, Performing arts medicine

* Correspondence: torresmc@mailbox.sc.edu
[1]University of South Carolina, Blatt PE Center 212, Columbia, SC 29208, USA
Full list of author information is available at the end of the article

Plain English summary

Marching band artists are a physically active population that faces similar physical and mental stressors as student athletes. The combination of rigorous physical activity, increased stress, and lack of medical oversight predisposes marching band artists to injury, illness, and mental health conditions including eating disorders. This study looks at the prevalence of eating disorder risk in university marching band artists using a multidimensional approach of eating disorder risk and psychosocial components (e.g., low self-esteem, personal alienation, interpersonal insecurity, emotional dysregulation, etc.). The results of this study found that eating disorder risk is highly prevalent in this population and can be attributed to the psychosocial components of eating disorders and pathogenic behaviors including dieting and excessive exercise to control weight.

Background

The marching arts is a popular activity across the United States; in 2015 it was reported to have approximately 27, 000 participants [1]. Marching arts is highly popular throughout the high school years, but many musicians continue marching through college as an extracurricular activity or as part of their major, if pursuing a music degree. Preparation for performance season typically includes introduction to fundamentals of music, marching styles, and placement drills making rehearsals lengthy and strenuous [2]. In general, performing artists (i.e., marching artists, dancers, aerial performers, actors, singers) are involved in highly structured, intense, and achievement-oriented activities. The 2018 Physical Activity Guidelines for Americans recommends 150–300 min of moderate-intensity activity for substantial health benefits [3]. While many may say marching band is not sufficient physical activity, an average of 6.5 h (390 min) per week (excluding performances) is spent doing physical practice with instruments or flags [4]. Furthermore, results from a study examining energy cost in marching band determine marching band met the criteria for moderate activity in adolescents and overall does contribute to physical activity [5]. Additionally, marching artists face mental stressors associated with performance anxiety, as many of them feel very critical and worry about their performance and constantly feel nervous [6, 7]. Therefore, marching artists are at risk for medical and mental health problems. Similar to Fall sport student athletes (football, soccer, and cross country), marching band artists are exposed to high temperatures and humidity and face similar physically active demands and mental stressors [8], that can lead to decreases in physical and mental performance. Additionally, similar to student athletes, artists lack knowledge on proper hydration and nutrition and have to manage stressors associated with class, rehearsal times, sleep deprivation, and long travel hours [8]. Given the increase in physical activity performed by marching band artists [4, 5], the combination of physical and mental stressors and decreased healthcare knowledge place marching band artists at risk for injury, illness and inadequate energy availability (energy deficiency) with or without risk for eating disorder (ED). However, unlike the competitive athletic population, marching bands typically do not have any allied healthcare professionals, such as a team physician or an athletic trainer, overseeing their care to prevent and/or recognize signs and symptoms for injuries, illnesses, and mental health conditions, including EDs.

Eating disorders are serious mental illnesses characterized by the persistent disturbance of eating or eating-related behaviors resulting in altered consumption or absorption of food and psychosocial and physical health impairments [9]. They can be a result of multiple factors including disordered and abnormal eating and compensatory behaviors, including restrictive eating, fasting, frequently skipped meals, diet pills, overeating, binge-eating and then purging (e.g., vomiting, excessive exercise, misuse of laxatives and medications, etc.). Elevated prevalence has been estimated across college students in the United States, with 2.2–30.5% of the studied population screening positive for an ED, with gradual increases over recent years [10–15]. Furthermore, 25.9–46.6% of US college students screened as "high risk" for an ED [11, 12]. While at times performing artists are not considered traditional athletes because of the differences in physical demands, similarities exist, and their demands include an aesthetic component during performances. Thus, marching artists potentially face some of the same risk factors for EDs as athletes. It is well researched and known the athletic population is at a higher risk for EDs compared to non-athletes [16–18]. Female athletes are more predisposed, especially those in aesthetic sports (e.g., gymnastics, cheerleading, swimming, dance) but approximately 10% of all ED cases are seen in males [19–21]. Similar to college students, ED prevalence in the athletic population has been on the rise since the 1990s and increased nearly by 10% in approximately 10 years [17, 18, 22, 23]. Aesthetics or "lean" sports, in which a thin/lean body or low body weight is perceived as the norm or as an advantage to performance, increases ED risk in athletes, most specifically in females [24].

The performing arts is aesthetically driven, from perfect uniforms/outfits to in unison dance moves, marching, and playing. Appearance is a priority, and for many artists this may put them at risk for EDs. In the marching arts we see an array of artists, including musicians in the horn line or drumline, and auxiliaries which are color guard, dancers, and twirlers, each of which may possess different risk factors or comorbidities of EDs. For example, auxiliary teams are extremely aesthetically driven and composed of predominately females who may be wearing revealing attire. We should also note that performing artists often report depression and anxiety, known comorbidities of EDs; 44% of artists reported depression as a health concern and 22% desired help for the problem [6, 7]. Mental health conditions are widely presented in college students including depression, anxiety, eating disorders, alcohol and other substance abuse problems, self-mutilation, and various other self-destructive and reckless behaviors. Multiple explanations exist for the increase in mental health needs for college students; students may not be prepared for the academic demands and adjustment needed to succeed in college; they face increased demands in managing studies, work, and extracurricular activities [25].

While some literature exists identifying ED prevalence in athletes and college students, to date no current research has been conducted examining the prevalence of EDs in university marching band artists. Therefore, the purpose of this study is to examine the prevalence of ED risk across sex in university marching band artists and to determine the type of risk based on the Eating Disorder Inventory-3 (EDI-3) and Eating Disorder Inventory-3 Symptom Check List (EDI-3 SC). A second aim is to examine the pathogenic behaviors (i.e., binge eating, self-induced vomiting; exercise patterns; use of laxatives, diet pills, and diuretics) used to control or lose weight, across marching band artists. We hypothesize there will be an increased prevalence of ED risk in marching band artists (similar to traditional athletes), compared with community norms and female artists will have a higher prevalence compared to males.

Methods

Study design

We utilized a cross sectional study design. The study is part of a larger field study and web-based survey examining exertional heat illness risk factors and energy needs in marching band. The portion used for this study was descriptive in nature and used the web-based survey developed from previously validated instruments for quantitative analysis. To best assess both eating attitudes, comorbid psychological constructs, and eating behaviors, we utilized both the Eating Disorder Inventory – 3 (EDI-3) and the EDI-3 Symptoms Checklist.

Ethics

Ethics approval for this study was approved by both the University of Kansas (IRB-STUDY00142728) and the University of South Carolina's (IRB-Pro00081581) Institutional Review Boards. All participants completed an online informed consent with the opportunity to decline participation.

Participants

Marching band artists were recruited for the study via in-person briefings at a marching band rehearsal by a member of the research team or band director. A total of 182 marching band artists began the study and 150 completed the study, yielding a relative completion rate of 82.4% (female: $n = 84$, male: $n = 66$,) age: (19.9 ± 1.1 years) from 3 NCAA Division I university marching bands. To be included in the study, all participants were enrolled in their respective university's marching band and between the ages of 18–30 years of age. No exclusion criteria were used for participation in the present study.

Instrumentation

Demographic and baseline medical history questionnaire

A questionnaire was used to acquire basic personal, demographic, and previous medical history data. The information collected included age, education level, sex, ethnicity, years of experience in marching band, and primary instrument/section. Participants also self-reported their height, current weight, lowest weight, highest weight, mental weight, and ideal weight. Mental weight is an individual's perceived weight if one does not consciously try to control their weight. For example, one may think they will weigh more if they do not exercise or eat healthy to control weight. Eliminating these behaviors such as exercise and eating healthy, may lead someone to feel like they will gain an unrealistic amount of weight.

Eating disorder inventory – 3 (EDI-3)

The EDI-3 was administered to screen for ED characteristics and behaviors. This is a 91-item self-reported questionnaire, used by clinicians to identify individuals with disordered eating patterns [26]. A Likert scale is composed of 6 ratings (always, usually, often, sometimes, rarely, never). The EDI-3 consists of 3 ED specific scales and 9 general psychological scales - that are highly relevant to ED patients. It yields 2 main composites, 1 ED specific (Eating Disorder Risk Composite-EDRC) and the overall Psychological Maladjustment composite (GPMC) which consist of 4 general integrative psychological composite constructs (Ineffectiveness-IC, Interpersonal Problems-IPC, Affective Problems-APC, Overcontrol-OC). Examples of statements consisted of: "I think that my stomach is to big"; "I feel ineffective as a person"; and "I trust others". The EDI-3 is a validated tool and has a high test-re-test reliability of .98 [26]. Two main composites consist of the EDRC (reliability range from .90 to .97 with a median of .95 [26]; current study was .83) and the GPMC (reliability range .93 to .97 and median of .93 [26]; and current study was .824). This instrument is copyrighted by Psychological Assessment

Resources, Inc. Permission for use is granted with purchase of inventory. The computer-based scoring program for the EDI-3 was used to assess the outcomes of each individual participants. The software generates individualized score reports with raw scores, T scores, percentiles, and qualitative classifications (Low Clinical, Typical Clinical, Elevated Clinical) for all EDI-3 scales [26]. Clinical ranges are based on percentile ranges for the U.S. Adult Combined Clinical sample (i.e., Low Clinical = 1st to 24th percentile; Typical Clinical = 25th to 66th percentile, Elevated Clinical = 37th to 99th percentile [26]. To account for response style (e.g., irregular, deviant, or anomalous response patterns, etc.; to be considered "at risk" for an ED on the EDI-3, participants had at least two or more composite scores at typical clinical or elevated clinical.

Eating disorder inventory – 3 symptom checklist (EDI-3 SC)

The EDI-3 SC is a screening tool used by allied healthcare professionals to identify individuals at risk for EDs and begin the appropriate referral plan. It is a self-reported measure that provides information regarding the frequency of symptoms/pathogenic behaviors (i.e., binge eating, self-induced vomiting; exercise patterns; use of laxatives, diet pills, and diuretics.) The assessment ranges depending on reporting yes or no to behaviors and ranges between 10 and 42 questions. If participant answers yes, they have follow-up questions regarding frequency of behaviors (e.g., not engaged in the behavior in the last 3 months, frequency daily, frequency weekly, frequency monthly). An example would be: have you ever had an episode of eating an amount of food that others would regard as usually large? If the answer is yes, then participants would be asked the following: how old were you when you first had an eating binge and how old were you when you began to binge eat on a regular basis; followed by during the last 3 months how often have you typically had an eating binge. Participants who reported "yes" but did not engage in the behavior in the last 3 months were not considered at risk. The EDI-3 SC is copyrighted by Psychological Assessment Resources, Inc. Permission for use is granted with purchase of inventory. To be considered "at risk" for ED on the EDI-3 SC, participants must meet the criteria for one pathogenic behavior.

Procedures

After approval from the institutional review boards, participants were notified of the study via in-person briefings at a marching band rehearsal by a member of the research team or band director. Following the briefings, all marching band members were contacted via e-mail. Participants who consented completed the basic demographic and baseline medical history questionnaire, EDI-3, and EDI-3 SC. All data was collected using an online platform, Qualtrics (Provo, UT). The surveys were open for 1 month, a reminder e-mail for participation was sent every 10 days, for a total of 3 reminders.

Statistical analysis

Data was analyzed using SPSS statistical software (version 26; SPSS Inc., Armonk, NY) with a significance level set at $p < .05$. A priori power analysis was conducted using G*Power statistical software (version 3.1.9.2., Heinrich Heine University, Dusseldorf Germany). Using a moderate effect size at .04, our power calculation indicated a sample size of 124 total participants was needed with estimated power being 0.95. Basic descriptive statistics, including means and standard deviations, were used for demographic information. Overall ED risk was considered if participants had at least two or more composite scores of either "typical clinical" or "elevated clinical" on the EDI-3, and/or met the criteria for at least one pathogenic behavior on the EDI-3 SC. Cross-tabulations and Chi-square analyses were used to examine the proportion of participants classified as "at risk" for an ED, using the EDI-3 only, or the EDI-3 SC only, and across ED Risk Type (EDI-3, EDI-3 SC or both EDI-3 and EDI-3 SC) and across sex.

Results

A total of 150 university marching band artists from 3 institutions participated in this study. Participants academic status was as follows: 22.7% freshmen/1st year college student ($n = 34$), 31.3% sophomores/2nd year college student ($n = 47$), 22.7% juniors/3rd year college student ($n = 34$), 23.3% seniors/4th year college student ($n = 35$) and ranged from 18 to 23 years of age (mean: 19.9 ± 1.1 years). They had participated in marching band 1 year or less (4.7%; $n = 7$), 2–3 years (4%; $n = 6$), 4–5 years (33.3%; $n = 50$), 6–7 years (42%; $n = 63$), or 8 or more years (16%; $n = 24$) and in the following sections: Brass (45.3%; $n = 68$), Woodwinds (36%; $n = 54$) Percussion (7.3%; $n = 11$), or Auxiliaries (11.3%; $n = 17$). Participants identified their ethnicity as White (80.7%; $n = 121$), Hispanic or Latino (2.7%; $n = 4$), Black or African American (5.3%; $n = 8$), American Indian or Alaska Native (0.7%; $n = 1$), or Other (8.7%; $n = 13$). Self-reported physical measures are demonstrated in Table 1.

Eating disorder risk

When assessing combined risk (i.e., EDI-3 Only, EDI-3 SC, or both EDI-3 and EDI-3 SC) 70.7% ($n = 106$) of marching band artists were at risk for EDs with no significant differences across sex (females: 41.3%; $n = 62$ vs. males: 29.3%; $n = 44$; $p = 0.340$). The ED risk per section was as follows: Brass (75%; $n = 51/68$), Woodwinds (63%; $n = 34/54$), Percussion (72.7%; $n = 8/11$), and Auxiliaries

Table 1 Self-reported physical measurements for marching band artists

	Females (n = 84) Mean ± SD	Males (n = 66) Mean ± SD
Age (yrs)	19.9 ± 0.9	19.8 ± 1.3
Current Height (cm)	165.9 ± 7.0	179.3 ± 9.4
Current Weight (kg)	68.7 ± 17.2	81.6 ± 22.6
Highest Weight (kg)	72.6 ± 17.5	87.5 ± 25.0
Lowest Weight (kg)	62.7 ± 14.6	75.7 ± 20.6
Mental Weight (kg)[a]	71.2 ± 18.1	86.4 ± 26.6
Ideal Weight (kg)	61.8 ± 13.8	77.7 ± 15.1
Current Weight-Ideal Weight (kg)	6.7 ± 10.1	3.9 ± 10.7
Current Weight-Mental Weight (kg)	−2.6 ± 5.8	−4.8 ± 7.1
Current BMI (kg/m^2)	25.0 ± 6.2	25.3 ± 5.9

[a]Mental Weight: Perceived weight if one did not consciously try to control weight

(76.5%; n = 13/17), no comparisons across section were made due to uneven distribution of sections in our sample. Table 2 demonstrates female and male within sample distribution. Using only the EDI-3, 45.3% (n = 68) were at risk, with females having a significant higher prevalence than males [χ^2 = 5.228, p = .022]. Using only the EDI-3 SC, 54.0% (n = 81) were at risk and no significant differences were found across sex. For all individuals with ED risk, we categorized their risk type as EDI-3 only, EDI-3 SC only, or being at risk based on both EDI-3 and EDI-3 scores (Table 2); and no significant differences were found across ED risk type and sex.

EDI-3 primary scales and composite scores

The primary scales and composite scores are displayed in Table 3. It is important to note that the typical clinical category reflect scores and characteristics of patients diagnosed with an ED. Marching band artists in this study had scores ranging from low clinical to elevated clinical across all scales and composites. Elevated clinical scores for ED risk scales were predominately seen in females; while elevated clinical scores for psychological trait scales were seen in both females and males. Overall females endorsed a stronger prevalence for Drive for Thinness (χ^2 = 8.541, p = .014), Bulimia (χ^2 = 7.215, p = .027), Interpersonal Insecurity (χ^2 = 12.258, p = .002), Interpersonal Alienation (χ^2 = 9.753, p = .008), and Maturity Fears (χ^2 = 7.410, p = .025) than males. Furthermore, significant differences were found between sex and the following composites: Eating Disorder Risk (χ^2 = 7.539, p = .023), Interpersonal Problems (χ^2 = 11.556, p = .003], and General Psychological Maladjustment (χ^2 = 6.962, p = .031).

Pathogenic behaviors

The EDI-3 SC examined marching band artists' pathogenic behavior risk (binging, purging, dieting, etc.) and is displayed in Table 4. Dieting was the most common behavior reported across the entire sample followed by exercise to control weight. Overall, significant differences were found between pathogenic behaviors and sex for purging to control weight (χ^2 = 3.94, p = .047) and laxative use (χ^2 = 4.064, p = .044).

Discussion

While different from traditional athletics, the marching arts is a physically demanding activity with similar challenges and health risk as organized sports. The purpose of this study was to examine ED risk among university marching band artists with respect to sex and examine the pathogenic weight control behaviors used by marching band artists. Findings suggest an increased risk for EDs among university marching band artists, with females facing higher risk compared to males. Additionally, and of concern, both female and male marching band artists are engaging in pathogenic behaviors to control their weight, including dieting, exercise, binge eating, and purging.

Eating disorder risk

Our study used a multidimensional approach (EDI-3, EDI-3 SC, and combination) to assess ED risk across

Table 2 Eating disorder risk type in marching band artists. Data is presented "within sex"

	All (n = 150) n (%)	Females (n = 84) n (%)	Males (n = 66) n (%)	p-value
EDI-3 Scale Risk				
EDI-3	68 (45.3)	45 (53.6)	23 (34.8)	0.022
EDI-3 SC	81 (54.0)	47 (56.0)	43 (51.5)	0.588
Overall, ED Risk (n = 150)	106 (70.7)	62 (41.3)	44(29.3)	0.340
ED Risk Type				0.108
EDI-3 only	25 (16.7)	15 (17.9)	10 (15.2)	
EDI-3 SC only	38 (25.3)	17 (20.2)	21 (31.8)	
Both EDI-3 and EDI-3 SC	43 (28.7)	30 (35.7)	13 (19.7)	

Table 3 Eating disorder characteristics among marching band artists. Data is presented "within sex"

	Females (n = 84)			**Males (n = 66)**			
	Classification			**Classification**			
	Raw Score[a]	**Typical Clinical**	**Elevated Clinical**	**Raw Score[a]**	**Typical Clinical**	**Elevated Clinical**	***p*-value**
	Mean ± SD	**n (%)**	**n (%)**	**Mean ± SD**	**n (%)**	**n (%)**	
Eating Disorders Risk Scale							
Drive for Thinness	9.0 ± 8.1	17 (20.2)	4 (4.8)	5.2 ± 5.8	5 (7.6)	0 (0)	0.014
Bulimia	5.5 ± 6.6	30 (35.7)	5 (6.0)	3.1 ± 3.5	16 (24.2)	0 (0)	0.027
Body Dissatisfaction	16.4 ± 10.6	20 (23.8)	4 (4.8)	11.1 ± 8.3	10 (15.2)	0 (0)	0.068
Eating Disorder Risk Composite	112.8 ± 27.6	12 (14.3)	4 (4.8)	99.7 ± 18.5	3 (4.5)	0 (0)	0.023
Psychological Scale							
Low Self-Esteem	7.0 ± 6.2	22 (26.2)	7 (8.3)	5.6 ± 5.6	11 (16.7)	5 (7.6)	0.348
Personal Alienation	8.1 ± 6.2	25 (29.8)	9 (10.7)	6.6 ± 5.4	16 (24.2)	4 (6.1)	0.380
Interpersonal Insecurity	10.7 ± 6.2	35 (41.7)	24 (28.6)	7.0 ± 5.5)	19 (28.8)	9 (13.6)	0.002
Interpersonal Alienation	7.7 ± 4.9	42 (50.0)	13 (15.5)	6.3 ± 10.6	25 (37.9)	3 (4.5)	0.008
Interceptive Deficits	10.1 ± 8.3	19 (22.6)	12 (14.3)	7.5 ± 6.6)	15 (22.7)	5 (7.6)	0.425
Emotional Dysregulation	4.0 ± 5.0	17 (20.2)	12 (14.3)	2.7 ± 2.9	13 (19.7)	3 (4.5)	0.131
Perfectionism	14.2 ± 5.2	38 (45.2)	29 (34.5)	12.5 ± 5.3	30 (45.5)	18 (27.3)	0.495
Asceticism	6.7 ± 4.8	16 (19.0)	6 (7.1)	6.2 ± 3.8	14 (21.2)	1 (1.5)	0.265
Maturity Fears	10.4 ± 5.9	36 (42.9)	29 (34.5)	7.8 ± 5.1	30 (45.5)	11 (16.7)	0.025
Composites							
Ineffectiveness Composite	81.1 ± 19.5	20 (23.8)	10 (11.9)	76.0 ± 17.3	9 (13.6)	5 (7.6)	0.152
Interpersonal Problems Composite	92.4 ± 19.1	41 (48.8)	14 (16.7)	82.6 ± 15.7	20 (30.3)	5 (7.6)	0.003
Affective Problems Composite	84.3 ± 17.6	18 (21.4)	9 (10.7)	78.2 ± 11.6	14 (21.2)	1 (1.5)	0.076
Over control Composite	90.0 ± 14.8	33 (39.3)	11 (13.1)	86.6 ± 12.9	25 (37.9)	4 (6.1)	0.307
General Psychological Maladjustment	404.7 ± 87.3	20 (23.8)	9 (10.7)	369.5 ± 47.2	11 (16.7)	1 (1.5)	0.031

[a]Raw scores calculated from the EDI-3 survey.

marching band artists, utilizing this approach yielded in 70.7% overall ED risk. However, it is important to note this risk may be inflated with the combination of the 2 instruments. When estimating ED risk across marching band artists using the questionnaires independently from each other (EDI-3: 45.3% vs. EDI-3 SC: 54%) findings reflect lower rates compared to the combined instrument approach. The utilization of independent questionnaires (EDI-3 or EDI-3 SC) still displayed similar and/or higher rates than those in undergraduate students, where "high risk" of EDs was found in 25.9–46.6% of the population [11, 12].

Table 4 Eating disorder pathogenic behaviors among marching band artists. Data presented "within sex"

Pathogenic Behavior	**All (n = 150)**	**Females (n = 84)**	**Males (n = 66)**	***p*-value**
	n (%)	**n (%)**	**n (%)**	
Dieting	72 (48.0)	43 (51.2)	29 (43.9)	0.378
Exercise	31 (20.7)	18 (21.4)	13 (19.7)	0.795
Binge Eating	28 (18.7)	16 (19.0)	12 (18.2)	0.893
Purging	18 (12.0)	14 (16.7)	4 (6.1)	0.047
Laxatives	5 (3.3)	5 (6.0)	0 (0)	0.044
Diet Pills	7 (4.7)	4 (4.8)	3 (4.5)	0.950
Diuretics	3 (2.0)	2 (2.4)	1 (1.5)	0.707

With regards to sex, both females and males were at risk for EDs with females displaying significantly higher prevalence than males. Studies that have examined ED risk in both female and male athletes demonstrate a lower risk, 7–13.5% [16, 17], than marching band artists in the current study. However, we should note that these studies conducted the gold standard of ED diagnosis, which is clinical interviews. Prior to interviews, Sundgot-Borgen et al. [17] and Martinsen et al. [16] conducted screenings using the EDI and EDI-2 respectively. Looking specifically at the results based on the screening, 14.5–25% of the participating athletes were classified at risk for an ED. Our study resulted in 45.3% of marching band artists being at risk utilizing only the EDI-3 tool, yielding close to two times the risk as athletes [16, 17]. We should also note, the evolution of the EDI, as the EDI-3 correctly identified a higher percentage (99%) of patients as positive for ED as compared to the EDI-2

(48%) [27]. Generally speaking, females have higher ED risk than males, but at least 10% of all cases are seen in males [20]. Studies that have looked specifically at the male population demonstrate ED risk in males ranging from 3.2 to 19.2% [16, 17, 19, 28–30], which is consistent with the prevalence of male marching band artists. The findings of this study are consistent with previous literature where female athletes have higher prevalence rates than males [16, 17]. It is important to note there may be some inconsistencies with our results compared to results presented on athletes [16–18, 28–30] One example is the instruments used in our study (EDI-3 and EDI-SC) to assess ED risk. Common instruments used to assess ED risk in athletes are the Eating Attitudes Test (EAT-26) [31], Eating Disorder Diagnostic Scale [32], and the Eating Disorder Examination Questionnaire (EDE-Q) [33]. These instruments range between 22 and 31 questions used to identify eating disorder risk associated with attitudes and behaviors. The EDI-3 is unique because it does assess other psychological comorbidities (e.g., self-esteem, maturity fears, interpersonal alienation, perfectionism, etc.), which may have led to the overall higher risk for EDs compared to athletes.

When looking specifically at female marching band artists, the prevalence rates of at risk are concerning. Typically, female athletes demonstrate increased prevalence of EDs, with rates ranging from 11 to 32.8% [16–18, 22, 28]. ED risk in female marching band artists appears to be higher than these rates, with over half of females being at risk using each tool independently. In the marching arts, a female may participate in the horn line or drum line, but others are in the color guard, dance team, or twirler group which are aesthetically driven and predominately composed of females. Auxiliary unit members have previously been assessed for ED risk, finding 29.7% of them at risk [34]. In our study a high prevalence of ED risk is present in the Auxiliaries section (76.5%; $n = 13/17$) and can be due to the aesthetic nature of these teams within the marching band. However, these findings should be taken with caution because of the very low sample size. Literature suggests athletes in aesthetic or leanness sports have higher ED prevalence rates than those in non-leanness sport [18, 19, 24]. Dancers can be considered aesthetic artists, the rates found in this study for Auxiliaries are closely related to those of dancers, where 69% of them were at risk for EDs [35]. However, we cannot disregard the high percentages of at risk band members in other sections, Brass, Woodwinds, and Percussion. To date, no literature has assessed ED risk in marching band, only the Auxiliary group and it is unknown if they may face some of the same aesthetic concerns and pressures. Special focus should be given to female marching band artists regarding nutrition and EDs, as ED risk may be the beginning of further medical and psychological complications.

EDI-3 primary scales and composite scores

Our study used a combination of both traditional and comorbid psychological factors related to EDs to assess marching band artists' ED risk. Evidence suggests that disordered eating attitudes and behaviors are multifactorial with interactions between personal, environmental/cultural, and genetic factors, with various psychosocial components and personality traits as risk factors or comorbidities [36]. While many of our participants did not display traditional ED risk (i.e., Drive for Thinness, Body Image Dissatisfaction, Bulimia), when examining the comorbid psychological risk, they were most prevalent for Interpersonal Insecurity, Interpersonal Alienation, Perfectionism, and Maturity Fears.

The Interpersonal Insecurity scale has a primary focus on assessing the difficulties of conveying one's personal thoughts and emotions, and the tendency of social inhibition. The Interpersonal Alienation scale assesses disappointment, disassociation, alienation and the distrust in relationships [26]. Previous studies have determined ED patients to have non-assertive interpersonal styles, higher social inhibition, and submissiveness [37, 38]. Furthermore, evidence exists that ED patients also experience social skill difficulties and less social competence than controls and difficulty adjusting in social situations along with social anxiety [39, 40]. Moreover, result indicated that over 50% of our participants had typical or elevated clinical risk for both Interpersonal Insecurity and Interpersonal Alienation. Those who displayed interpersonal insecurity may have thoughts of discomfort, apprehension and are reserved in social situations. In turn, these behaviors may lead to difficulty expressing feelings and personal thoughts with others which may lead to withdrawal and isolation from others. It is also concerning; interpersonal alienation was displayed in half the marching band artists. Interpersonal alienation may lead one to have lack of trust in relationships with people and/or they may feel trapped in relationships. Both of these constructions may lead marching band artists to experience stress and anxiety, which has been previously reported in performing artists which can potentially increase their risk for EDs [6–8].

We observed a large percentage (79.7%) of marching band artists in the typical and elevated clinical classification for Perfectionism. Perfectionism is assessed through evaluating the extent of an individual's drive to meet high goals and standards, whether that is for personal achievement or to meet others' expectations [26]. Performing artists often perform in front of large groups and/or at events that are televised or streamed online, this makes artists want to not make mistakes that can constantly be replayed or criticized by their instructors, peers, and friends/family. Perfectionism in the performing arts is widely common, and evidence suggest that it can in fact be a hindering personality trait in the music industry [41]. For marching band artists specifically, the recollection of a perfect performance is extremely meaningful, they are praised for playing the perfect tune while maintaining perfect marching lines and choreography. On the other hand, failed routines are often talked about as examples of what not to do, which may be hindering to the marching band artists' confidence. At times, the relentless pursuit of perfection can be debilitating psychologically and a contributing factor to mental health conditions including EDs in athletes and performing artists [42, 43]. While many may see perfectionism as an asset in the performing arts, it can also hamper an artists' health and well-being.

Lastly, we observed a majority of marching band artists displayed typical and elevated clinical classifications for Maturity Fears. Maturity Fear is a desire to return to the security of childhood and the avoidance of developmental demands and weight gains [26]. Given the stressors faced by marching band artists, we can attribute the higher percentages in maturity fears to the avoidance in demands of being college students and performers along with the desire to be a certain weight. While in the later years in college (3rd and 4th year) marching band artists may try to maintain an unrealistic middle school or high school weight which tends to be lower due to maturation. We do observe this with the differences in current and ideal weight, where both females and males self-report their ideal weight as lower than their current weight. Additionally, both females and males have the perception that their weight would be higher if they did not try to control for it, as depicted by their mental weight.

Pathogenic behaviors

When assessing the pathogenic behaviors to control weight, dieting, excessive exercise, binge eating, and purging were most commonly used by marching band artists. Though females displayed higher percentages than males for all behaviors, only purging was significantly greater. These same pathogenic behaviors are commonly used by collegiate and elite athletes [29, 30, 44]. Specifically looking at females, our study demonstrates higher rates in marching artists than athletes for dieting (51.2% vs 15.6%) and purging (16.7% vs 2.9%), but close similarities in exercise (21.4% vs 25.5%) and binge eating (19% vs 18.6%) [44]. Similar to female athletes, these female artists may experience weight-related pressures, including pressures from instructors, teammates, and oneself to maintain a lean physique for performance, or that of performing in front of hundreds of fans and being on the media. Moreover, revealing attire specific for color guard and dancers may encourage them to engage in behaviors, like dieting and restricting, to rapidly decrease weight. These periods of dieting may also be followed by periods of binge eating or vice-versa.

For male marching band artists, we demonstrate 18.2% engage in binge eating and 6.4% engage in purging, which is consistent with the literature on athletes, 16.7–21.4% for binge eating and 1.6–6.6% for purging [29, 30]. However, rates are two times higher for dieting in male artists as compared to male athletes [29, 30]. Potential reasons for higher rates for dieting may be because athletes in the US may have more resources and access to a dining hall composed of healthier foods planned by a team sport dietitian. Whereas marching band artists who may be trying to adjust their weight may follow fad diets or guidelines found on the internet or from word of mouth and may only have access to university/college dining halls. Male athletes do report higher percentages of exercise to control weight than male artists, but this may be due to the nature of their participation in exercise with the belief that it may increase performance [29, 30].

Clinical implications

Marching band artists face similar physical and mental stressors as student athletes, with similar predisposition to mental health conditions. While actively participating in marching band rehearsals, performances, and travel, artists also complete the traditional academic workload, ranging from 12 to 20 h per week. Depending on their academic discipline they may need to complete supervised instructional experiences, internships, or full immersion clinical practicums, and some engage in additional physical activity or recreational sports. Ultimately, they must find a balance between being a student and a marching artist and staying physically and mentally healthy. However, while facing similar demands and stressors, an important difference between marching band artists and athletes is that compared to organized athletics most marching band artists do not have medical, psychological, nutritional, or sports performance professionals readily available to discuss best practices of overall health and wellness, including energy intake and exercise expenditure. Having immediate access to healthcare professionals, like a team physician or an athletic trainer, is imperative to this population as these professionals can educate and provide adequate instruction on nutrition and performance to minimize the risk of EDs and injuries and provide immediate referral upon the recognition of mental health conditions. While it is important to take the multidimensional approach, if resources do not permit assessment using multiple forms and/or interviews, clinicians should at least try to use one short ED assessment (e.g., EAT-26, EDE-Q, etc). In this study, using either the EDI-3 or the EDI-SC would also be appropriate, but should be examined independently vs. risk combined as we saw in this study it was over inflated. It is also important to note these assessments only identify risk and if a more thorough evaluation needs to take place, marching band artists should be referred to a physician.

Limitations and future research

Our study demonstrated increased ED risk in marching band artists; however, some limitations exist. The instruments utilized in this study are self-reported, we assume they were completed entirely, and participants provided accurate and truthful answers. Additionally, these instruments served as an assessment for disordered eating behaviors and ED risk, not as a diagnostic tool. The gold standard for diagnosis would include an interview with the participant; given that participants were anonymous, this interview process was not conducted, and authors were unable to validate our methods of identifying risk for ED compared to the gold standard. Furthermore, participation in our study was limited to 3 U.S university marching bands only. University marching bands vary in performance styles, traditions, and demands and are also associated outside the college setting (e.g., International Drum Corp.). Therefore, these results cannot be generalized to the entire marching band population. Future research should utilize a larger sample size, with a larger distribution of sex and with participants from across states, inclusive to various NCAA divisions, and international marching bands. It is also recommended future research examines college marching band artists to the general college student population to seek any potential risk differences. Researchers should consider conducting follow-up interviews with participants to determine validate the methodology of identifying risk for ED in this study, as well as examine the type of health care available to marching band artists to determine if availability of health care minimizes the risk of EDs and its comorbidities.

Conclusion

Our study indicates ED risk was highly prevalent for both female and male marching band artists; and females displayed higher risk for ED than males. It is a concern that both female and male marching band artists are engaging in pathogenic behaviors to control their weight, with females displaying higher risk for purging and laxative use. Our findings ultimately reveal crucial information regarding the health and wellness of marching band artists and the importance of medical oversight in this population to be able to educate, prevent and provide adequate treatment or referral for any injury, illness, or mental health condition. Although our findings are novel, yet important, additional research exploring a larger sample size and distribution around the country and world would provide physicians, athletic trainers and other healthcare providers working in this setting more awareness of the risk factors and characteristics of EDs displayed in marching band artists. Additionally, marching band administrators should be aware of all medical risk factors associated with the marching arts and the benefit of having medical oversight, such as a physician and/or an athletic trainer, to oversee the health and wellness of marching band artists.

Abbreviations

ED: Eating disorder; EDI-3: Eating disorder inventory-3; EDI-3 SC: Eating disorder inventory-3 symptoms check; IRB: Institutional review board; NCAA: National Collegiate Athletic Association

Acknowledgements

The authors would like to thank Dr. Cormac Cannon (University of South Carolina Director of Bands), Dr. Jay Jacobs (University of South Carolina Director of Athletic Bands), Matthew Smith (University of Kansas Director of Marching Band), and Dr. Kevin Kloesel (Director of Oklahoma Climate Survey) for their support in this project. We would also like to thank all the individuals who participated in this study.

Informed consent

Informed consent was obtained from all individual participants in the study.

Authors' contributions

DME and TTM were involved in the design of the study; NAU, ABS, and MRK collected the data. NAU and TTM analyzed the data. All authors contributed to drafted and approved the final manuscript.

Competing interests

NAU, DME, ABS, MRK, TTM declare that they have no conflict of interest.

Author details

[1]University of South Carolina, Blatt PE Center 212, Columbia, SC 29208, USA. [2]University of Kansas, 1301 Sunnyside Avenue, Robinson 161, Lawrence, KS 66045, USA.

References

1. Beckett S, Seidelman L, Hanney WJ, Liu X, Rothschild CE. Prevalence of musculoskeletal injury among collegiate marching band and color guard members. Med Probl Perform Art. 2015;30(2):106–10.
2. Kilanowski JF. Marching athletes: injuries and illnesses at band camp. MCN Am J Matern Child Nurs. 2008;33(6):338–45.
3. Services UDoHaH, editor. Physical Activity Guidelins for Americans. 2nd ed. Washington, DC: Services UDoHaH; 2018.
4. Harman SE. Medical problems of marching musicians. Med Probl Perform Art. 1993;50:41.
5. Erdmann LD, Graham RE, Radlo SJ, Knepler PL. Adolescents' energy cost in marching band. Percept Mot Skills. 2003;97(2):639–46.
6. Castille CM. An investigation of musical performance anxiety in the marching arts. Med Probl Perform Art. 2011;26(1):30–4.
7. Werner MJ, Rosenthal SL, Biro FM. Medical needs of performing arts students. J Adolesc Health. 1991;12(4):294–300.
8. Hatheway M, Chesky K. Epidemiology of health concerns among collegiate student musicians participating in marching band. Med Probl Perform Art. 2013;28(4):242–51.

9. Association AP. Diagnostic and statistical manual of mental disorders. Arlington: American Psychiatric Publishing; 2013.
10. Eisenberg D, Nicklett EJ, Roeder K, Kirz NE. Eating disorder symptoms among college students: prevalence, persistence, correlates, and treatment-seeking. J Am Coll Heal. 2011;59(8):700–7.
11. Fitzsimmons-Craft EE, Balantekin KN, Eichen DM, Graham AK, Monterubio GE, Sadeh-Sharvit S, et al. Screening and offering online programs for eating disorders: reach, pathology, and differences across eating disorder status groups at 28 US universities. Int J Eat Disord. 2019;52(10):1125–36.
12. Jones M, Kass AE, Trockel M, Glass AI, Wilfley DE, Taylor CB. A population-wide screening and tailored intervention platform for eating disorders on college campuses: the healthy body image program. J Am Coll Heal. 2014; 62(5):351–6.
13. Kronfol Z, Khalifa B, Khoury B, Omar O, Daouk S, Dewitt JP, et al. Selected psychiatric problems among college students in two Arab countries: Comparison with the USA. BMC Psychiatry. 2018;18(1):147.
14. Lipson SK, Jones JM, Taylor CB, Wilfley DE, Eichen DM, Fitzsimmons-Craft EE, et al. Understanding and promoting treatment-seeking for eating disorders and body image concerns on college campuses through online screening, prevention and intervention. Eat Behav. 2016;25:68.
15. White S, Reynolds-Malear JB, Cordero E. Disordered eating and the use of unhealthy weight control methods in college students: 1995, 2002, and 2008. Eat Disord. 2011;19(4):323–34.
16. Martinsen M, Sundgot-Borgen J. Higher prevalence of eating disorders among adolescent elite athletes than controls. Med Sci Sports Exerc. 2013; 45(6):1188–97.
17. Sundgot-Borgen J, Torstveit MK. Prevalence of eating disorders in elite athletes is higher than in the general population. Clin J Sport Med. 2004; 14(1):25–32.
18. Torstveit MK, Rosenvinge JH, Sundgot-Borgen J. Prevalence of eating disorders and the predictive power of risk models in female elite athletes: a controlled study. Scand J Med Sci Sports. 2008;18(1):108–18.
19. Bratland-Sanda S, Sundgot-Borgen J. Eating disorders in athletes: overview of prevalence, risk factors and recommendations for prevention and treatment. Eur J Sport Sci. 2013;13(5):499–508.
20. Joy E, Kussman A, Nattiv A. 2016 update on eating disorders in athletes: a comprehensive narrative review with a focus on clinical assessment and management. Br J Sports Med. 2016;50(3):154–62.
21. Torres-McGehee TM, Leaver-Dunn D, Green JM, Bishop PA, Leeper JD, Richardson MT. Knowledge of eating disorders among collegiate administrators, coaches, and auxiliary dancers. Percept Mot Skills. 2011; 112(3):951–8.
22. Sundgot-Borgen J. Prevalence of eating disorders in elite female athletes. Int J Sport Nutr Exerc Metab. 1993;3(1):29–40.
23. Sundgot-Borgen J, Torstveit MK. Aspects of disordered eating continuum in elite high-intensity sports. Scand J Med Sci Sports. 2010;20(s2):112–21.
24. Thompson R. Dissecting the disorders: eating disorders. In: Brown GT, editor. Mind, body, and sport: understanding and Supporthing student-athlete mental wellness. Indianapolis: National Collegiate Athletic Association; 2014. p. 25–8.
25. Cook LJ. Striving to help college students with mental health issues. J Psychosoc Nurs Ment Health Serv. 2007;45(4):40–57.
26. Garner DM. EDI-3, eating disorder inventory-3: professional manual: psychological assessment resources, Incorporated; 2004.
27. Segura-García C, Aloi M, Rania M, Ciambrone P, Palmieri A, Pugliese V, et al. Ability of EDI-2 and EDI-3 to correctly identify patients and subjects at risk for eating disorders. Eat Behav. 2015;19:20–3.
28. Abbott W, Brett A, Brownlee TE, Hammond KM, Harper LD, Naughton RJ, et al. The prevalence of disordered eating in elite male and female soccer players. Eat Weight Disord. 2020.
29. Chatterton JM, Petrie TA. Prevalence of disordered eating and pathogenic weight control behaviors among male collegiate athletes. Eat Disord. 2013; 21(4):328–41.
30. Petrie TA, Greenleaf C, Reel J, Carter J. Prevalence of eating disorders and disordered eating behaviors among male collegiate athletes. Psychol Men Masculinity. 2008;9(4):267–77.
31. Garner D, Olmsted M, Bohr Y, Garfinkel P. The eating attitudes test: psychometric features. Psychol Med. 1982;12:871–8.
32. Stice E, Fisher M, Martinez E. Eating disorder diagnostic scale: additional evidence of reliability and validity. Psychol Assess. 2004;16(1):60.
33. Berg KC, Peterson CB, Frazier P, Crow SJ. Psychometric evaluation of the eating disorder examination and eating disorder examination-questionnaire: a systematic review of the literature. Int J Eat Disord. 2012;45(3):428–38.
34. Torres-McGehee TM, Green JM, Leeper JD, Leaver-Dunn D, Richardson M, Bishop PA. Body image, anthropometric measures, and eating-disorder prevalence in auxiliary unit members. J Athl Train. 2009;44(4):418–26.
35. Robbeson JG, Kruger HS, Wright HH. Disordered eating behavior, body image, and energy status of female student dancers. Int J Sport Nutr Exerc Metab. 2015;25(4):344.
36. Striegel-Moore RH, Bulik CM. Risk factors for eating disorders. Am Psychol. 2007;62(3):181.
37. Hartmann A, Zeeck A, Barrett MS. Interpersonal problems in eating disorders. Int J Eat Disord. 2010;43(7):619–27.
38. Troop NA, Allan S, Treasure JL, Katzman M. Social comparison and submissive behaviour in eating disorder patients. Psychol Psychother. 2003; 76(3):237–49.
39. Grisset NI, Norvell NK. Perceived social support, social skills, and quality of relationships in bulimic women. J Consult Clin Psychol. 1992;60(2):293.
40. Striegel-Moore RH, Seeley JR, Lewinsohn PM. Psychosocial adjustment in young adulthood of women who experienced an eating disorder during adolescence. J Am Acad Child Adolesc Psychiatry. 2003;42(5):587–93.
41. Zwaan K, ter Bogt TFM. Research note: breaking into the popular record industry: an insider's view on the career entry of pop musicians. Eur J Commun. 2009;24(1):89–101.
42. Anshel MH. Sources of disordered eating patterns between ballet dancers and non-dancers. J Sport Behav. 2004;27(2):115.
43. Haase AM, Prapavessis H, Owens RG. Perfectionism, social physique anxiety and disordered eating: a comparison of male and female elite athletes. Psychol Sport Exerc. 2002;3(3):209–22.
44. Greenleaf C, Petrie TA, Carter J, Reel JJ. Female collegiate athletes: prevalence of eating disorders and disordered eating behaviors. J Am Coll Heal. 2009;57(5):489–95.

17

Believing emotions are uncontrollable is linked to eating disorder psychopathology via suppression and reappraisal

Laura Vuillier[1*†], Jemma Joseph[1†], Matthew P. Somerville[2] and Amy Harrison[2]

Abstract

Objective: Research suggests that beliefs about emotional controllability influence the use of emotion regulation strategies, which in turn impact psychological health and illness. However, no research has yet investigated whether emotional controllability is linked to eating psychopathology. The current study investigates whether these concepts are related, as individuals with eating disorders have problems with emotion regulation.

Method: We collected self-report data from 718 participants from a community sample using validated questionnaires, and ran mediational analyses to assess the relationship between emotional controllability and eating psychopathology, via reappraisal and suppression, two emotion regulation strategies.

Results: Our mediational analyses suggest that believing emotions to be uncontrollable relates to high levels of suppression ($\beta = -.08$), low levels of reappraisal ($\beta = .19$) and poorer eating disorder psychopathology ($\beta = -.11$). Reappraisal and suppression were found to partially mediate the relationship between emotional controllability and eating psychopathology.

Discussion: The current study has demonstrated relationships that support investigations relating emotional controllability, emotion regulation and psychological health. This research has potential implications for developing interventions to target beliefs about emotions in order to help improve emotion regulation skills and eating psychopathology.

Keywords: Emotional controllability, Emotion regulation, Reappraisal, Suppression, Eating psychopathology

Plain English summary

Everyone holds beliefs about the world and themselves. One of these beliefs concerns the ability to regulate emotions. Some people believe that they can control their emotions, while others believe that emotions are not changeable. Research into emotional controllability has found that believing emotions to be controllable is linked to better abilities to regulate them, and higher wellbeing. We also know from other research that people with eating disorders have difficulties regulating their emotions. However no research has looked at whether people with eating disorder behaviours view their emotions as uncontrollable and whether this has an influence on their abilities to regulate them. With the aid of 718 participants we found that, indeed, believing emotions to be uncontrollable was linked to poorer eating disorder behaviours. We also found that this relationship was partially explained by poorer emotion regulation strategies use. Our findings are important as they suggest practical implications for improving eating disorder psychopathology by changing beliefs about emotional controllability. However they are limited by

* Correspondence: lrenshawvuillier@bournemouth.ac.uk
†Laura Vuillier and Jemma Joseph should be considered joint first authors.
[1]Faculty of Science and Technology, Department of Psychology, Bournemouth University, Poole, UK
Full list of author information is available at the end of the article

the cross-sectional nature of the study, meaning we cannot imply causality. We recommend that further research replicate our findings in people with diagnosed eating disorders using a longitudinal design.

Introduction

Emotional controllability refers to an individual's beliefs about whether emotions are controllable or uncontrollable [1]. Recent studies suggest that beliefs about emotional controllability influence how people regulate their emotions, which in turn impacts psychological health [1, 2]. Emotional controllability is an area of emotional functioning that has been relatively under-researched in relation to eating disorders (EDs), yet we think these concepts could be related as individuals with EDs have problems with emotion regulation [3]. Identifying and exploring factors that relate to ED psychopathology is important due to the high comorbidity of EDs with other psychopathologies including mood, anxiety, personality, impulse-control, self-harm, and substance use disorders [4–6], and the high mortality associated with EDs [7]. This study seeks to contribute to this understanding by exploring relationships between emotional controllability and ED psychopathology, through emotion regulation.

Emotional controllability

Believing that emotions are uncontrollable has been linked to experiencing more negative emotions, greater depression and lower levels of well-being. In a sample of male ($n = 192$) and female ($n = 245$) college students, Tamir et al. [1] found that, just before starting college, nearly 40% of the students believed emotions to be uncontrollable. After one academic year, individuals who held these beliefs had experienced more negative emotions and reported greater depression than those who had considered emotions to be controllable. These results were replicated by De Castella et al. [2] who revealed that increased stress and depression, and decreased self-esteem and satisfaction with life were reported by those who believed that emotions cannot be controlled.

Emotion regulation and emotional controllability

Emotion regulation is a form of self-regulation that influences which emotions we experience, when they occur, how they are experienced, and how they are expressed [8]. While there are many strategies for regulating emotions, cognitive reappraisal and expressive suppression have received the most attention (e.g., [9]). Cognitive reappraisal (changing the way one *thinks* about emotion eliciting events) has been hypothesised to protect against psychopathology and is generally considered an adaptive strategy, while suppression (changing the way one *behaviourally responds* to the emotion) is thought to be a maladaptive strategy that has been considered a risk factor for psychopathology [10].

Emotional controllability has been found to influence an individual's use of emotion regulation strategies like reappraisal [11]. Studies have consistently shown that individuals are less likely to reappraise their emotions when they believe them to be uncontrollable [1, 2, 11–13]. Ford et al. [12] noted this relationship fits with investigations into self-regulation that have suggested that engagement in self-regulation requires motivation, and the belief that it is achievable. As such, an individual who believes emotions are uncontrollable may not think that modifying them is achievable, and may, therefore, lack the motivation to use adaptive strategies like reappraisal.

King et al. [13] conducted recent research into emotional controllability, well-being and reappraisal, using a sample of 355 Filipino college students (females = 259, males = 82). Believing emotions to be uncontrollable was negatively related to life satisfaction and positive emotions (positive indicators of well-being), and positively related to negative emotions, depression and anxiety (negative indicators of well-being). The effect of emotional controllability on well-being was found to be partially mediated by reappraisal. This suggests that emotional controllability influences an individual's reappraisal use, which then impacts their wellbeing.

Research into the relationship between emotional controllability and suppression has generated mixed results. Tamir et al. [1] and Ford et al. [12] found no difference in the use of suppression in individuals who viewed emotions as controllable vs uncontrollable. This suggests that emotional controllability is associated with strategies like reappraisal that aim to alter emotional *experiences*, not strategies like suppression that aim to alter emotional *expression* [12]. Yet this position is inconsistent with one of Schroder et al.'s [11] studies which did find a relationship between emotional controllability and suppression. However, this relationship was not consistent across their two experiments, rendering the significance of the relationship unclear. Further exploration of emotional controllability and suppression would be beneficial in providing clarity for the kind of strategies emotional controllability is associated with.

Emotions and eating disorders

Problems with emotion regulation have been suggested to play a role in the development and maintenance of ED psychopathology [14–16]. The cognitive interpersonal maintenance model [17] has identified important predisposing roles of cognitive and socio-emotional factors in EDs. This model, with accumulating evidence to support it [18], suggests that EDs such as anorexia nervosa are maintained by difficulties surrounding emotional functioning. Examples of problems with emotional functioning that have been seen in individuals with EDs include alexithymia (the inability to identify and describe one's feelings) [19, 20], increased negative emotionality [21], and difficulties regulating emotions [3, 21]. Importantly, difficulties with emotion regulation have been shown to correlate with the severity of ED psychopathology [15, 21–23].

Findings from Svaldi et al. [22] and Danner et al. [24] revealed that the severity of ED psychopathology in women negatively correlates with reappraisal use, and positively correlates with suppression use. However, Dixon-Gordon et al. [25] found that individuals who report a low use of all strategies (including reappraisal and suppression) experience amplified bulimia symptoms, making the use of suppression in EDs unclear and worthy of further exploration.

The present study

The aforementioned literature suggests that emotional controllability influences the way people regulate their emotions, which then has an impact upon psychological health [1, 2, 13]. While emotional controllability has not yet been explored in relation to ED psychopathology, difficulties regulating emotions are known to play an important role in eating disordered behaviours [20, 21]. This raises the question of whether emotional controllability is associated with EDs via the use of emotion regulation strategies.

The main aim of the current study is to examine the relationship between emotional controllability, ED psychopathology and two emotion regulation strategies, namely suppression and reappraisal. We hypothesised a significant negative relationship between beliefs about emotional controllability and ED psychopathology mediated by the use of reappraisal and suppression independently. We also predicted relationships between reappraisal and ED psychopathology, as well as between suppression and ED psychopathology. That is, we expected those who report a high use of reappraisal to display less severe ED psychopathology as the use of adaptive strategies has been thought to protect against psychopathology [10] and is associated with better interpersonal functioning and well-being [9]. In addition, drawing on theories which suggest maladaptive strategies are a risk factor for psychopathology [10] and have been found to negatively correlate with interpersonal functioning and well-being [9], we expected more severe ED psychopathology to be displayed by those who report a high use of suppression.

Method

Participants

Originally, 884 participants completed the survey. However, 166 participants were excluded from the data set due to several missing responses in one or more questionnaires. The final sample included 718 participants ($n = 556$ females, $n = 156$ males, $n = 6$ other) from a range of ethnic groups ($n = 398$ Whites; n = 15 Blacks; $n = 204$ Asians; $n = 35$ Mixed; $n = 59$ Other; $n = 7$ not provided), with a mean age of 23.01 (SD = 8.18, age range = 56). Of the sample, 260 participants were students recruited from Bournemouth University, and the other participants ($n = 458$) were recruited online through a link distributed through email and social media (Facebook and Reddit).

Measures

The predictor variable (emotional controllability) was operationalised using scores from two scales, the Implicit Beliefs about Emotion scale [1] and the Personal Beliefs about Emotion scale [2]. The outcome variable (ED psychopathology) was operationalised using the total score from the Eating Disorder Examination Questionnaire (EDE-Q [26];). The mediating variables (reappraisal and suppression) were operationalised using the scores from the Emotion Regulation Questionnaire (ERQ [9];).

Implicit beliefs about emotion scale

To assess general beliefs about the nature of emotion, we used Tamir et al.'s [1] Implicit Beliefs about Emotion Scale (IBES). The scale has shown good internal consistency in previous studies (α = .75, [1]; α = .77, [2]) and also in the current sample (α = .74). This scale correlates with the general controllability component of the Emotion Beliefs Questionnaire ($r = -.45$) [27], suggesting good external validity.

Personal beliefs about emotion scale

To assess personal beliefs about the nature of emotion, De Castella et al.'s [2] Personal Beliefs about Emotion Scale– an adapted version of the Implicit Beliefs about Emotion Scale [1] was used. The scales differ in terms of item wording, such that items embodying general beliefs use indefinite and third-person pronouns (e.g. "Everyone can learn to control their emotions"), whereas, personal beliefs are embodied by the use of first-person pronouns (e.g. "I can learn to control my emotions"). This scale shows good internal consistency (α = .79) [2],which was also confirmed in the current sample (α = .80). This scale correlated highly with the IBES in our sample ($r = .70$) and the results remained consistent across both scales. We report the results from the general belief scale (IBES) in the manuscript and the ones from the personal belief scale in the supplementary material.

Eating disorder examination questionnaire

Participants completed the Eating Disorder Examination Questionnaire (EDE-Q [26];) to assess their ED psychopathology severity. The EDEQ contains 28 questions referring to the past 28 days, such that high scores indicate severe ED psychopathology. The EDE-Q total score has strong internal consistency (α = .90) [28], which was confirmed in our sample (α = .96). This measure has also been shown to have good external validity in a community sample, (r = .84 with the Eating Disorder Examination Interview) [29], suggesting good external validity. Only the EDE-Q total score was examined as this study's main aim was to investigate emotional controllability in relation to general ED psychopathology. As per Table 1, our sample was within the community norms reported in Carey et al. [30].

Emotional regulation questionnaire

Participants completed the Emotion Regulation Questionnaire (ERQ [9];) to evaluate their use of reappraisal and suppression. The scale consists of 10 questions with responses rating the agreeability of statements scored on a 7-point scale (1 = strongly disagree, 7 = strongly agree). The ERQ has demonstrated good external validity [31] as well as good internal consistency (reappraisal, α = .79; suppression, α = .73) [9], which was also confirmed in our sample (reappraisal, α = .86; suppression, α = .77).

Procedure

The questionnaires were presented through the online platform Qualtrics (Qualtrics, Provo, UT) and began with demographic information, followed by the ERQ, the Emotional Controllability questionnaire and the EDE-Q. Participants also answered other questionnaires not reported in the current paper. This study received ethical approval from the Research Ethics Panel at Bournemouth University and University College London.

Data analysis

A mediational analysis was conducted with all variables represented by continuous data. The PROCESS regression macro was used (via SPSS, version 25) as it uses bootstrapping, which is a nonparametric method that does not rely upon normally distributed data. It involves resampling the data set (5000 times) and estimating the indirect effect in each sample [32]. Research supports the use of bootstrapping as it provides accurate confidence limits [33], has good Type I error control and high power levels [34]. The effect size was calculated by means of percent mediation (P_M = (a*b)/c), to determine the degree to which the mediating variable is responsible for the total effect (c). This standardised method is independent of sample size, and the absence of a better alternative makes this a commonly used measure despite its limitations [35]. Model 1 looked at the relationship between personal emotional controllability and eating psychology through reappraisal while Model 2 looked at this relationship through suppression. We also ran these models with general rather than personal emotional controllability; results can be found in the supplementary material (Figs. 3 and 4).

Table 1 Descriptive statistics of the five scales used

	Mean	SD	Range (Min-Max)
General EC (IBES)	3.2	0.80	4 (1–5)
Personal EC	3.4	0.87	4 (1–5)
EDE-Q	2.09	1.60	6 (0–6)
EDE-Q N clinical range	n = 121		
Reappraisal	4.60	1.5	6 (1–7)
Suppression	3.92	1.39	6 (1–7)

Results

The range, mean and standard deviations of the scores for each variable are presented in Table 1.

Average scores, followed by standard deviation, range and min-max (in brackets) on the Implicit Beliefs about Emotions scale (General EC), Personal Beliefs about Emotions scale (Personal EC), Eating Disorder Examination Questionnaire total score (EDE-Q), Reappraisal, and Suppression. For the EDE-Q, we added a row indicating the number of participants scoring in the clinical range (i.e. scoring above 4; EDE-Q N in clinical range).

Mediation analysis of model 1

As predicted, there was a significant negative relationship between general emotional controllability and the severity of ED psychopathology (path c: $\beta = -.11$, $t(716) = -3.09$, $p = .002$).

The results for the mediation analysis of Model 1 are displayed in Fig. 1. The positive relationship between general emotional controllability and reappraisal was significant (path a: $\beta = .19$, $t(716) = 5.10$, $p < .001$), as was the negative relationship between reappraisal and ED psychopathology (path b: $\beta = -.29$, $t(715) = -5.63$, $p < .001$). In addition, there was a significant indirect effect of emotional controllability on ED psychopathology through the use of reappraisal ($ab = -0.05$, BCa CI [−0.13, −0.04]). When controlling for the mediating variable of reappraisal, the direct effect of emotional controllability on ED psychopathology was reduced but remained significant suggesting partial mediation (path c': $\beta = -.15$, $t(715) = -2.04$, $p = .041$). There was a moderate effect of reappraisal, $P_M = .48$, showing that reappraisal accounted for 48% of the effect of general emotional controllability on ED psychopathology.

Mediation analysis of model 2

The mediation analysis of Model 2 (Fig. 2) demonstrated a significant negative relationship between general emotional controllability and ED psychopathology through

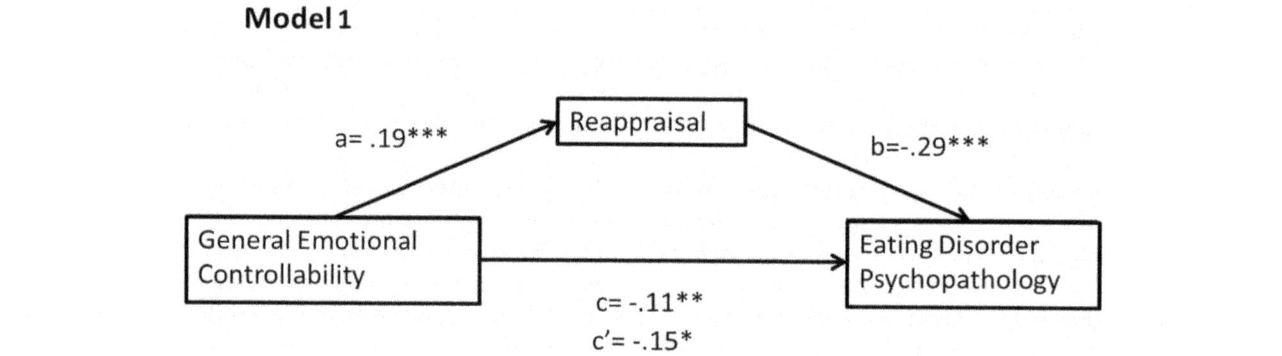

Fig. 1 Mediation of Model 1, displaying standardised regression coefficients with their significance and the absolute value of c' (* = $p < .05$, ** = $p < .010$, *** = $p < .001$)

the mediation of suppression ($ab = -0.02$, BCa CI [−0.07, −0.002]). There was a significant negative relationship between emotional controllability and suppression (path a: $\beta = -.08$, $t(716) = -2.12$, $p = .035$), and a significant positive relationship between suppression and ED psychopathology (path b: $\beta = .25$, $t(715) = 5.83$, $p < .001$). Additionally, the direct effect of emotional controllability and ED psychopathology was reduced when controlling for suppression (path c': $\beta = -.10$, $t(715) = -2.69$, $p = .007$), but remained significant indicating partial mediation. There was a moderate effect of suppression, $P_M = .17$, showing that suppression accounted for 17% of the effect of general emotional controllability on ED psychopathology.

Discussion

The aim of the present study was to explore the relationships between emotional controllability and ED psychopathology, and whether these relationships were mediated by emotion regulation. Through mediation analyses conducted on the self-report data from 718 participants, we found that (a) emotional controllability is linked to ED psychopathology, and (b) the relationship between emotional controllability and ED psychopathology is partially mediated by both reappraisal and suppression.

As predicted, the results demonstrated a significant negative relationship between emotional controllability and ED psychopathology severity. This supports the idea that viewing emotions as uncontrollable relates to poorer psychological health and well-being [1, 2, 12, 13], as individuals who held this view displayed greater severity of ED psychopathology. Moreover, the mediation analysis showed that this relationship was partially mediated by the use of reappraisal, partially confirming our hypothesis. Consistent with the findings from Tamir et al. [1], De Castella et al. [2], Schroder et al. [11], King et al. [13], and Ford et al. [12], results from the mediation analysis of Model 1 indicate a reduced use of reappraisal in individuals who perceived emotions as uncontrollable. The pattern of these findings suggests individuals who held the view that emotions are uncontrollable indicated a lack of reappraisal, and also more severe ED psychopathology. As discussed previously, an individual who believes emotions are uncontrollable may not think altering them was achievable, and in turn, may lack the motivation to use reappraisal. The insufficient use of adaptive strategies like reappraisal means an

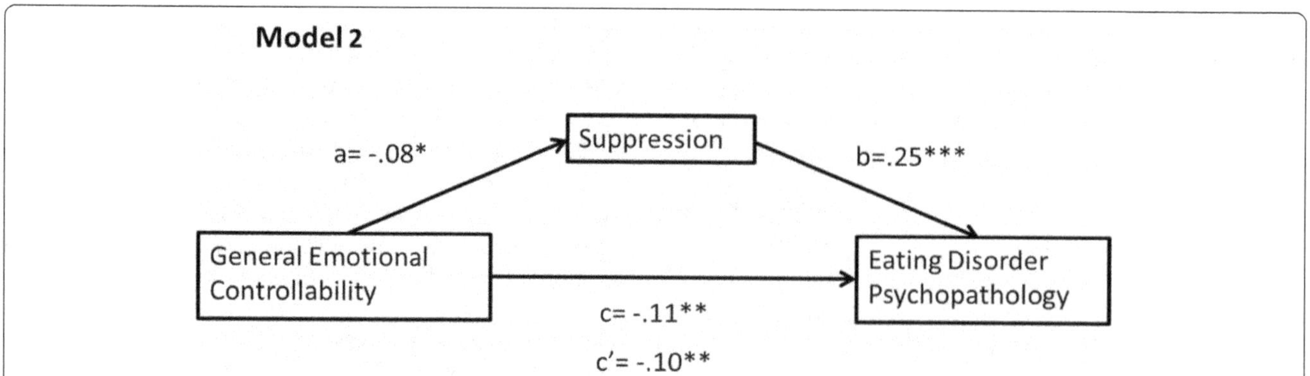

Fig. 2 Mediation of Model 2, displaying standardised regression coefficients with their significance and the absolute value of c' (* = $p < .05$, ** = $p < .010$, *** = $p < .001$)

individual may not be able to effectively modify their emotional experiences, leading to emotion dysregulation [36]. This, in turn, may worsen the psychological and behavioural aspects of EDs, as previous research has demonstrated an association between emotion dysregulation and the severity of ED symptoms [21].

Interestingly, the results from the mediation analysis of Model 2 showed the use of suppression partially mediated the relationship between emotional controllability and ED psychopathology. A small negative relationship was found between emotional controllability and suppression, suggesting individuals who believe emotions to be uncontrollable display a *greater* use of suppression than those who believe emotions to be controllable. This challenges the findings that suggest emotional controllability only relates to strategies that target emotional *experience* [1, 12]. The current study also challenges the findings from Schroder et al. [11], which is the only known study to find an association between emotional controllability and suppression. Their findings suggest the belief that emotions are uncontrollable links to *little* use of suppression, whereas the findings in our study suggest this belief links to *high* use of suppression. It must again be noted that Schroder et al.'s [11] findings were inconsistent, with only their second study - conducted in a small and female only sample - finding a significant relationship between these concepts. Our findings suggest that an individual who views emotions as uncontrollable may not feel it is possible to change the negative emotions they experience, so may use suppression more frequently in order to alter the expression of emotions yet avoid having to engage with their emotional reactions.

Limitations

A first limitation is that the findings are restricted to non-clinical samples, and may not be representative of the general population due to recruitment through opportunity sampling. As such, future studies could expand upon our findings by investigating whether our results replicate in a clinical sample. Ideally, this could be tested in a sample presenting a range of eating disorders (e.g. anorexia nervosa, bulimia nervosa and binge eating disorder) to explore potential differences between ED pathologies, and understand whether some eating disorder behaviours (e.g. dieting, bingeing or purging) may particularly correlate with emotional controllability. That being said, using non-clinical samples and investigating emotional functioning in ED psychopathology is beneficial. Firstly, in its own right, due to many individuals engaging in these behaviours [37], their higher prevalence compared to threshold eating disorders [38], and their links with psychopathology [39]. Secondly, some individuals exhibiting ED psychopathology may develop a full-threshold ED [38], meaning investigations with non-clinical samples could provide insight into the contribution of emotional functioning in the development of EDs [21].

Another limitation is the lack of generalisability arising from a predominately female sample, with a relatively young average age. As such, the findings may not be applicable to male dominated samples and older populations. In addition, the samples' disproportionate female to male ratio may have impacted upon the findings given the higher prevalence of ED symptoms in females [40] and gender differences in emotion and emotion regulation. Generally, females are thought to be more emotional than males, expressing and experiencing them more regularly [41]. Moreover, while there are inconsistencies in the research surrounding gender differences in reappraisal and suppression use [12, 42–45], engagement in most forms of emotion regulation is more likely to be reported in females than males [46]. However, it is theorised that emotion regulation in males may be unconscious and automatic, and that their emotion regulation processes may as a consequence be inadequately informed in research [47], therefore suggesting fewer differences than originally thought. Future work may wish to investigate these gender differences, as well as explore a wider range of emotion regulation strategies such as avoidance, which is another strategy that has been related to both EDs [48] and emotional controllability [49].

Due to the cross-sectional nature of this study, interpretation of the results is also limited. Firstly because mediation tested in cross-sectional data may not always be replicated in longitudinal data [50, 51], so it is important to treat our current results with caution until such study is conducted. Second because our results cannot be interpreted in a way that suggests causation. The proposed models hypothesise the directions of the relationships between these variables, however, the directional relationships theorised may not be correct. For example, severe ED psychopathology may impact an individual's ability to effectively regulate their emotions, which would guide their belief about their emotions. A longitudinal study would need to be conducted in order to confirm our findings and establish relationships of cause and effect. Nonetheless, the contributions of the current study should not be overlooked. This study has indeed challenged previous research into emotional controllability and suppression, supported existing research into emotion regulation strategies and ED psychopathology, and examined a link between emotional controllability and ED psychopathology that had not previously been investigated.

Practical implications

The relationships and ideas suggested in this study have practical implications for improving ED psychopathology.

Research has shown treatment addressing emotion regulation strategies decreases the rate of ED behaviours [52, 53]. In addition, Ford et al. [12] suggested targeting the belief that emotions are uncontrollable "may be a key 'early' step in the process of employing effective forms of emotion regulation" (p.1186). Blackwell et al.'s [54] findings suggest this approach can be successful as they demonstrated improvement in educational outcomes after interventions to improve adolescents' beliefs about intelligence. Similar results have also been found in undergraduates [55]. Gutentag et al. [56] also found – in natural and unnatural settings – that the belief that emotions can be controlled relates to successful emotion regulation and more frequent use of effective emotion regulation strategies. From these findings, it could be reasoned that challenging the belief that emotions are uncontrollable may improve the use of effective emotion regulation strategies, which in turn may improve the psychological and behavioural aspects of EDs. Gutentag et al.'s [56] findings as well as ours will need replication, and further research is required, but support for this theory may have implications for ED treatments. If replicated and supported in a clinical sample, our results suggest that challenging emotional controllability beliefs may be an important component to add to the Emotional and Social Mind module of the Maudsley Anorexia Nervosa Treatment for Adults (MANTRA [49];) for example.

Conclusion

The current study has demonstrated relationships that support investigating emotional controllability, emotion regulation and psychological health. Our findings suggest that one's beliefs about emotional controllability has important outcomes with regards to eating psychopathology. While our results need to be replicated and tested in a clinical sample, our study lays the foundations for future research and possible treatment options in this area.

Abbreviations

EC: Emotional Controllability; ED: Eating Disorder; EDE-Q: Eating Disorder Examination Questionnaire; ERQ: Emotion Regulation Questionnaire

Acknowledgements

The authors would like thank the students who collected the data which was used in this study for their dissertation projects, including Samantha Sewell, Daniel Pearson, Louise Presant, Katie McGuire, Amatullah Khuzaima, Elizabeth Tilbrook, Alexandra Tepper, Aniqua Amir, Forhad Alom, Helen Lai, Levi Spence, Natalie Wong, Yuk Ching, Samuel Hass, Xing Liu, Faranak Mohammadzadeh Shaghouei, Baasma Valiya Parambil, Carla Deplancke, Wanyi Ma, Sandra Shamu, Sergey Ershikov, and Eleni Desypri. We also would like to thank the participants who took part in this study.

Authors' contributions

LV, AH and MS designed the study. JJ collected the data. LV and JJ analysed the data. LV and JJ wrote the manuscript. All authors contributed to the final version of the manuscript. The author(s) read and approved the final manuscript.

Competing interests

The authors declare that they have no competing interests.

Author details

[1]Faculty of Science and Technology, Department of Psychology, Bournemouth University, Poole, UK. [2]UCL Institute of Education, University College London, London, UK.

References

1. Tamir M, John OP, Srivastava S, Gross JJ. Implicit theories of emotion: affective and social outcomes across a major life transition. J Personal Soc Psychol. 2007;92(4):731-744. Available from: https://doi.org/https://doi.org/10.1037/0022-3514.92.4.731.
2. De Castella K, Goldin P, Jazaieri H, Ziv M, Dweck CS, Gross JJ. Beliefs about emotion: links to emotion regulation, well-being, and psychological distress. Basic Appl Soc Psychol. 2013;35(6):497-505. Available from: https://doi.org/https://doi.org/10.1080/01973533.2013.840632.
3. Harrison A, Sullivan S, Tchanturia K, Treasure J. Emotional functioning in eating disorders: attentional bias, emotion recognition and emotion regulation. Psychol Med. 2010;40(11):1887-1897. Available from: https://doi.org/https://doi.org/10.1017/S0033291710000036.
4. Hudson JI, Hiripi E, Pope HG, Jr., Kessler RC. The prevalence and correlates of eating disorders in the National Comorbidity Survey Replication. . Biol Psychiatry. 2007;61(3):348-358. Available from: https://doi.org/https://doi.org/10.1016/j.biopsych.2006.03.040.
5. Keski-Rahkonen A, Mustelin L. Epidemiology of eating disorders in Europe: prevalence, incidence, comorbidity, course, consequences, and risk factors. Curr Opin Psych. 2016;29(6):340–5. https://doi.org/10.1097/YCO.0000000000000278.
6. Solmi F, Hotopf M, Hatch SL, Treasure J, Micali N. Eating disorders in a multi-ethnic inner-city UK sample: prevalence, comorbidity and service use. Soc Psychiatry Psychiatr Epidemiol. 2016;51(3):369-381. Available from: https://doi.org/https://doi.org/10.1007/s00127-015-1146-7.
7. Smink FR, van Hoeken D, Hoek HW. Epidemiology of eating disorders: incidence, prevalence and mortality rates. Curr Psychiatry Rep. 2012;14(4):406-414. Available from: https://doi.org/https://doi.org/10.1007/s11920-012-0282-y.
8. Gross JJ. Antecedent-and response-focused emotion regulation: divergent consequences for experience, expression, and physiology. J Pers Soc Psychol. 1998;74(1):224–37. https://doi.org/10.1037/0022-3514.74.1.224.
9. Gross JJ, John OP. Individual differences in two emotion regulation processes: implications for affect, relationships, and well-being. J Pers Soc Psychol. 2003;85(2):348-62. Available from: https://doi.org/https://doi.org/10.1037/0022-3514.85.2.348.
10. Aldao A, Nolen-Hoeksema S, Schweizer S. Emotion-regulation strategies across psychopathology: a meta-analytic review. Clinical psychology review. 2010;30(2):217-37. Available from: https://doi.org/https://doi.org/10.1016/j.cpr.2009.11.004.
11. Schroder HS, Dawood S, Yalch MM, Donnellan MB, Moser JS. The role of implicit theories in mental health symptoms, emotion regulation, and hypothetical treatment choices in college students. Cognitive therapy and research. 2015;39(2):120-39. Available from: https://doi.org/https://doi.org/10.1007/s10608-014-9652-6.
12. Ford BQ, Lwi SJ, Gentzler A, Hankin B, Mauss IB. The cost of believing emotions are uncontrollable: youths' beliefs about emotion predict emotion regulation and depressive symptoms. J Exp Psychol Gen. 2018;147(8):1170–90. https://doi.org/10.1037/xge0000396.
13. King RB, Dela Rosa ED. Are your emotions under your control or not? Implicit theories of emotion predict well-being via cognitive reappraisal. Personality and individual differences. 2019;138:177-82. Available from: https://doi.org/https://doi.org/10.1016/j.paid.2018.09.040.
14. Dingemans A, Danner U, Parks M. Emotion regulation in binge eating disorder: a review. Nutrients. 2017;9(11). Available from: https://doi.org/https://doi.org/10.3390/nu9111274.
15. Harrison A, Tchanturia K, Treasure J. Attentional bias, emotion recognition, and emotion regulation in anorexia: state or trait? Biol psychiatry. 2010;68(8):755-61. Available from: https://doi.org/https://doi.org/10.1016/j.biopsych.2010.04.037.

16. Leehr EJ, Krohmer K, Schag K, Dresler T, Zipfel S, Giel KE. Emotion regulation model in binge eating disorder and obesity--a systematic review. Neurosci Biobehav rev. 2015;49:125-34. Available from: https://doi.org/https://doi.org/10.1016/j.neubiorev.2014.12.008.
17. Schmidt U, Treasure J. Anorexia nervosa: valued and visible. A cognitive-interpersonal maintenance model and its implications for research and practice. Br J Clin Psychol. 2006;45(Pt 3):343-66. Available from: https://doi.org/https://doi.org/10.1348/014466505X53902.
18. Treasure J, Schmidt U. The cognitive-interpersonal maintenance model of anorexia nervosa revisited: a summary of the evidence for cognitive, socio-emotional and interpersonal predisposing and perpetuating factors. Journal of eating disorders. 2013;1(13). Available from: https://doi.org/https://doi.org/10.1186/2050-2974-1-13.
19. Brewer R, Cook R, Cardi V, Treasure J, Bird G. Emotion recognition deficits in eating disorders are explained by co-occurring alexithymia. R Soc open Sci. 2015;2(1):140382. Available from: https://doi.org/https://doi.org/10.1098/rsos.140382.
20. Westwood H, Kerr-Gaffney J, Stahl D, Tchanturia K. Alexithymia in eating disorders: systematic review and meta-analyses of studies using the Toronto alexithymia scale. J Psychosom res. 2017;99:66-81. Available from: https://doi.org/https://doi.org/10.1016/j.jpsychores.2017.06.007.
21. Lavender JM, Wonderlich SA, Engel SG, Gordon KH, Kaye WH, Mitchell JE. Dimensions of emotion dysregulation in anorexia nervosa and bulimia nervosa: a conceptual review of the empirical literature. Clin Psychol rev. 2015;40:111-22. Available from: https://doi.org/https://doi.org/10.1016/j.cpr.2015.05.010.
22. Svaldi J, Griepenstroh J, Tuschen-Caffier B, Ehring T. Emotion regulation deficits in eating disorders: a marker of eating pathology or general psychopathology? Psychiatry res. 2012;197(1-2):103-11. Available from: https://doi.org/https://doi.org/10.1016/j.psychres.2011.11.009.
23. Whiteside U, Chen E, Neighbors C, Hunter D, Lo T, Larimer M. Difficulties regulating emotions: do binge eaters have fewer strategies to modulate and tolerate negative affect? Eat Behav. 2007;8(2):162-9. Available from: https://doi.org/https://doi.org/10.1016/j.eatbeh.2006.04.001.
24. Danner UN, Sternheim L, Evers C. The importance of distinguishing between the different eating disorders (sub)types when assessing emotion regulation strategies. Psychiatry res. 2014;215(3):727-32. Available from: https://doi.org/https://doi.org/10.1016/j.psychres.2014.01.005.
25. Dixon-Gordon KL, Aldao A, De Los Reyes A. Repertoires of emotion regulation: a person-centered approach to assessing emotion regulation strategies and links to psychopathology. Cogn Emot. 2015; 29(7):1314-25. Available from: https://doi.org/https://doi.org/10.1080/02699931.2014.983046.
26. Fairburn CG, Beglin SJ. Assessment of eating disorders: interview or self-report questionnaire?. The International Journal of Eating Disorders. 1994;16(4):363–70. Available from: https://doi.org/https://doi.org/10.1002/1098-108X.
27. Becerra R, Preece DA, Gross JJ. Assessing beliefs about emotions: development and validation of the emotion beliefs questionnaire. PLoS one. 2020;15(4):e0231395. Available from: https://doi.org/https://doi.org/10.1371/journal.pone.0231395.
28. Peterson CB, Crosby RD, Wonderlich SA, Joiner T, Crow SJ, Mitchell JE, et al. Psychometric properties of the eating disorder examination-questionnaire: factor structure and internal consistency. Int J eat Disord. 2007;40(4):386-9. Available from: https://doi.org/https://doi.org/10.1002/eat.
29. Mond JM, Hay PJ, Rodgers B, Owen C, Beumont PJV. Validity of the eating disorder examination questionnaire (EDE-Q) in screening for eating disorders in community samples. Behaviour research and therapy. 2004; 42(5):551-67. Available from: https://doi.org/https://doi.org/10.1016/S0005-7967(03)00161-X.
30. Carey M, Kupeli N, Knight R, Troop NA, Jenkinson PM, Preston C. Eating disorder examination questionnaire (EDE-Q): norms and psychometric properties in U.K. females and males. Psychol assess. 2019;31(7):839-50. Available from: https://doi.org/https://doi.org/10.1037/pas0000703, .
31. Preece DA, Becerra R, Robinson K, Gross JJ. The emotion regulation questionnaire: psychometric properties in general community samples. Journal of personality assessment. 2019;102(3):348-56. Available from: https://doi.org/https://doi.org/10.1080/00223891.2018.1564319.
32. Preacher KJ, Hayes AF. Asymptotic and resampling strategies for assessing and comparing indirect effects in multiple mediator models. Behav res methods. 2008;40(3):879-91. Available from: https://doi.org/https://doi.org/10.1037/a0022658
33. Mackinnon DP, Lockwood CM, Williams J. Confidence limits for the indirect effect: distribution of the product and resampling methods. Multivariate Behav res. 2004;39(1):99. Available from: https://doi.org/https://doi.org/10.1207/s15327906mbr3901.
34. Hayes AF. Beyond baron and Kenny: statistical mediation analysis in the new millennium. Communication monographs. 2009;76(4):408-20. Available from: https://doi.org/https://doi.org/10.1080/03637750903310360.
35. Preacher KJ, Kelley K. Effect size measures for mediation models: quantitative strategies for communicating indirect effects. Psychol methods. 2011;16(2):93-115. Available from: https://doi.org/https://doi.org/10.3758/BRM.40.3.879.
36. Fruzzetti AE, Crook W, Erikson KM, Lee JE, Worrall JM. Emotion Regulation. In: Fisher WTODJE, editor. General principles and empirically supported techniques of cognitive behaviour therapy Wiley. J & Sons, Inc.; 2009. p. 272–84.
37. Eisenberg D, Nicklett EJ, Roeder K, Kirz NE. Eating disorder symptoms among college students: prevalence, persistence, correlates, and treatment-seeking. J am Coll health. 2011;59(8):700-7. Available from: https://doi.org/https://doi.org/10.1080/07448481.2010.546461.Eating.
38. Stice E, Marti CN, Shaw H, Jaconis M. An 8-year longitudinal study of the natural history of threshold, subthreshold, and partial eating disorders from a community sample of adolescents. J Abnorm Psychol. 2009;118(3):587-97. Available from: https://doi.org/https://doi.org/10.1037/a0016481.An.
39. Patton GC, Coffey C, Carlin JB, Sanci L, Sawyer S. Prognosis of adolescent partial syndromes of eating disorder. Br J psychiatry. 2008;192(4):294-9. Available from: https://doi.org/https://doi.org/10.1192/bjp.bp.106.031112.
40. Striegel-Moore RH, Rosselli F, Perrin N, DeBar L, Wilson GT, May A, et al. Gender difference in the prevalence of eating disorder symptoms. Int J eat Disord. 2009;42(5):471-4. Available from: https://doi.org/https://doi.org/10.1002/eat.20625.
41. Plant EA, Hyde JS, Keltner D, Devine PG. The gender stereotyping of emotions. Psychology of women quarterly. 2000;24(1):81-92. Available from: https://doi.org/https://doi.org/10.1111/j.1471-6402.2000.tb01024.x.
42. Haga SM, Kraft P, Corby E-K. Emotion regulation: antecedents and well-being outcomes of cognitive reappraisal and expressive suppression in cross-cultural samples. Journal of happiness studies. 2009;10(3):271-91. Available from: http://doi.org/https://doi.org/10.1007/s10902-007-9080-3.
43. John OP, Gross JJ. Healthy and unhealthy emotion regulation: personality processes, individual differences, and life span development. Journal of personality. 2004;72(6):1201-334. Available from: https://doi.org/https://doi.org/10.1111/j.1467-6494.2004.00298.x.
44. Nolen-Hoeksema S, Aldao A. Gender and age differences in emotion regulation strategies and their relationship to depressive symptoms. Personality and individual differences. 2011;51(6):704-8. Available from: https://doi.org/https://doi.org/10.1016/j.paid.2011.06.012.
45. Zimmermann P, Iwanski A. Emotion regulation from early adolescence to emerging adulthood and middle adulthood. International journal of behavioral development. 2014;38(2):182-94. Available from: https://doi.org/https://doi.org/10.1177/0165025413515405.
46. Tamres LK, Janicki D, Helgeson VS. Sex differences in coping behavior: A meta-analytic review and an examination of relative coping. Personality and Social Psychology Review,. 2002;6(1):2–30. Available from: https://doi.org/https://doi.org/10.1207/S15327957PSPR0601_1.
47. Nolen-Hoeksema S. Emotion regulation and psychopathology: the role of gender. Annu rev Clin Psychol. 2012;8:161-87. Available from: http://doi.org/https://doi.org/10.1146/annurev-clinpsy-032511-143109
48. De Castella K, Platow MJ, Tamir M, Gross JJ. Beliefs about emotion: implications for avoidance-based emotion regulation and psychological health. Cogn Emot. 2018;32(4):773–95. https://www.tandfonline.com/doi/full/10.1080/02699931.2017.1353485?src=recsys.
49. Schmidt U, Renwick B, Lose A, Kenyon M, DeJong H, Broadbent H, et al. The MOSAIC study - comparison of the Maudsley model of treatment for adults with anorexia nervosa (MANTRA) with specialist supportive clinical management (SSCM) in outpatients with broadly defined anorexia nervosa: a randomized controlled trial. Journal of consulting and clinical psychology. 2015;83(4):796. Available from: https://doi.org/https://doi.org/10.1186/1745-6215-14-160.
50. Cole DA, Maxwell SE. Testing mediational models with longitudinal data: questions and tips in the use of structural equation modeling. Journal of abnormal psychology. 2003;112(4):558. Available from: http://doi.org/https://doi.org/10.1037/0021-843X.112.4.558.

51. Maxwell SE, Cole DA. Bias in cross-sectional analyses of longitudinal mediation. Psychological Methods,. 2007;12(1). Available from: http://doi.org/https://doi.org/10.1037/1082-989X.12.1.23.
52. Safer DL, Telch CF, Agras SW. Dialectical behavior therapy for bulimia nervosa. Am J Psychiatr. 2001;158(4):632–4. https://doi.org/10.1176/appi.ajp.158.4.632.
53. Telch CF, Agras WS, Lineham MM. Dialectical behavior therapy for binge eating disorder. J Consult Clin Psychol. 2001;69(6):1061–5. https://doi.org/10.1037/0022-006X.69.6.1061.
54. Blackwell LS, Trzesniewski KH, Dweck CS. Implicit theories of intelligence predict achievement across an adolescent transition: a longitudinal study and an intervention. Child Dev. 2007;78(1):246–63. https://doi.org/10.1111/j.1467-8624.2007.00995.x.
55. Aronson J, Fried CB, Good C. Reducing the effects of stereotype threat on African American college students by shaping theories of intelligence. Journal of experimental social psychology. 2002;38(2):113-25. Available from: https://doi.org/https://doi.org/10.1006/jesp.2001.1491.
56. Gutentag T, Halperin E, Porat R, Bigman YE, Tamir M. Successful emotion regulation requires both conviction and skill: beliefs about the controllability of emotions, reappraisal, and regulation success. Cogn Emot. 2017;31(6):1225-33. Available from: https://doi.org/https://doi.org/10.1080/02699931.2016.1213704.

18

Beyond difficulties in self-regulation: the role of identity integration and personality functioning in young women with disordered eating behaviours

Marko Biberdzic*, Josephine Tang and Junhao Tan

Abstract

Background: Past research has established individual relationships between disordered eating behaviours (DEB) and both self-regulation difficulties and identity disturbance. However, no research has looked at the shared influence of these constructs on DEB nor at personality functioning in individuals with DEB.

Methods: In the present study, self-regulation was explored in terms of effortful control, impulsivity and emotion regulation while identity integration was measured in terms of impairments in self-functioning using a sample of 247 undergraduate students.

Results: Significant associations were found between all components of self-regulation and DEB, with the exception of impulsivity. Identity instability was also associated with self-regulation difficulties and DEB. Structural Equation Modelling analyses indicated that identity instability partially mediated the relationship between self-regulation and DEB. Lastly, disordered eating was associated with difficulties in personality functioning, with young women presenting with DEB reporting significantly greater difficulties in both self and interpersonal personality functioning.

Conclusion: Behavioural eating anomalies should be considered as epiphenomena secondary to a possible deeper issue that reflects difficulties related to identity integration and potential personality functioning. The clinical implications of these findings are discussed.

Keywords: Disordered eating behaviours, Identity integration, Personality functioning, Eating disorders, Self-regulation

Plain English summary

Eating disorders involve patterns of problematic eating and behaviours aimed at reducing body weight and/or preventing weight gain. Since early disordered eating behaviours such as dietary restraint and binge-eating are highly predictive of a later development of eating disorders, it is important to investigate the roots of these behaviours. This study aimed to compare different contributing factors, previously suggested to play a role in disordered eating behaviors, such as emotion regulation, impulsivity, and identity disturbance. We also aimed to examine the unique role of identity disturbance in explaining the relation between difficulties in emotion regulation and disordered eating behaviours. By using different questionnaires and a sample of 218 university women, we found that both emotion regulation and identity instability predicted disordered eating behaviours.

* Correspondence: markob@uow.edu.au
School of Psychology, University of Wollongong, Wollongong, NSW 2522, Australia

However, part of the impact of poor emotion regulation was explained by identity disturbance, which suggests that the latter plays a more central role in the development of disordered eating behaviours. Our results therefore suggest that young women who present with disordered eating may have underlying difficulties related to their sense of identity, i.e. a more unstable sense of self, and may benefit from targeting this specific area in psychotherapy.

Eating disorders and disordered eating behaviours are estimated to affect over 16% of the Australian population [36], and are one of the most prevalent disorders in youth [24]. Although the aetiology of eating pathology is complex [13], it has been argued that several variables involved in self-regulation and associated inhibitory processes – such as impulsivity [52], emotion regulation [38] and effortful control [11] – play an important role in the manifestation of these behaviours. More recently, an increased amount of literature has also re-emphasized the role of identity impairment in the development of disturbed eating, with an unclear sense of self being considered as the main underlying factor and contributor to eating disorder symptomatology [51]. However, despite general consensus in the theoretical literature, very few studies have empirically tested the role of identity pathology as a pathway to disordered eating, and no study has investigated the combined relation between impulsivity, emotion regulation, effortful control and identity disturbance in predicting disordered eating behaviours.

Eating disorders and disordered eating behaviours

Eating disorders (EDs) are characterized by continuous patterns of problematic eating and engagement in behaviours aimed at reducing body weight and/or preventing weight gain [1]. Disordered eating can include behaviours that reflect many but not all of the symptoms of feeding and eating disorders [1]. These disordered eating behaviours (DEB) are the most common indicators of the development of an eating disorder, with disordered eating being linked to a reduced ability to cope with stressful situations, as well as an increased incidence of suicidal thoughts and behaviours, particularly in youth [36]. Both eating disorders and DEB involve considerable psychological impairment and distress, and are associated with a range of serious medical complications [36]. The mortality rate for people with eating disorders is also one of the highest among all psychiatric illnesses [3], with these difficulties considered to be a serious public health concern [42].

Self-regulation: emotion regulation, effortful control and impulsivity

While self-regulation is known to be a multi-dimensional construct, it is broadly characterised as the ability to have emotional, behavioural and cognitive control over contextual demands. Self-regulation also encompasses a whole range of terms and functions including behavioural inhibition, impulsivity, effortful control, emotion control and cognitive control [5]. These regulatory mechanisms allow the individual to make relevant responses through processes such as initiation, adjustment, interruption or inhibition of thoughts and behaviours [4]. Effective self-regulation is reflected in appropriate management of situations and impulses and is related to beneficial outcomes in all age groups [7]. Conversely, failure to self-regulate is associated with a range of unfavourable outcomes including the development of many psychological disorders.

In the context of eating disorders, it has been suggested that DEB such as dietary restraint and purging/binging are used to regulate emotion [43]. More specifically, in the affect regulation model, DEB is understood as a coping and compensatory strategy for temporary reduction of negative affect or increase in positive affect [30]. This in turn is believed to reinforce poor self-regulation as the binges reduce the intensity of the negative affect, making it more difficult to regulate eating impulses. For individuals in the restrictive subtype, it has been postulated that diet restraint can help in affect regulation by using hunger to temporarily decrease one's reactivity towards emotional stimuli ([19]; for a review of the affect regulation model and escape theory, see [22, 23]). A recent meta-analysis by Prefit et al. [38] also reported medium-to-large effect sizes for the associations between maladaptive emotion regulation and EDs and eating-related symptoms. Emotion regulation difficulties did not differ across EDs, further supporting the transdiagnostic character of emotion regulation problems in eating pathology.

Numerous studies on eating disorders have also underlined the contribution of temperamental factors involved in self-regulation, especially effortful control (e.g., [10]). Effortful control is described by Rothbart and Bates [40] as the 'capacity to inhibit dominant responses so as to activate sub-dominant ones', and thus pertains to the ability to wilfully inhibit, activate, or change attention and behaviour. The capacity for effortful control has been linked with the modulation of emotional reactivity and behaviour in general [7], and has been identified more specifically as an important risk factor for eating disorders [50]. Associations between DEB and low effortful control have been consistently reported in both non-clinical [10] and clinical [11] samples.

Similarly, several studies have shown associations between DEB and impulsivity (e.g. [41]). Although clinically associated with the presence of binge eating, impulsivity and impulsive behaviour are not uncommon among other ED subtypes, including restricting anorexia nervosa [18], with impulsivity being more recently considered as a transdiagnostic characteristic of individuals with EDs [31]. Considering that impulsivity in EDs has also been associated with poorer prognosis [33], the importance of further investigating the role of impulsivity in the development and onset of DEB has recently been called upon.

Identity integration and sense of self

Identity consolidation is not only a crucial developmental milestone in youth, but also a salient challenge experienced by many patients with EDs [51]. The association between identity pathology and disordered eating has its roots in early psychodynamic thinking where EDs have traditionally been characterized as disorders of the self [8].

Bruch [9], among others, argued that identity impairment was the main predictor of EDs. Limited opportunities for autonomous functioning in childhood were posited to interfere with the development of a clear and coherent sense of self, which in turn contributed to feelings of incompetency, self-doubt and fear of losing control [8]. In concurrence with the corresponding feeling of powerlessness, an unstable sense of self is argued to lead to body weight and eating behaviours which are salient and more controllable [9]. Engagement in DEB would thus provide short-term relief from more pervasive and intolerable inner experiences.

Furthermore, Bruch [8] observed that patients with anorexia manifest difficulties in accurately perceiving or interpreting stimuli arising in their bodies, such as hunger and satiety, as well as often being unable to describe their emotions. She argued that one's lack of awareness of inner experiences and failure to rely on feelings, thoughts, and bodily sensations to guide behaviour, may contribute to an overwhelming sense of ineffectiveness and an overall lack of agency [8]. The DEBs that follow could therefore be understood as the patient's effort to compensate for these underlying deficits.

Consistent with the theory, several studies have investigated the association between dimensions of the self-concept (including global self-esteem, unclear sense of self, attitudes toward body image) and ED symptomatology. For example, individuals with bulimia were shown to have greater identity disturbance than controls as reflected through greater confusion, enmeshment and overall instability of sense of self [43]. These results were found to be consistent with the findings of Stein and Corte [48] who reported overall identity disturbances in women with AN and BN. More recently, similar difficulties with identity integration in a clinical sample of women with EDs were also associated with borderline personality symptomatology [51].

Identity consolidation as an indicator of personality functioning

Considering that identity disturbance is considered to be a core indicator of personality pathology as defined in the DSM-5's Alternative Model of Personality Disorders ([AMPD], [1]), the high prevalence and comorbidity of personality disorders in individuals with EDs should not come as a surprise (for a review see [34]). On the contrary, disturbance in personality functioning has been found to contribute to poor treatment outcome and to contribute to the persistence of ED symptomatology in some patients [16]. Nonetheless, although research has established a link between eating pathology and identity problems, and despite many suggesting that identity disturbance may contribute to ED development [54], few studies have empirically investigated the role of identity pathology as a potential pathway to DEB.

Present study

Since early DEBs such as dietary restraint, bingeing and purging are highly predictive of a later onset of EDs, it is imperative to investigate the contributing factors of these behaviours and their potential associations with other indicators of psychopathology. Known for its multifactorial origin, extensive research has been done on the etiology of DEB [39]. In particular, psychological factors involved in self-regulation – namely emotion regulation [32], effortful control [12] and impulsivity [31] – and impairments in identity and self-functioning [51] have consistently been associated with ED symptomatology. While extensive research has been done on the individual contributions of these variables, the existing study is the first to investigate the role of identity disturbance in explaining the relation between core deficits in self-regulation and DEBs. In addition, the current study also aimed to investigate impairments in personality functioning in individuals presenting with DEB. It was hypothesized that: 1) poor self-regulation, as defined by greater difficulties with emotion regulation, impulsivity and effortful control, would be associated with higher occurrences of DEB; 2) identity disturbance would mediate the relationship between self-regulation and DEB; and 3) individuals presenting with DEB would have greater impairments in personality functioning than those not engaging in disordered eating.

Methods

Participants and procedure

A total of 247 undergraduate psychology students from the University of Wollongong were initially recruited for this study, with 28 males (11.3%) and 218 females (88.7%). Considering the significantly uneven distribution and poor representation of males, only the female population was included in the final sample. Participants' age ranged from 18 to 25 years old (M = 19.39, SD = 1.70). Amongst these, 94 participants (43.1%) had a mental health diagnosis while nearly half of the total sample reported a mental health diagnosis in their immediate family members (107 participants; 49.1%). These mental health diagnoses included depressive disorders, anxiety disorders, eating disorders, bipolar I and II disorder, schizoaffective disorder, obsessive-compulsive disorder, post-traumatic stress disorder, and borderline personality disorder. Participation was voluntary and consent was obtained through the consent form after reviewing the study's information found in the participant information sheet. As we were interested in assessing DEB in youth, participants were required to be of age 18 to 25 years old and proficient in English. Upon giving their consent, participants completed the demographic information sheet before proceeding on to complete the self-report measures described below. Participants took on average about 20 min to complete the survey and were awarded 0.5 credit for research participation. Items within the survey were presented in random order and were not part of a larger survey battery.

Measures

Adult temperament questionnaire (ATQ)

The ATQ-short form [15] consists of a total of four scales, including Negative Affect, Extraversion/Surgency, Effortful Control and Orienting Sensitivity. Only the Effortful Control scale of the ATQ-short form was used in the present study. The scale comprises 19 items to be rated in a 7-point Likert scale (1 = *extremely untrue of you*; 7 = *extremely true of you*) and is divided into three subscales: inhibitory control (i.e. capacity to inhibit inappropriate behaviour; 7 items), attentional control (i.e. capacity to focus attention as well as to shift attention when desired; 5 items) and activation control (i.e. capacity to perform an action when there is a strong tendency to avoid it; 7 items). Internal consistency for the Effortful Control scales was adequate in the current study (α= .75).

Barratt impulsiveness scale-15 (BIS-15)

The BIS-15 [45] is a brief version of one of the most commonly used scales to assess impulsivity. Similar to its predecessor, the BIS-11 [37], this instrument assessed overall impulsivity across three domains: non-planning, motor, and attention impulsivity. Participants respond on a 4-point Likert scale. Within the current study, these three subscales indicated adequate reliabilities of α = .71, α = .79, and α = .74 respectively.

Severity indices of personality problems-118 (SIPP-118)

The SIPP-118 is a self-report questionnaire that assesses the core components of (mal) adaptive personality functioning. It contains 118 items that are answered on a 4-point Likert scale, and cover 5 domains including 16 facets of personality functioning. Only the Identity Integration domain and Emotional Regulation facet of the SIPP-118 were used in this study. The Emotional regulation facet measures the capacity for emotional tolerance and control, whereas the Identity Integration domain encompasses five facets reflecting an integrated sense of self, including: Self-respect, Stable self-image, Self-reflexive functioning, Enjoyment and Purposefulness. Both Identity Integration and Emotional regulation indicated adequate reliabilities of α = .94 and α = .74 respectively.

Levels of personality functioning scale-brief form 2.0 (LPFS-BF 2.0)

The LPFS-BF 2.0 [53] is a brief self-report questionnaire, which assesses the LPFS as described in Section III of the DSM-5 [1]. The LPFS-BF 2.0 consists of 12 items, clustered into two higher order domains: self-functioning and interpersonal functioning. Participants are asked to rate the 12 items on a 4-point Likert scale from 1 (completely untrue) to 4 (completely true). Both domains had satisfactory reliability in this study (Self-functioning α = .82; Interpersonal funtioning α = .74).

Eating disorder examination questionnaire 6.0 (EDE-Q 6.0)

The EDE-Q 6.0 was designed to assess the key behaviour-oriented aspects of eating disorders over the past 4 weeks (28 days) and consists of four main subscales (Restraint, Eating concern, Shape concern and Weight concern). Frequencies relating to DEB such as binging and purging were also assessed with items surrounding overeating and attempts at losing weight with extreme measures. Participants responded on a 7-point Likert scales that differed depending on the question (e.g. 1 'No days' to 7 'Every day'). All individual subscales had good to excellent reliabilities (α = .84 for restraint, α = .84 for eating concern, α = .92 for shape concern and α = .88 for weight concern). According to the DSM-5 [1], binge eating and inappropriate compensatory behaviours both occur, on average, at least once a week for 3 months for individuals diagnosed with Bulimia Nervosa. In order to distinguish individuals presenting with DEB from those without, the presence of DEB was defined as individuals with at least four occurrences of either binge eating or inappropriate compensatory behaviours or both over the last month.

Data analysis strategy

The Statistical Package for Social Sciences (SPSS Version 25.0; [26]) software and Amos [2] were used in the present study for all analyses including regression and structural equation modelling (SEM). A bivariate correlations analysis was conducted between effortful control, emotional regulation, impulsivity, identity integration, personality functioning, and DEB. Following that, the current study examined the mediating effect of identity integration and personality functioning in the relationship between self-regulation and DEB in two separate SEM analyses. Based on the recommendation by Shrout and Bolger [44], mediation was examined via bootstrapping, by estimating the confidence intervals of the indirect effects to test their significance. Finally, by using the six behavioural items of the EDE-Q, personality functioning scores of participants with presence of DEB was compared with those without.

Results

Preliminary analyses

Preliminary analyses were conducted to determine the confounding effects of age and previous history of mental health conditions on the variables of interest. No effects of age were found through correlational analysis. However, young women with a prior history of mental health conditions scored significantly higher on all variables of interest when compared with those without a previous history. As such, history of mental health conditions was controlled for.

Bivariate Pearson's correlation coefficients were calculated to test for the direction and strength of the linear relationships between all individual components of the main variables as shown in Table 1. Results showed DEB to significantly and positively correlate with effortful control, emotional regulation, identity integration, and personality functioning, but not impulsivity. Out of the four subscales of the EDE-Q, eating, shape, and weight concerns also correlated significantly with effortful control, emotional regulation, identity integration, and personality functioning. Notably, restrain correlated with only identity integration and personality functioning. Due to impulsivity's lack of significant associations with other variables, it was excluded from further analyses.

Structural equation modelling

SEM analyses were conducted to investigate the mediating effect of identity integration on the relationship between self-regulation and DEB as illustrated in Fig. 1. All analyses were done with 5000 bootstrapped samples with a 95% confidence interval for each indirect effect. We challenged the obtained results by running a second mediation model using personality functioning as the mediating variable. Results for both of these analyses are presented in Tables 2 and 3.

In the first mediation model, modelling prior mental health conditions as a confounding variable showed that it is not significantly related to both DEB and identity integration. Further results showed that self-regulation had significant indirect effects on DEB through identity integration (β = .555, p < .001 : CI = [1.563, 5.037]). Hence, results indicated a mediating effect of identity integration on the relationship between DEB and self-regulation as measured by both emotional regulation and effortful control. Furthermore, since the resulting direct effects between both components of self-regulation and DEB were significant, results suggest a partial mediating effect of identity integration. Per Kline [27] and Hooper et al. [25], the recommended cut-offs of

Table 1 Correlations between main variables

	1	2	3	4	5	6	7	8	9	10	11	12
1. Effortful Control-ATQ	–											
2. Emotional Regulation-SIPP	.407**	–										
3. Impulsivity-BIS-15	.400**	.348**	–									
4. Identity Integration-SIPP	.427**	.598**	.363**	–								
5. Personality Functioning-LPFS	.456**	.592**	.398**	.836**	–							
6. Restraint-EDE-Q 6.0	.100	.023	.106	.220**	.175*	–						
7. Eating Concerns-EDE-Q 6.0	.201*	.150*	.080	.471**	.354**	.639**	–					
9. Shape Concerns-EDE-Q 6.0	.150*	.164*	.111	.443**	.335**	.642**	.746**	–				
9. Weight Concerns-EDE-Q 6.0	.165*	.149*	.100	.423**	.317**	.642**	.732**	.939**	–			
10. Global Score-EDE-Q 6.0	.171*	.147*	.111	.448**	.339**	.775**	.856**	.963**	.951**	–		
11. Binging behaviours	.173*	.143*	.038	.264**	.230**	.273**	.477**	.388**	.362**	.419**	–	
12. Purging behaviours	.009	.018	−.001	.130	.134	.517**	.526**	.397**	.418**	.495**	.152*	–

N = 218

ATQ Adult Temperament Questionnaire, *SIPP* Severity Indices of Personality Problems-118, *BIS-15* Barratt Impulsiveness Scales-15, *LPFS* Levels of Personality Functioning Scale-Brief Form 2.0, *EDE-Q 6.0* Eating Disorder Examination-Questionnaire 6.0

* = p < .05, ** = p < .001

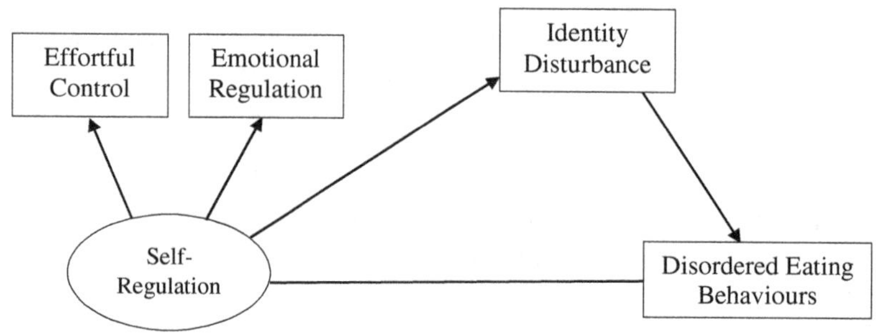

Fig. 1 Mediation model with main variables of interest. Note. Confounding variable (history of mental health) was not included in the figure

goodness of fit indices indicative of a good model fit are as follow: χ^2 $p > .05$, CFI > .90, CFI > .95, NFI > .95, RMSEA < .08, SRMR < .08. The goodness of fit indices ($\chi^2(2) = 2.816$, $p = .245$, CFI = .996, GFI = .995, NFI = .987, RMSEA = .043, SRMR = .024) suggest an excellent fit between the observed data and the current model.

When looking more broadly at personality functioning as the mediating variable, self-regulation was shown to have significant indirect effects on DEB through self-functioning ($\beta = .348$, $p < .001 : \text{CI} = [.671, 2.906]$). However, interpersonal functioning did not have any significant effect on DEB ($\beta = .076$, $p > .05$). Because the resulting direct effects between self-regulation and DEB were nonsignificant, results suggest a complete mediating effect (full mediation). Contrary to the first analysis, prior history of mental health conditions as a confounder had a significant relationship with DEB ($\beta = .149$, $p < .05$), but not with the other two mediators. Similar to the first model, fit indices suggested excellent fit: $\chi^2(4) = 4.010$, $p = .405$, CFI = .999, GFI = .994, NFI = .986, RMSEA = .003, SRMR = .019.

Independent samples *T*-test

Finally, independent samples *t*-tests were conducted to investigate whether young women presenting with DEB would have greater impairments in personality functioning compared to those not engaging in disordered eating (see Table 4). Results show that there were significant differences between the two groups on both self- and interpersonal-functioning scores. Specifically, young women who presented with DEB scored significantly higher on both self- ($t(216) = 3.464$, $p < .01$, $d = .474$) and interpersonal functioning ($t(216) = 2.924$, $p < .01$, $d = .397$) impairments than their counterparts, both with small to medium effect sizes.

Discussion

The present study aimed to investigate the shared contribution of difficulties in self-regulation and identity disturbance to DEB. More specifically, this study aimed to investigate the role of identity instability as a mediator of the relationship between effortful control, impulsivity, emotion regulation and DEB. Significant associations were found between all components of self-regulation and DEB, with the exception of impulsivity. Both identity instability and personality dysfunction were also associated with DEB. Binging behaviours more specifically were associated with effortful control deficits, emotional regulation difficulties, identity instability and personality dysfunction. Eating restraint was however only associated with identity instability and personality dysfunction. Moreover, findings suggest that the effect of both

Table 2 Path standardized coefficients and indirect effects for identity integration as mediator

	Path Coefficients		Estimate	Indirect Effects	
				95% Confidence Interval	
	to Identity Integration	to Disordered Eating Behaviours		Lower	Upper
Mental Health Hx	.038	.129			
Self-Regulation	.780***	−.374*			
Identity Integration		.711***			
SR → II → DEB			.555***	1.563	5.037

$N = 246$
Mental Health Hx Mental Health History, *SR* Self-Regulation, *II* Identity Integration, *DEB* Disordered Eating Behaviours
* = $p < .05$, *** = $p < .001$

Table 3 Path standardized coefficient and indirect effects for personality functioning as mediator

	Path Coefficient			Estimate	Indirect Effects	
					95% Confidence Interval	
	to Self-Functioning	to Interpersonal Functioning	to Disordered Eating Behaviour		Lower	Upper
Mental Health Hx	−.009	.013	.149*			
Self-Regulation	.772***	.703***	−.201			
Self-Functioning			.450**			
Interpersonal Functioning			.076			
SR → SF → DEB				.348***	.671	2.906
SR → IF → DEB				.053	−.315	.495

N = 246
Mental Health Hx Prior history of Mental Health Conditions, *SR* Self-Regulation, *SF* Self-Functioning, *IF* Interpersonal-Functioning, *DEB* Disordered Eating Behaviours
* = $p < .05$, ** = $p < .01$, *** = $p < .001$

emotion regulation and effortful control on DEB was non-significant once identity instability was introduced in the model, as it fully mediated the relationship between both variables and DEB.

The significant association between disordered eating and both poor effortful control and emotion regulation difficulties are consistent with results from previous studies that have highlighted the role of these variables in the manifestation of DEB (e.g. [30]). However, these associations were not as strong as those between DEB and difficulties in identity integration and personality functioning. In fact, our findings suggest that difficulties in both effortful control and emotion regulation only impact disordered eating through the effect of identity disturbance. These results were further supported when comparing participants who engaged in DEB with those who did not, with the former group displaying significantly more difficulties in both self and interpersonal domains of personality functioning. However, difficulties in interpersonal functioning were not significant predictors of DEB.

Most importantly, our findings suggest that behavioural eating anomalies may best be understood as epiphenomena secondary to a potentially deeper psychopathological core that reflects difficulties related to identity integration and personality functioning. This is in line with findings from Stanghellini et al. [46] who found that the central psychopathological features of shape and weight concerns in EDs are the result of a disturbance in the way these individuals experience their own body and difficulties in defining their identity. From a developmental perspective, the body plays an important role in the process of identity development and integration, and self-organization initially entails the integration of body-related experiences [49]. It is therefore not surprising that individuals with ED pathology have difficulty recognizing and making sense of internal bodily sensations as this reflects the basic form of self-awareness [47].

Although emotional regulation difficulties were included in our model as preceding identity integration, we acknowledge the bi-directional relationship between these two variables, and that both may reinforce each other through a vicious circle. For example, it is possible that difficulties with affect regulation may be secondary to unclear and unstable representations of self in individuals who engage in DEB, and that individuals who have difficulty making sense of their internal world may resort to behaviours like bingeing and purging to decrease the intensity of negative emotional states. As previously suggested, DEB can thus be understood as specific strategies of affect regulation [43], linked to an inability to contain, metabolize and mentalize affects. Likewise, as argued by many, DEB could also represent attempts to "take care of one's self, a search for a sense of subjectivity and interpersonal efficacy through the control of eating behaviours" ([21], p.53).

Table 4 Comparing individuals with and without presence of DEB on personality functioning

Variable	DEB Presence	*N*	*M*	*SD*	*t*	*P*	Cohen's D
Self-Functioning	Y	91	14.517	4.031	3.464	.001	.474
	N	127	12.638	3.889			
Interpersonal Functioning	Y	91	12.506	3.573	2.924	.004	.397
	N	127	11.181	3.087			

N = 218

Lastly, our findings related to the potential difficulties in personality functioning in young women who present with DEB echo the high resistance to treatment that has been reported in patients with EDs [17]. Indeed, research has shown that the treatment of EDs is often of modest effect and that significant difficulties persist after treatment [29]. More specifically, existing studies show that personality pathology is one of the most comorbid presentations in EDs [14]. As a recent meta-analysis of 87 studies has shown, more than half of ED patients have comorbid PD diagnoses [34]. Individuals with EDs also often present with ego-syntonic features and a chronic course of illness occurs in a considerable number of these individuals, as is the case in individuals with PDs [28]. It is therefore possible that variance in the onset, clinical course, symptomatic profile, and maintenance of ED symptomatology can be explained by underlying difficulties related to personality functioning and identity integration more specifically. The importance of considering personality functioning more broadly was also further supported by the significant differences observed between young women presenting with DEB and those without on the LPFS (despite interpersonal functioning not being a significant mediator in the tested models). Our findings thus support the argument that EDs should be considered as developmental disorders [17] and difficulties around identity integration and personality functioning as crucial issues involved in treatment resistance.

Our findings should however be interpreted in light of certain limitations. First, all analyses were cross-sectional and therefore, causal relationships cannot be directly inferred. Although the use of SEM has been found to have sound psychometric value in comparison to simple mediation analysis (see [6]), fitting the data does not "prove" the causal assumptions and a strong mediator in a cross-sectional analysis is not guaranteed to be a significant mediator in a longitudinal design [35]". Second, our sample consisted of self-selected, female psychology students and was relatively small. In addition, the racial breakdown of our participants was unknown. Although this proportion is to be expected considering that DEB and EDs are more prevalent in women [20], future studies that include a larger, male, and more age-diverse sample are needed to ensure generalizability of the results and assess the roles of ethnicity in these models. Lastly, the measures used in this study were exclusively self-reports. It would have been desirable to have access to structured clinical interview data, especially considering the ego-syntonic nature of these difficulties. Future studies should therefore look to replicate these findings in clinical populations using a longitudinal framework as well as investigate how some of the well-documented etiological factors (e.g. abuse and negative family experiences) may specifically relate to the development of identity disturbance and personality functioning in individuals with EDs.

Conclusion

Taken together, our results support early theoretical understandings [8] and extend findings from recent empirical work [51] that suggest that eating disorders are essentially disorders of the *self*. Unfortunately, in the current bio-psycho-social paradigm, the focus remains directed at external factors such as body mass index, food behaviors, or weight and shape comparisons. Our findings support previously suggested models (e.g. [17]) where the profound nature and meaning underlying the symptomatology of these disorders should be prioritized over the previously mentioned surface-level behaviours. It is possible that another reason for the limited effectiveness of treatment in these patients, is in fact the extensive focus on DEB rather than on the underlying issues that underpin these behaviours and the frequent secondary gain associated with disordered eating symptomatology. Moreover, our findings highlight the importance of assessing personality (dys) function and identity disturbance when working with individuals who engage in DEB, considering the clinical implications of personality-related difficulties (e.g. greater resistance, negative transference, tenuous therapeutic relationship). Although patients with EDs may present at times with symptomatology so severe that it becomes tempting to focus solely on the maladaptive eating, clinicians should not forget the interpersonal nature of these difficulties and that the core of the disorder may still lie in difficulties related to identity integration with different etiological factors potentially interfering with healthy personality development, especially in youth.

Abbreviations

APA: American Psychological Association; AN-BP: Anorexia Nervosa – Binge/Purge; AN-R: Anorexia Nervosa – Restricting; ATQ: Adult Temperament Questionnaire; BED: Binge-Eating Disorder; BIS: Barratt Impulsiveness Scale; BN: Bulimia Nervosa; CFI: Comparative Fit Index; DEB: Disordered Eating Behaviour(s); ED: Eating Disorder(s); EDE-Q: Eating Disorder Examination Questionnaire; GFI: Goodness of Fit Index; LPFS: Level of Personality Functioning Scale; NEDC: National Eating Disorders Collaboration; NFI: Normed Fit Index; RMSEA: Root Mean Square Error of Approximation; SEM: Structural Equation Modelling; SIPP: Severity Indices of Personality Problems

Authors' contributions

MB was responsible for the conceptualization and rewriting of the manuscript for publication. JoT was responsible for collecting the data and running the initial analyses. JuT was responsible for running the analyses and contributed to the writing. The author(s) read and approved the final manuscript.

Competing interests

The authors declare that they have no competing interests.

References

1. American Psychiatric Association. Diagnostic and statistical manual of mental disorders. 5th ed. Arlington: American Psychiatric Publishing; 2013. https://doi.org/10.1176/appi.books.9780890425596
2. Arbuckle JL. Amos (version 24.0) [computer program]. Chicago: IBM SPSS; 2014.
3. Arcelus J, Mitchell AJ, Wales J, Nielsen S. Mortality rates in patients with anorexia nervosa and other eating disorders: a meta-analysis of 36 studies. Arch Gen Psychiatry. 2011;68(7):724–31 https://doi.org/10.1001/archgenpsychiatry.2011.74.
4. Baumeister RF, Heatherton TF. Self-regulation failure: An overview. Psychol Inq. 1996;7(1):1–15.
5. Bénard M, Bellisle F, Kesse-Guyot E, Julia C, Andreeva V, Etilé F, et al. Impulsivity is associated with food intake, snacking, and eating disorders in a general population. Am J Clin Nutr. 2018;109:117–26.
6. Bollen KA, Pearl J. Eight myths about causality and structural equation models. In: Handbook of causal analysis for social research. Dordrecht: Springer; 2013. p. 301–28.
7. Bridgett DJ, Oddi KB, Laake LM, Murdock KW, Bachmann MN. Integrating and differentiating aspects of self-regulation: effortful control, executive functioning, and links to negative affectivity. Emotion. 2013;13(1):47–63 https://doi.org/10.1037/a0029536.
8. Bruch H. Eating disorders. Eating disorders: Obesity, anorexia nervosa, and the person within. New York: Basic Books; 1973.
9. Bruch H. Developmental considerations of anorexia nervosa and obesity. Can J Psychiatr. 1981;26(4):212–7 https://doi.org/10.1177/070674378102600402.
10. Claes L, Bijttebier P, Mitchell JE, de Zwaan M, Mueller A. The relationship between compulsive buying, eating disorder symptoms, and temperament in a sample of female students. Compr Psychiatry. 2011;52(1):50–5 https://doi.org/10.1016/j.comppsych.2010.05.003.
11. Claes L, Müller A, Norré J, Van Assche L, Wonderlich S, Mitchell JE. The relationship among compulsive buying, compulsive internet use and temperament in a sample of female patients with eating disorders. Eur Eat Disord Rev. 2012;20(2):126–31 https://doi.org/10.1002/erv.1136.
12. Claes L, Robinson MD, Muehlenkamp JJ, Vandereycken W, Bijttebier P. Differentiating bingeing/purging and restrictive eating disorder subtypes: the roles of temperament, effortful control, and cognitive control. Personal Individ Differ. 2010;48(2):166–70 https://doi.org/10.1016/j.paid.2009.09.016.
13. Culbert KM, Racine SE, Klump KL. Research Review: What we have learned about the causes of eating disorders–a synthesis of sociocultural, psychological, and biological research. J Child Psychol Psychiatry. 2015; 56(11):1141–64.
14. De Bolle M, De Clercq B, Pham-Scottez A, Mels S, Rolland JP, Guelfi JD, et al. Personality pathology comorbidity in adult females with eating disorders. J Health Psychol. 2011;16(2):303–13 https://doi.org/10.1177/1359105310374780.
15. Evans DE, Rothbart MK. Developing a model for adult temperament. J Res Pers. 2007;41(4):868–88 https://doi.org/10.1016/j.jrp.2006.11.002.
16. Farstad SM, McGeown LM, von Ranson KM. Eating disorders and personality, 2004–2016: a systematic review and meta-analysis. Clin Psychol Rev. 2016; 46:91–105 https://doi.org/10.1016/j.cpr.2016.04.005.
17. Fassino S, Abbate-Daga G. Resistance to treatment in eating disorders: a critical challenge. BMC Psychiatry. 2013;13(1):282–5 https://doi.org/10.1186/1471-244X-13-282.
18. Favaro A, Santonastaso P. Self-injurious behavior in anorexia nervosa. J Nerv Ment Dis. 2000;188(8):537–42 https://doi.org/10.1097/00005053-200008000-00010.
19. Fischer S, Munsch S. Self-regulation in eating disorders and obesity–implications for treatment. Verhaltenstherapie. 2012;22(3):158–64 https://doi.org/10.1159/000341540.
20. Galmiche M, Déchelotte P, Lambert G, Tavolacci MP. Prevalence of eating disorders over the 2000–2018 period: a systematic literature review. Am J Clin Nutr. 2019;109(5):1402–13 https://doi.org/10.1093/ajcn/nqy342.
21. Granieri A, Schimmenti A. Mind–body splitting and eating disorders: a psychoanalytic perspective. Psychoanal Psychother. 2014;28(1):52–70 https://doi.org/10.1080/02668734.2013.872172.
22. Hawkins RC, Clement PF. Binge eating: measurement problems and a conceptual model. In: The binge purge syndrome: diagnosis, treatment, and research; 1984. p. 229–51.
23. Heatherton TF, Baumeister RF. Binge eating as escape from self-awareness. Psychol Bull. 1991;110(1):86–108 https://doi.org/10.1037/0033-2909.110.1.86.
24. Herpertz-Dahlmann B. Adolescent eating disorders. Child Adolesc Psychiatr Clin N Am. 2014;24:177–96.
25. Hooper D, Coughlan J, Mullen M. Structural equation modelling: guidelines for determining model fit. Electron J Bus Res Methods. 2008;6:53–60.
26. IBM Corp. IBM SPSS statistics for windows, version 25.0. Armonk: IBM Corp; 2017.
27. Kline RB. Principles and practice of structural equation modelling. 3rd ed. New-York: Guilford Publications; 2011.
28. Klump KL, Bulik CM, Kaye WH, Treasure J, Tyson E. Academy for eating disorders position paper: eating disorders are serious mental illnesses. Int J Eat Disord. 2009;42(2):97–103 https://doi.org/10.1002/eat.20589.
29. Kotilahti E, West M, Isomaa R, Karhunen L, Rocks T, Ruusunen A. Treatment interventions for severe and enduring eating disorders: systematic review. Int J Eat Disord. 2020;53(8):1280–302 https://doi.org/10.1002/eat.23322.
30. Leehr EJ, Krohmer K, Schag K, Dresler T, Zipfel S, Giel KE. Emotion regulation model in binge eating disorder and obesity-a systematic review. Neurosci Biobehav Rev. 2015;49:125–34 https://doi.org/10.1016/j.neubiorev.2014.12.008.
31. Mallorquí-Bagué N, Testa G, Lozano-Madrid M, Vintró-Alcaraz C, Sánchez I, Riesco N, et al. Emotional and non-emotional facets of impulsivity in eating disorders: from anorexia nervosa to bulimic spectrum disorders. Eur Eat Disord Rev. 2020;28(4):410–22 https://doi.org/10.1002/erv.2734.
32. Mallorquí-Bagué N, Vintró-Alcaraz C, Sánchez I, Riesco N, Agüera Z, Granero R, et al. Emotion regulation as a transdiagnostic feature among eating disorders: cross-sectional and longitudinal approach. Eur Eat Disord Rev. 2018;26(1):53–61 https://doi.org/10.1002/erv.2570.
33. Manasse SM, Goldstein SP, Wyckoff E, Forman EM, Juarascio AS, Butryn ML, et al. Slowing down and taking a second look: inhibitory deficits associated with binge eating are not food-specific. Appetite. 2016;96:555–9 https://doi.org/10.1016/j.appet.2015.10.025.
34. Martinussen M, Friborg O, Schmierer P, Kaiser S, Øvergård KT, Neunhoeffer AL, et al. The comorbidity of personality disorders in eating disorders: a meta-analysis. Eat Weight Disord. 2017;22(2):201–9 https://doi.org/10.1007/s40519-016-0345-x.
35. Maxwell SE, Cole DA. Bias in cross-sectional analyses of longitudinal mediation. Psychol Methods. 2007;12(1):23.
36. National Eating Disorder Collaboration. Eating Disorders - A Current Affair. An Introduction. An Integrated Response to Complexity: National Eating Disorders Framework 2012; 2012. Retrieved from: https://nedc.com.ou/ossets/NEDC-Publicotions/Appendix-Eoting-Disorders-A-Current-Affair.pdf
37. Patton JH, Stanford MS, Barratt ES. Factor structure of the Barratt impulsiveness scale. J Clin Psychol. 1995;51(6):768–74.
38. Prefit AB, Cândea DM, Szentagotai-Tătar A. Emotion regulation across eating pathology: a meta-analysis. Appetite. 2019;143:104438.
39. Rosen D. Eating disorders in children snd Young Adolscents: etiology, classification, clinical features, and treatment. Adolesc Med. 2003;14(1):49–59.
40. Rothbart MK, Bates JE. Temperament. In: Damon W, Lerner RM, editors. Handbook of child psychology, N. Eisenberg (Vol. Ed.), Social, emotional, and personality development. New York: Wiley; 2006. p. 99–166.
41. Schag K, Schönleber J, Teufel M, Zipfel S, Giel KE. Food-related impulsivity in obesity and binge eating disorder–a systematic review. Obes Rev. 2013; 14(6):477–95 https://doi.org/10.1111/obr.12017.
42. Schmidt U, Adan R, Böhm I, Campbell IC, Dingemans A, Ehrlich S, et al. Eating disorders: the big issue. Lancet Psychiatry. 2016;3(4):313–5 https://doi.org/10.1016/S2215-0366(16)00081-X.
43. Schupak-Neuberg E, Nemeroff C. Disturbances in identity and self-regulation in bulimia nervosa: implications for a metaphorical perspective of "body as self". Int J Eat Disord. 1993;13(4):335–47 https://doi.org/10.1002/1098-108X(199305)13:4<335::AID-EAT2260130402>3.0.CO;2-M.
44. Shrout PE, Bolger N. Mediation in experimental and nonexperimental studies: new procedures and recommendations. Psychol Methods. 2002;7(4): 422–45 https://doi.org/10.1037/1082-989X.7.4.422.
45. Spinella M. Normative data and a short form of the Barratt Impulsiveness Scale. Int J Neurosci. 2007;117(3):359–68 https://doi.org/10.1080/00207450600588881.
46. Stanghellini G, Castellini G, Brogna P, Faravelli C, Ricca V. Identity and eating disorders (IDEA): a questionnaire evaluating identity and embodiment in eating disorder patients. Psychopathology. 2012;45(3):147–58 https://doi.org/10.1159/000330258.

47. Stanghellini G, Trisolini F, Castellini G, Ambrosini A, Faravelli C, Ricca V. Is feeling extraneous from one's own body a core vulnerability feature in eating disorders? Psychopathology. 2015;48(1):18–24 https://doi.org/10.1159/000364882.
48. Stein KF, Corte C. Identity impairment and the eating disorders: content and organization of the self-concept in women with anorexia nervosa and bulimia nervosa. Eur Eat Disord Rev. 2007;15(1):58–69 https://doi.org/10.1002/erv.726.
49. Stern DN. Interpersonal world of the infant: a view from psychoanalysis and developmental psychology. New-York: Basic Books; 1985.
50. Verschueren M, Claes L, Palmeroni N, Bogaerts A, Gandhi A, Moons P, et al. Eating disorder symptomatology in adolescent boys and girls: identifying distinct developmental trajectory classes. J Youth Adolesc. 2020;49(2):410–26 https://doi.org/10.1007/s10964-019-01174-0.
51. Verschueren M, Luyckx K, Kaufman EA, Vansteenkiste M, Moons P, Sleuwaegen E, et al. Identity processes and statuses in patients with and without eating disorders. Eur Eat Disord Rev. 2017;25(1):26–35 https://doi.org/10.1002/erv.2487.
52. Waxman SE. A systematic review of impulsivity in eating disorders. Eur Eat Disord Rev. 2009;17(6):408–25 https://doi.org/10.1002/erv.952.
53. Weekers LC, Hutsebaut J, Kamphuis JH. The level of personality functioning scale-brief form 2.0: update of a brief instrument for assessing level of personality functioning. Personal Ment Health. 2019;13(1):3–14 https://doi.org/10.1002/pmh.1434.
54. Wheeler HA, Wintre MG, Polivy J. The association of low parent-adolescent reciprocity, a sense of incompetence, and identity confusion with disordered eating. J Adolesc Res. 2003;18(4):405–29 https://doi.org/10.1177/0743558403018004005.

19

Overcontrolled, undercontrolled and resilient personality styles among patients with eating disorders

Martina Isaksson[1*], Ata Ghaderi[2,3], Martina Wolf-Arehult[1,4] and Mia Ramklint[1]

Abstract

Background: Personality has been suggested to be an important factor in understanding onset, maintenance, and recovery from eating disorders (ED). The objective of the current study was to evaluate personality style in different ED diagnostic groups as classified in the Diagnostic and Statistical Manual of Mental Disorders, Fifth edition (DSM-5).

Methods: The overcontrolled, undercontrolled, and resilient personality styles were compared in four groups of patients with EDs: anorexia nervosa restricting (ANr) ($n = 34$), anorexia nervosa binge eating/purging (ANbp) ($n = 31$), atypical anorexia nervosa (AAN) ($n = 29$), and bulimia nervosa (BN) ($n = 76$). These groups were compared with a group of patients with borderline personality disorder (BPD) ($n = 108$), and a non-clinical group (NC) ($n = 444$). Patient data were collected at two outpatient clinics in Uppsala, Sweden. NC control data were collected through convenience sampling. Participants filled out questionnaires assessing personality style.

Results: The main findings were more pronounced overcontrol reported by the ANr and AAN groups compared with the BN, BPD, and NC groups, and no significant difference in resilience between the ED and the NC groups. Considerable variability of over- and undercontrol was also found within each group.

Conclusions: The results replicate previous findings when EDs are classified according to current diagnostic criteria (DSM-5). Taking personality styles into account may improve our understanding of certain characteristics in EDs, such as social deficits and rigidity that are attributed to poor treatment outcome.

Keywords: Eating disorders, Anorexia, Bulimia, Overcontrol, Undercontrol, Resilience

Plain English summary

To increase our understanding of eating disorders (ED), we need to know more about risk factors for developing as well as maintaining EDs. In this study, we evaluated if overcontrol (characterized by rigidity, perfectionism, and inhibition of feelings), is more common in certain eating disorder difficulties compared to undercontrol (characterized by impulsivity and immediate expression of feelings). We also evaluated if the groups differed when contrasted to a group in the community and to patients with borderline personality disorder (BPD; characterized by excessive undercontrol). Finally, we evaluated if resilience, such as being able to flexibly adapt to changing demands in the environment, differed between those with EDs and the community group. Our results showed that restricting and atypical anorexia nervosa had the highest levels of overcontrol, that BPD had the highest level of undercontrol, and that bulimia and the community sample were in between. Further, there were no differences in resilience between the ED group and the community sample. Our findings may help us understand more about factors that are contributing to poor treatment

* Correspondence: martina.isaksson@neuro.uu.se
[1]Department of Neuroscience, Psychiatry, Uppsala University, Entrance 10, Floor 3B, SE-751 85 Uppsala, Sweden
Full list of author information is available at the end of the article

outcome in anorexia, such as rigidity and social difficulties.

Introduction

Researchers studying the etiology of eating disorders (ED) have suggested that personality is an important factor in the understanding of EDs, likely to affect how symptoms are exhibited and maintained [1, 2]. Knowledge of personality characteristics contributes to better prediction of level of functioning, clinical course, and treatment outcome – beyond specific ED diagnoses [1, 3, 4].

Several studies have identified three personality subtypes in the ED field [3–6]: one constricted overcontrolled, one emotionally dysregulated undercontrolled, and one high-functioning perfectionistic. Most commonly, personality constructs related to overcontrol or high self-control such as introversion and constraint have been related to anorexia nervosa (AN) and restricting ED subtypes, whereas personality constructs related to undercontrol and low self-control such as impulsiveness have been related to bulimia nervosa (BN) or binge eating/purging ED subtypes [1, 5, 7]. The high-functioning subtype has been found to be more diverse, yet somewhat overrepresented in BN [4]. In a recent, systematic, review by Farstad and von Ranson [1], it was highlighted that almost all research on personality in EDs had been done based on outdated diagnostic criteria from DSM-IV. Also, findings on distinctions between different ED groups have been limited [1], and some have not been able to replicate e.g., overcontrolled and high-functioning personality subgroups in AN [1, 8]. Further, when studying personality constructs in the ED group, subthreshold diagnoses such as atypical AN (AAN; i.e., patients with significant weight loss, but whose weight is still within or above normal range), have rarely been included [1]. Thus, the field is in need of further evaluation and replication.

A personality theory with specific emphasis on emotional control, first developed by Block and Block [9], have identified three recurrent personality styles in different populations [10–12]: the overcontrolled (characterized by high self-control, inhibitory control, and persistence, and low impulsiveness and emotional expression), the undercontrolled (characterized by high levels of impulsivity and emotional expression, with low levels of self-control and inhibition), and the resilient (characterized by an ability to modify the level of control to ever changing demands in the environment) [9, 12–14]. These styles resembles the personality constructs previously identified among EDs, but differs e.g., in terms of the definition of high functioning versus resilience. To our knowledge, the occurrence of resilience in ED groups has only been evaluated by Tsigkaropoulou and colleagues [15]. They found significant differences in resilience between a non-clinical (NC) group and the ED group, but not between ED subgroups.

In sum, identification of personality subtypes has shown clinical utility in predicting e.g., treatment outcome [3], and it has been suggested that identification of personality may be one way to individualize the interventions to improve treatment effectiveness [2]. However, knowing what differs and what is shared between diagnoses, might also facilitate the possibility of adapting the treatments on a group level, to better fit the more common personality style identified in each group.

The aim of the current study was to investigate personality style in restricting AN (ANr), binge eating/purging AN (ANbp), AAN, and BN, classified according to DSM-5. These were to be compared with a group with borderline personality disorder (BPD), expected to be undercontrolled, and a NC group, expected to be high in resilience and intermediate in over–/undercontrol. Replicating findings of personality styles in different ED according to current diagnostic criteria is important, especially as the current classification is more inclusive, which may reduce the somewhat limited distinctions in personality that has previously been identified across diagnoses [1]. Also, including the AAN group provides information about an ED group that is commonly left out [1]. Moreover, by contrasting the ED groups to a NC group and a relevant clinical group (i.e., BPD), the specific characteristics of the ED group in terms of personality will be easier to contextualize. In the current study, we hypothesized: 1) A difference in over- and undercontrol between ED groups, with higher levels of overcontrol in the ANr compared to the BN group, 2) higher levels of overcontrol in the ANr group in comparison with the NC and BPD group, and 3) lower levels of resilience in the ED groups when compared with the NC group.

Materials and methods

Procedure

Data were collected at two outpatient clinics, the ED clinic and the BPD clinic, at Uppsala University Hospital. ED patients were recruited between October 2014 and December 2019. The ED clinic treats patients with AN, atypical AN, moderate and severe BN, and other EDs in cases with complex comorbidity or suicidality. Patients with binge eating disorder (BED) and obesity are referred to the obesity unit at the medical clinic, whereas less severe EDs such as subclinical BN are referred to primary care or private practices, and could therefore not be included in the study.

Patients underwent a diagnostic evaluation, including the semi-structured Eating Disorder Examination interview (EDE) [16]. Fifteen psychologists were trained in performing the interview by an expert and co-rated six filmed interviews performed by the expert. All assessors showed complete agreement in all ratings with a prevalence and bias adjusted kappa (PABAK) [17] of 1.0. Diagnoses were initially based on the Diagnostic and Statistical Manual of Mental Disorders 4th ed., Text Revision (DSM-IV-TR) [18], but later recoded based on the DSM-5. Hence, patients not diagnosed with AN under DSM-IV-TR, due to higher weight (17.5 kg/m^2 < BMI < 18.5 kg/m^2) and no amenorrhea, were included in AN. Patients fulfilling all criteria from AN except having weight within or above normal, i.e. BMI ≥ 18.5, but with significant weight loss, were included in AAN. Those with a lower frequency of binge eating and compensation (both at least once per week, in contrast to twice per week in previous versions) were included in BN. If a patient was not weighed at the clinic, an approximation of the weight was estimated to enable accurate diagnostics; this was done in one case.

EDs were grouped so that patients diagnosed with AN *without* episodes of binge eating or purging were included in the ANr group, patients diagnosed with AN *with* episodes of binge eating or purging in the ANbp group, patients diagnosed with AAN in the AAN group, and patients diagnosed with BN in the BN group.

Patients with BPD were recruited at the BPD clinic between October 2014 and November 2017. Diagnosis was based on the Structured Clinical Interview for DSM-IV Axis II Personality Disorders, general and borderline criteria (SCID-II) [19], performed by psychologists. All psychologists were trained by an expert in performing the interview, with co-ratings showing a kappa (PABAK) ranging from .6–1.0 between assessors. No recoding was necessary for the BPD group, as diagnostic criteria are the same in both DSM versions.

Patients were informed about the study through verbal and written information at their first meeting during the psychological assessment phase. Participants signed an informed consent and filled out the questionnaires. Weight and height were measured at the clinic.

The NC sample was recruited between October 2014 and June 2016 through information in classes at Uppsala University and advertisement on the web and in social media. Interested participants received more information and a link to the questionnaires online. Participants received two scratch cards or one movie ticket, or could donate the corresponding amount to a charity of their choice.

Participants

In total, 170 ED patients (ANr: $n = 34$, ANbp: $n = 31$, AAN = 29, BN: $n = 76$), 108 BPD patients, and 444 NC individuals participated in the study. Inclusion criterion for the NC sample was minimum age of 18 years. For the clinical sample, inclusion was restricted to patients represented at the ED and BPD clinics. Inclusion criteria for patients were 1) minimum age 18 years, and 2) being diagnosed with AN, AAN, BN, or BPD. Excluded were patients 1) already participating in the study at a prior referral, 2) too ill to participate, 3) with insufficient cognitive abilities or knowledge in Swedish 4) with BED ($n = 8$), and 5) with other EDs ($n = 55$), e.g., BN with lower frequency or unspecified feeding or eating disorder. Because all ED patients were 50 years or younger, all participants over 50 years of age ($n = 31$) were excluded from the NC and BPD comparison groups. Subjects not defining an education level ($n = 8$) or not defining gender ($n = 4$) were also excluded from the comparison groups. Recruitment and demographic characteristics are presented in Fig. 1 and Table 1.

The instruments

The Ego Undercontrol-13 and Ego resilience scales

The Ego Undercontrol (EUC) scale is originally a 37-item self-report questionnaire [9] designed to assess over- and undercontrolled personality styles. Since the original scale has shown insufficient psychometric properties, a short version (the EUC-13) was developed and evaluated in a Swedish study, showing improved psychometrics [20]. The short version had not been developed at the beginning of the study. Therefore, items from the EUC-13 were extracted and a sum was calculated for the EUC-13 for subjects who completed the original EUC. The Ego Resilience (ER) scale is a 14-item questionnaire [9, 21] designed to assess the ability to adapt the level of control based on the circumstances.

Both scales have shown acceptable to high internal consistency (EUC-13: $\alpha = .71$; ER: $\alpha = .84$) and test-retest reliability (EUC-13: $r = .86$, $p < .001$; ER $r = .85$, $p < .001$), and acceptable factor structure and validity [20]. Items are reported on a four-point Likert scale ranging from "Disagree very strongly" (1) to "Agree very strongly" (4). For the EUC-13, low scores indicate high levels of overcontrol, and high scores indicate high levels of undercontrol. High scores on the ER indicate high adaptive control. In the present study, internal consistency was .75 for the EUC-13 and .81 for the ER.

Data analysis

Power analyses were performed to estimate a desired sample size. To detect small changes, the recommended number of participants in each group were estimated at $n = 35$ (given an eta effect size of $\eta^2 = .25$, power = .80, $\alpha = .05$). However, because of the low prevalence of AN, and because the AN group was divided in to three separate groups, we needed to consider limitations in achieving large samples. Thus, sample size was a bit smaller for some groups, which may imply that it was not possible detect small differences in terms of significance.

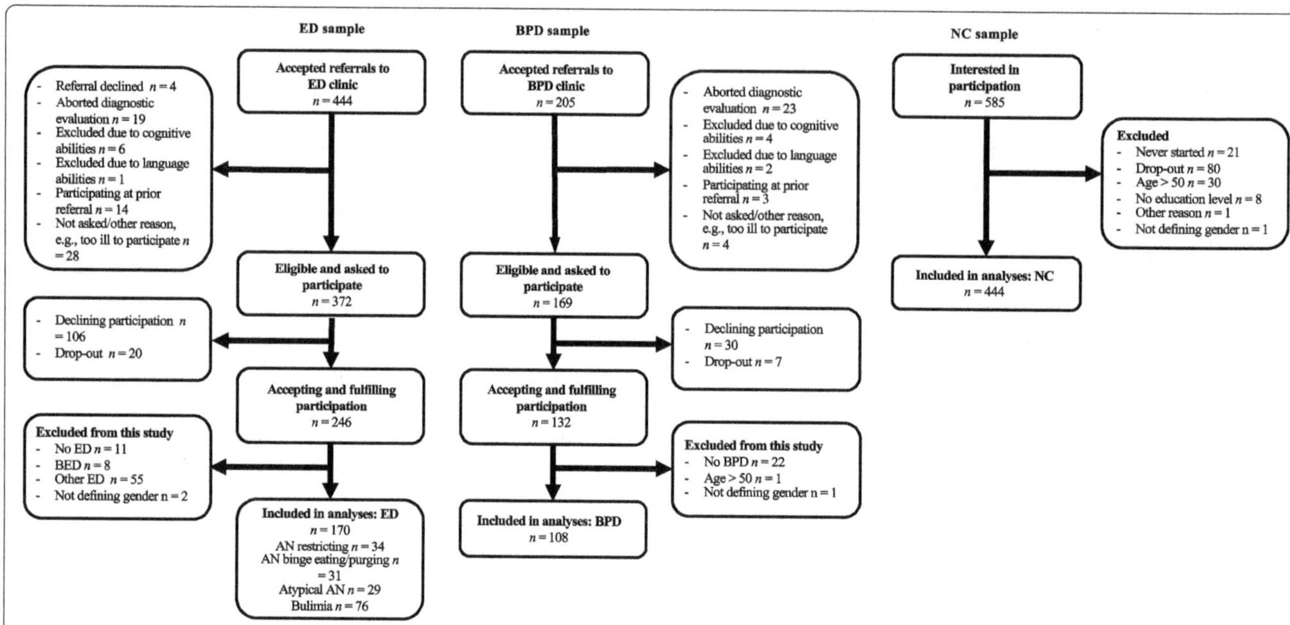

Fig. 1 Flowchart of participant recruitment

Moderate to large differences could, however, be detected, and measures of effect are presented to enable interpretation of group differences beyond the issue of significance.

Normal distribution was checked with skewness ratio (skewness/SE (skewness)). All measures were below the recommended value of 2.0, supporting the use of linear models. Missing values were rare (< 0.1% of participants), and were imputed with the mean of that subscale. In case of more than one missing value per subscale or two missing for the whole scale, that person was omitted from the analysis. Group differences of overcontrol and resilience were analyzed using a generalized linear model (GZLM). A GLZM is preferred to a general linear model (GLM, e.g., ANOVA) when group sizes are unequal, as it allows specification of a model in which the outcome variable follows different kinds of distributions. We applied two separate crude analyses in the GLZM with the diagnostic group as the independent variable. Overcontrol/undercontrol (measured with the EUC-13) was used as the dependent variable in one analysis and resilience (measured with the ER) in the other. Next, we performed adjusted analyses to see if results were stable when adding gender, age, marital status, and level of education as covariates to the model. Both crude and adjusted results are presented in Table 2. Due to multiple comparisons, we used the Bonferroni post hoc test to adjust the significance level. Because only small differences were seen when adjusting for covariates, crude results were used for all succeeding analyses. To test if the extraction of items from EUC 37 affected the outcome, we performed additional analyses when groups were separated based on what version of the EUC they conducted (the EUC 37 or the EUC-13). No significant differences were identified. Effect sizes were estimated with Cohen's d, with SD derived from the standard error and pooled to correct for differences in sample size. To illustrate the spread of over- and undercontrol, group medians with dispersion were visualized for the EUC-13 and the ER (Fig. 2). Analyses were performed using IBM SPSS Statistics version 25 and R version 3.5.1.

Results

Group differences in personality style

Distribution and dispersion are presented in Fig. 2; unadjusted and adjusted group means with standard errors are presented in Table 2. All significant effects in the crude model were stable when adjusted for relevant covariates.

Measures of effect in personality style

Investigation of the differences in over- and undercontrol between ED groups showed that the ANr reported higher levels of overcontrol than the BN ($d = 0.75$), as hypothesized. The AAN also reported higher levels of overcontrol than the BN ($d = 0.74$). No other differences were identified between the ED groups in terms of overcontrol. Further, the magnitudes of effects were generally small to moderate, as reflected in the corresponding effect sizes: ANr vs. ANbp ($d = 0.19$), ANr vs. AAN ($d = 0.00$), ANbp vs. AAN ($d = 0.18$), or ANbp vs. BN ($d = 0.56$).

When over- and undercontrol was contrasted to the comparison groups, the ANr group reported significantly higher levels of overcontrol than the BPD group ($d =$

Table 1 Demographic characteristics of study participants

	ANr (n = 34)	ANbp (n = 31)	AAN (n = 29)	BN (n = 76)	BPD (n = 108)	NC (n = 444)
Mean age (SD)	24.2 (5.1)	24.5 (6.8)	22.7 (3.7)	27.3 (7.8)	26.5 (6.4)	28.7 (8.2)
Mean BMI (SD)[a]	16.7 (1.2)	17.3 (1.0)	20.0 (1.8)	24.7 (4.7)	–	–
Gender						
Female	31 (91.2%)	30 (96.8%)	27 (93.1%)	74 (97.4%)	96 (88.9%)	340 (76.6%)
Male	3 (8.8%)	1 (3.2%)	2 (6.9%)	2 (2.6%)	12 (11.1%)	104 (23.4%)
Marital status[b]						
Married or in relationship	7 (21.2%)	9 (30.0%)	12 (41.4%)	26 (34.2%)	56 (51.9%)	270 (60.8%)
Single	24 (72.7%)	19 (63.3%)	16 (55.2%)	46 (60.5%)	51 (47.2%)	163 (36.7%)
Other (e.g., living with parents)	2 (6.1%)	2 (6.7%)	1 (3.4%)	4 (5.3%)	1 (0.9%)	11 (2.5%)
Highest level of education						
Elementary school	5 (15.2%)	7 (22.6%)	4 (13.8%)	9 (11.8%)	16 (14.8%)	14 (3.2%)
High school	17 (51.5%)	14 (45.2%)	14 (48.3%)	36 (47.4%)	68 (63.0%)	152 (34.2%)
Higher education	11 (33.3%)	10 (32.3%)	11 (37.9%)	31 (40.8%)	24 (22.2%)	278 (62.6%)
Main occupation[c]						
Paid work	8 (25.0%)	9 (29.0%)	7 (25.0%)	33 (44.0%)	36 (33.6%)	189 (42.6%)
Student	16 (50.0%)	17 (54.8%)	11 (39.3%)	27 (36.0%)	21 (19.6%)	197 (44.4%)
Unemployed	2 (6.3%)	0 (0.0%)	2 (7.1%)	0 (0.0%)	6 (5.6%)	20 (4.5%)
Sick leave	5 (15.6%)	4 (12.9%)	8 (28.6%)	14 (18.7%)	41 (38.3%)	17 (3.8%)
Other (e.g., housewife, internship, parental leave)	1 (3.1%)	1 (3.2%)	0 (0.0%)	1 (1.3%)	3 (2.8%)	21 (4.7%)

ANr Anorexia nervosa restricting, *ANbp* Anorexia nervosa binge eating/purging, *AAN* atypical anorexia nervosa, *BPD* borderline personality disorder, *NC* non-clinical
[a]One patient with AAN was missing BMI
[b]one patient with ANr and one with ANbp were missing marital status
[c] two patients with ANr, one with AAN, one with BN, and one with BPD were missing main occupation

1.40) and the NC group ($d = 0.78$), as hypothesized. All other ED groups also showed higher levels of overcontrol when compared with the BPD groups: BPD vs. ANbp ($d = 1.20$), BPD vs. AAN ($d = 1.39$), and BPD vs. BN ($d = 0.63$). The AAN group showed significantly higher levels of overcontrol than the NC group ($d =$ 0.78), while the differences between the NC group and the other ED groups were non-significant: NC vs. ANbp ($d = 0.56$), NC vs. BN ($d = 0.11$).

In contrast to our hypotheses, there were no significant differences between the NC group and any of the ED groups regarding resilience: ANr vs. NC ($d = 0.30$); ANbp vs. NC ($d = 0.42$), AAN vs. NC ($d = 0.33$), and BN vs. NC ($d = 0.25$).

Discussion

The main findings were a higher level of overcontrol in the ANr and ANN groups compared with the BN, BPD, and NC groups, with medium to large effect sizes. The ANr and AAN groups showed the highest levels of overcontrol, the BPD group showed the highest level of undercontrol, and the BN and NC groups were at the same intermediate level. No significant difference in overcontrol was found when comparing the ANbp group with other ED groups or the NC group. This was, however, probably an effect of the relatively small n in the ANbp group, and effect sized provides information of at least small differences between both the ANbp and the BN, and the ANbp and the NC groups – with higher overcontrol in ANbp. Lastly, there were no significant group differences of resilience between the ED and the NC groups.

Our results add strength to the previously identified patterns of over- and undercontrolled personality styles [13, 22], supporting their occurrence in different EDs [3–6, 23]. As we included a BPD comparison group, we were able to conclude that the pattern displayed by the BN group more closely resembled that of the BPD undercontrolled group than did the patterns of any of the other ED groups assessed in the study. An interesting finding, adding information to this field of research, is that the AAN group showed large similarities to the ANr group with regard to levels of overcontrol.

Resilience has previously been associated with well-being and functional control, which is often seen in NC

Table 2 Differences between eating disorder and comparison groups on overcontrol/undercontrol and resilience

		ANr (*n* = 34) Mean (SE)	ANbp (*n* = 31) Mean (SE)	AAN (*n* = 29) Mean (SE)	BN (*n* = 76) Mean (SE)	BPD (*n* = 108) Mean (SE)	NC (*n* = 444) Mean (SE)	Bonferroni post hoc
EUC-13	Crude	2.05 (0.08)	2.14 (0.09)	2.05 (0.09)	2.43 (0.06)	2.76 (0.05)	2.38 (0.02)	ANr < BN**, ANr < BPD***, ANr < NC** ANbp < BPD*** AAN < BN**, AAN < BPD***, AAN < NC**, BN < BPD***, BPD > NC***
	Adjusted	2.08 (0.09)	2.17 (0.09)	2.11 (0.10)	2.47 (0.07)	2.79 (0.06)	2.42 (0.05)	ANr < BN**, ANr < BPD***, ANr < NC**, ANbp < BPD***, AAN < BN*, AAN < BPD***, AAN < NC*, BN < BPD***, BPD > NC***
ER	Crude	2.45 (0.09)	2.40 (0.10)	2.44 (0.09)	2.47 (0.06)	2.33 (0.05)	2.58 (0.02)	BPD < NC***
	Adjusted	2.50 (0.09)	2.46 (0.10)	2.47 (0.10)	2.52 (0.07)	2.41 (0.06)	2.60 (0.05)	BPD < NC**

Measures of estimated means (crude/unadjusted) and estimated marginal means (adjusted for covariates) with standard errors (SEs) *for the Ego Undercontrol scale – 13 (EUC-13) and the Ego Resiliency scale (ER)*. Significant differences between groups are calculated using the Bonferroni post hoc test, adjusting for multiple comparisons, * $p < 0.05$, ** $p < 0.01$, *** $p < 0.001$

ANr anorexia nervosa restricting, *ANbp* AN binge eating/purging, *AAN* atypical AN, *BN* bulimia nervosa (BN), *BPD* borderline personality disorder (BPD), *NC* non-clinical

samples and in less severe psychiatric disorders [6, 22]. Hence, as identified in one previous study [15] the NC group was expected to report higher level of resilience, compared with ED groups. Our results did not confirm this expectation. Lack of significant differences might be partly due to low rating of resilience in the NC group. Their ratings were in fact lower than the University students from the original evaluation of the scale [22]. It is also worth emphasizing that the occurrence of a separate resilient high functioning/perfectionistic group, previously identified within EDs [4], was not investigated in this study. Hence, because the high-functioning individuals were included in the over- or undercontrolled groups, resilience ratings were supposedly higher than if they would have been represented by a separate high-functioning group.

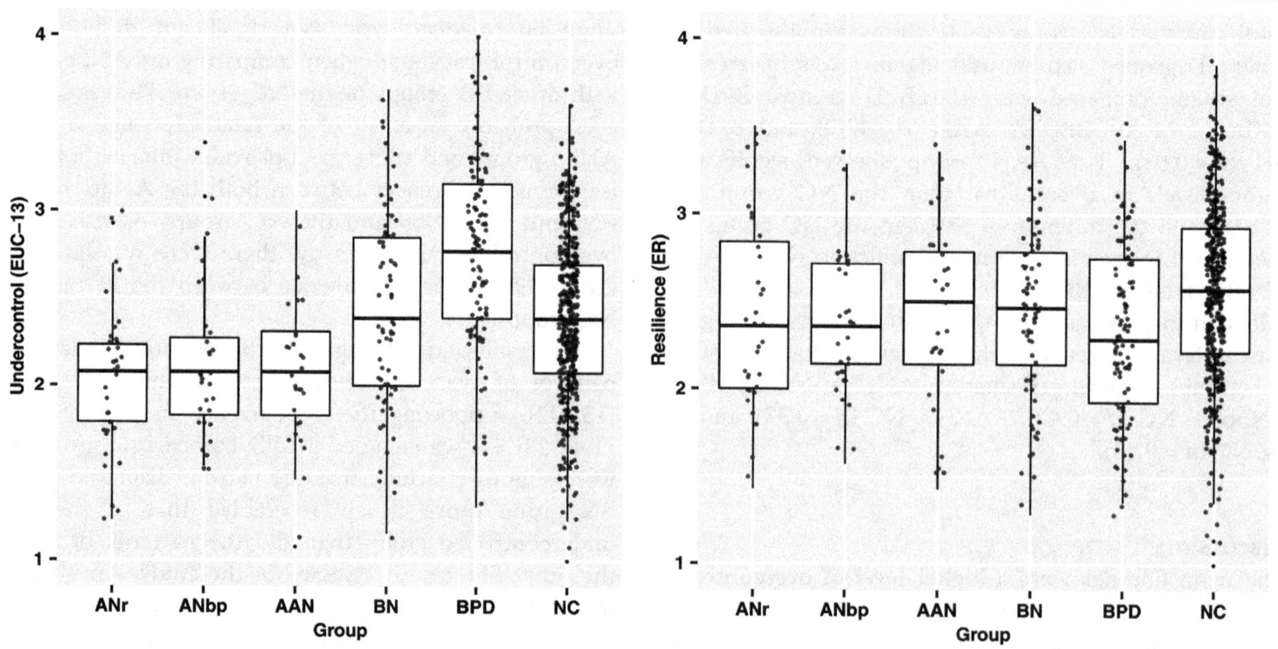

Fig. 2 Boxplot and jittered scatterplot of overcontrol, undercontrol, and resilience. *Note.* Group differences on Ego Undercontrol scale – 13 (EUC-13) and Ego Resilience scale (ER) are illustrated for anorexia nervosa restricting (ANr), AN binge eating/purging (ANbp), atypical AN (AAN), bulimia nervosa (BN), borderline personality disorder (BPD), and non-clinical (NC)

Implications

The present study offers an important contribution to research on EDs, as previous research could be replicated and refined with a thorough diagnostic assessment procedure (i.e., a semi-structured interview) and diagnoses based on DSM-5. Our results, together with previous findings, have several implications. For example, some researchers have suggested that personality should be taken into consideration when planning treatment [2, 14]. Fairburn's Enhanced Cognitive-Behavioral Therapy for ED (CBT-E) [24] includes ways of individualizing treatment to address personality traits, such as perfectionism. Also, impulsivity could be added as a treatment target for BN patients with an undercontrolled personality style [25], whereas rigidity could be targeted for AN patients with an overcontrolled personality style [26].

Results in the present study also showed a high variability of personality style within each ED group, as illustrated by the individual ratings in the scatterplot. Thus, the relationship between different ED subtypes and personality styles may be more complex than simply describing individuals with restrictive AN as overcontrolled and those with BN as undercontrolled [4, 23]. Heterogeneity within the AN and BN subgroups, and frequent migration between diagnoses [2, 27], highlights the need for improved precision in ED assessments. Other measures, improving prognostic accuracy (e.g., assessing personality style), should be considered.

Finally, behavioral and neurobiological similarities have been found between AN and common comorbid conditions, such as cluster C personality disorder and autism spectrum disorder [28, 29]. Considering personality style might give us a better understanding of the shared social deficits and behavioral rigidity within these groups, and possibly also help us understand at least some of the poor treatment outcomes for both AN and autism [30, 31].

Limitations

The study has several limitations. First, conclusions cannot be drawn about causality, since the design is cross-sectional. Some studies have shown that traits like obsessive-compulsiveness and perfectionism predict the risk of developing EDs [1, 32]. Others have shown that starvation is a state which alters an individual's thoughts, feelings, and behaviors, which also may affect the personality assessment [33]. However, rigid behaviors seem to persist even after recovery from AN with weight restoration [34]. This supports the idea of overcontrol as, at least partially, a personality style rather than a consequence of starvation. Second, even though our sample was large enough to detect meaningful differences in most pairwise comparisons, it was probably insufficient to detect smaller, yet clinically meaningful differences. However, sample size in our study is larger than many other studies investigating personality style in EDs [4, 6, 23]. Also, effect sizes provide a valid indication of the strength of the relation, beyond the issue of power and significance. Third, some of the participants in the comparison groups might also suffer from EDs, which was not assessed in this study. Levels of EDs among those with BPD have been reported to be as high as 50% [35], limiting the precision in our findings. However, excluding these individuals would make the group less representative of the actual clinical BPD group, and it is important to remember that BPD is their main diagnosis. Also, while the prevalence of EDs in BPD is high, the prevalence of BPD among those with EDs is lower: around 2% in ANr, 16% in ANbp, and 26% in BN [1, 36]. Fourth, recoding might call into question the validity of the DSM-5 diagnoses. However, due to the concrete parameters used for recoding (weight, amenorrhea, and instances of binge eating/compensation), the potential errors due to this recoding are considered to be minimal. Finally, the thirteen items included in the EUC-13 were in some cases extracted from the full version of the EUC administered at the beginning of the study. This could have some impact on how those participants rated the items. However, additional analyses showed that there were no significant differences in outcome regardless of the version of the EUC, reducing the risk for measurement error.

Conclusion and future research

Classified according to current diagnostic criteria (DSM-5), overcontrol is higher in ANr and ANN than in BN, NC, and BPD. In addition, AAN show clear similarities with ANr in terms of overcontrol. Taking personality styles into account may improve our understanding of certain characteristics in EDs, such as social deficits and rigidity that are attributed to poor treatment outcome. Future research should evaluate the stability of these personality styles after remission from ED, and evaluate the presence of these styles in a larger variety of ED groups such as BED and subclinical BN.

Abbreviations

AAN: Atypical anorexia nervosa; AN: Anorexia nervosa; ANbp: Anorexia nervosa binge eating/purging subtype; ANr: Anorexia nervosa restricting subtype; BED: Binge eating disorder; BMI: Body mass index; BN: Bulimia nervosa; BPD: Borderline personality disorder; DSM: Diagnostic and statistical manual of mental disorders; ED: Eating disorder; EDE: Eating disorder examination; ER: Ego resilience; EUC: Ego undercontrol; GLZM: Generalized linear model; NC: Non-clinical; PABAK: Prevalence and bias adjusted kappa; SCID: Structured clinical interview; SE: Standard error

Acknowledgments

We thank region Uppsala for providing salary to the first author and Hans Arinell for providing statistical advice. Additionally, we thank Erica Nyström, Mimmi Edgren, participants, and co-workers for their contributions.

Authors' contributions
All authors contributed substantially to each part of the manuscript. The first draft of the manuscript was written by Martina Isaksson and all authors commented on previous versions of the manuscript. All authors read and approved the final manuscript.

Competing interests
The authors declare that they have no conflict of interest.

Author details
[1]Department of Neuroscience, Psychiatry, Uppsala University, Entrance 10, Floor 3B, SE-751 85 Uppsala, Sweden. [2]Division of Psychology, Department of Clinical Neuroscience, Karolinska Institutet, SE-171 77 Stockholm, Sweden. [3]Stockholm Centre for Eating Disorders, Stockholm Health Care Services, Stockholm County Council, SE-171 77 Stockholm, Sweden. [4]Psychiatry Northwest, Region Stockholm, Clinical Management, PO Box 98, SE-191 22 Sollentuna, Sweden.

References
1. Farstad SM, McGeown LM, von Ranson KM. Eating disorders and personality, 2004-2016: a systematic review and meta-analysis. Clin Psychol Rev Elsevier Ltd. 2016;46:91–105. https://doi.org/10.1016/j.cpr.2016.04.005.
2. Martinez MA, Craighead LW. Toward person (ality)-centered treatment: how consideration of personality and individual differences in anorexia nervosa may improve treatment outcome. Clin Psychol Sci Pract. 2015;22(3):296–314. https://doi.org/10.1111/cpsp.12111.
3. Wildes JE, Marcus MD, Crosby RD, Ringham RM, Dapelo MM, Gaskill JA, et al. The clinical utility of personality subtypes in patients with anorexia nervosa. J Consult Clin Psychol. 2011;79(5):665–74. https://doi.org/10.1037/a0024597.
4. Westen D, Harnden-Fisher J. Personality profiles in eating disorders: rethinking the distinction between Axis I and Axis II. Am J Psychiatry American Psychiatric Association. 2001;158(4):547–62. https://doi.org/10.11 76/appi.ajp.158.4.547.
5. Lavender JM, Wonderlich SA, Crosby RD, Engel SG, Mitchell JE, Crow SJ, et al. Personality-based subtypes of anorexia nervosa: examining validity and utility using baseline clinical variables and ecological momentary assessment. Behav Res Ther Elsevier Ltd. 2013;51(8):512–7. https://doi.org/1 0.1016/j.brat.2013.05.007.
6. Turner BJ, Claes L, Wilderjans TF, Pauwels E, Dierckx E, Chapman AL, et al. Personality profiles in eating disorders: further evidence of the clinical utility of examining subtypes based on temperament. Psychiatry Res Elsevier. 2014;219(1):157–65. https://doi.org/10.1016/j.psychres.2014.04.036.
7. Keel PK, Brown TA, Holland LA, Bodell LP. Empirical classification of eating disorders. Annu Rev Clin Psychol. 2012;8(1):381–404. https://doi.org/10.114 6/annurev-clinpsy-032511-143111.
8. Jennings KM, Bodell LP, Crosby RD, Haynos AF, Wildes JE. Mixture modeling to characterize anorexia nervosa: integrating personality and eating disorder psychopathology. J Am Psychiatr Nurses Assoc. 2019:107839031986202. https://doi.org/10.1177/1078390319862029.
9. Block JH, Block J. The role of ego-control and ego-resiliency in the organization of behavior. In: Collins WA, editor. Dev Cogn Affect Soc relations Minnesota Symp child Psychol. Hillsdale: NJ: Erlbaum; 1980. p. 39–101.
10. Robins RW, John OP, Caspi A, Moffitt TE, Stouthamer-Loeber M. Resilient, overcontrolled, and undercontrolled boys: three replicable personality types. J Pers Soc Psychol. 1996;70(1):151–71. https://doi.org/10.1037/0022-3514.70.1.157.
11. Meeus W, Van de Schoot R, Klimstra T, Branje S. Personality types in adolescence: change and stability and links with adjustment and relationships: a five-wave longitudinal study. Dev Psychol. 2011;47(4):1181–95. https://doi.org/10.1037/a0023816.
12. Chapman BP, Goldberg LR. Replicability and 40-year predictive power of childhood ARC types. J Pers Soc Psychol. 2011;101:593–606. https://doi.org/10.1037/a0024289
13. Alessandri G, Vecchione M, Donnellan BM, Eisenberg N, Caprara GV, Cieciuch J. On the Cross-Cultural Replicability of the Resilient, Undercontrolled, and Overcontrolled Personality Types. J Pers. 2013;82:340–53. https://doi.org/10.1111/jopy.12065
14. Lynch TR, Hempel RJ, Dunkley C. Radically open-dialectical behavior therapy for disorders of over-control: signaling matters. Am J Psychother. 2015;69(2): 141–62. https://doi.org/10.1176/appi.psychotherapy.2015.69.2.141.
15. Tsigkaropoulou E, Ferentinos P, Karavia A, Gournellis R, Gonidakis F, Liappas I, et al. Personality dimensions could explain resilience in patients with eating disorders. Eat Weight Disord Springer International Publishing. 2020. https://doi.org/10.1007/s40519-020-01012-4.
16. Cooper Z, Fairburn CG. The eating disorder examination: a semi-structured interview for the assessment of the specific psychopathology of eating disorders. Int J Eat Disord. 1987;6(1):1–8. https://doi.org/10.1002/1098-108X(1 98701)6:1<1::AID-EAT2260060102>3.0.CO;2-9.
17. Byrt T, Bishop J, Carlin JB. Bias, prevalence and kappa. J Clin Epidemiol. 1993; 46(5):423–9. https://doi.org/10.1016/0895-4356(93)90018-V.
18. American Psychiatric Association. Diagnostic and statistical manual of mental disorders. 4th ed. Washington, DC: Author: American Psychiatric Association; 2000.
19. First MB, Gibbon M, Spitzer RL, Williams JBW, Benjamin LS. Structured Clinical Interview for DSM-IV Axis II Personality Disorders, (SCID-II). Washington, D.C: American Psychiatric Press, Inc; 1997.
20. Isaksson M, Ghaderi A, Wolf-Arehult M, Ramklint M. Psychometric properties of the Swedish version of the Ego resilience scale (ER) and a new shortened version of the Ego Undercontrol scale (EUC). Curr Psychol. 2021;40(3):1498–506. https://doi.org/10.1007/s12144-018-0069-3.
21. Block J, Kremen AM. IQ and ego-resiliency: conceptual and empirical connections and separateness. J Pers Soc Psychol. 1996;70(2):349–61. https://doi.org/10.1037/0022-3514.70.2.349.
22. Letzring TD, Block J, Funder DC. Ego-control and ego-resiliency: Generalization of self-report scales based on personality descriptions from acquaintances, clinicians, and the self. J Res Pers. 2005;39:395–422. https://doi.org/10.1016/j.jrp.2004.06.003.
23. Gazzillo F, Lingiardi V, Peloso A, Giordani S, Vesco S, Zanna V, et al. Personality subtypes in adolescents with anorexia nervosa. Compr Psychiatry Elsevier Inc. 2013;54:702–12. https://doi.org/10.1016/j.compsych.2013.03.006.
24. Fairburn CG. Cognitive behavior therapy and eating disorders. New York: Guilford Publications; 2008.
25. Safer DL, Telch CF, Chen EY. Dialectical behavior therapy for binge eating and bulimia. New York: Guilford Press; 2009.
26. Lynch TR. Radically open dialectical behavior therapy: theory and practice for treating disorders of Overcontrol. Oakland, CA: New Harbinger Publications; 2018.
27. Eddy KT, Dorer DJ, Franko DL, Tahilani K, Thompson-Brenner H, Herzog DB. Diagnostic crossover in anorexia nervosa and bulimia nervosa: Implications for DSM-V. Am J Psychiatry. 2008;165(2):245–50. https://doi.org/10.1176/a ppi.ajp.2007.07060951.
28. Wentz Nilsson E, Gillberg C, Gillberg IC, Råstam M. Ten-year follow-up of adolescent-onset anorexia nervosa: personality disorders. J Am Acad Child Adolesc Psychiatry. 1999;38(11):1389–95. https://doi.org/10.1097/00004583-1 99911000-00013.
29. Björnsdotter M, Davidovic M, Karjalainen L, Starck G, Olausson H, Wentz E. Grey matter correlates of autistic traits in women with anorexia nervosa. J Psychiatry Neurosci. 2018;43(2):79–86. https://doi.org/10.1503/jpn.170072.
30. Schulte-Rüther M, Mainz V, Fink GR, Herpertz-Dahlmann B, Konrad K. Theory of mind and the brain in anorexia nervosa: Relation to treatment outcome. J Am Acad Child Adolesc Psychiatry Elsevier Inc. 2012;51:832–841.e11. https://doi.org/10.1016/j.jaac.2012.06.007.
31. Treasure J. Coherence and other autistic spectrum traits and eating disorders: building from mechanism to treatment. The Birgit Olsson lecture. Nord J Psychiatry. 2013;67(1):38–42. https://doi.org/10.3109/08039488.2012.674554.
32. Lilenfeld LRR, Wonderlich S, Riso LP, Crosby R, Mitchell J. Eating disorders and personality: a methodological and empirical review. Clin Psychol Rev. 2006;26(3):299–320. https://doi.org/10.1016/j.cpr.2005.10.003.
33. Vitousek KM, Stumpf RE. Difficulties in the assessment of personality traits and disorders in eating-disordered individuals. Eat Disord. 2005;13(1):37–60. https://doi.org/10.1080/10640260590893638.
34. Lindner SE, Fichter MM, Quadflieg N. Set-shifting and its relation to clinical and personality variables in full recovery of anorexia nervosa. Eur Eat Disord Rev. 2014;22(4):252–9. https://doi.org/10.1002/erv.2293.

35. Zanarini M, Frankenburg F, Hennen J, Reich D, Silk K. Axis I comorbidity in patients with borderline personality disorder: 6-year follow-up and prediction of time to remission. Am J Psychiatry. 2004;161(11):2108–14. https://doi.org/10.1176/appi.ajp.161.11.2108.
36. Ramklint M, Jeansson M, Holmgren S, Ghaderi A. Assessing personality disorders in eating disordered patients using the SCID-II: influence of measures and timing on prevalence rate. Personal Individ Differ. 2010;48(2): 218–23. https://doi.org/10.1016/j.paid.2009.10.014.

20

Identity processes and eating disorder symptoms during university adjustment

Aoife-Marie Foran*, Orla T. Muldoon and Aisling T. O'Donnell

Abstract

Background: Young people with eating disorders (EDs) and ED symptoms are at risk during university adjustment, suggesting a need to protect their health. The social identity approach proposes that people's social connections – and the identity-related behaviour they derive from them – are important for promoting positive health outcomes. However, there is a limited understanding as to how meaningful everyday connections, supported by affiliative identities, may act to reduce ED symptoms during a life transition.

Methods: Two hundred eighty-one first year university students with an ED or ED symptoms completed an online survey during the first month of university. Participants completed self-reported measures of affiliative identity, social support, injunctive norms and ED symptoms. Path analysis was used to test a hypothesised mediated model, whereby affiliative identity has a significant indirect relation with ED symptoms via social support and injunctive norms.

Results: Results support the hypothesised model. We show that affiliative identity predicts lower self-reported ED symptoms, because of its relation with social support and injunctive norms.

Conclusions: The findings imply that affiliative identities have a positive impact on ED symptoms during university adjustment, because the social support derived from affiliative identity is associated with how people perceive norms around disordered eating. Our discussion emphasises the possibility of identity processes being a social cure for those at risk of ED symptoms.

Keywords: Affiliative identity, Eating disorder symptoms, Social support, Injunctive norms

Plain English summary

Adjustment to university is a major challenge for many young people, as it often involves a change in meaningful connections. Young people with eating disorders (EDs) and ED symptoms are at risk during this transition. Research outside the ED field shows that people's social connections can have important implications for health behaviours. This study aimed to explore how meaningful everyday connections may help reduce ED symptoms during university adjustment. Two hundred eighty-one first year university students with an ED or ED symptoms completed an online survey during the first month of university. Meaningful everyday connections were shown to have positive implications for ED symptoms during university adjustment. This is because the social support received from these connections is associated with how people perceive group norms around disordered eating. Health professionals working with people with EDs or at risk of an ED, may profit from this research as it speaks to the benefits of incorporating

* Correspondence: aoife.marie.foran@ul.ie
Centre for Social Issues Research, Department of Psychology, University of Limerick, Castletroy, Limerick, Republic of Ireland

connections that are important to each person during periods of adjustment or life change.

Identity processes and eating disorder symptoms during university adjustment: a cross-sectional study

Adjustment to university is a major challenge for young people. This is because for many, a transition to university involves a natural change in meaningful connections [1]. Therefore, it is not surprising that young people with disordered eating are at risk during this transition and may report compromised health outcomes [2]. Understanding how to manage such transitions may allow people with EDs and ED symptoms to protect their health. Speaking to this issue, the social identity approach suggests that people's social connections – and the identity-related behaviour they derive from them – are important for improving health [3]. Researchers have also shown how identity continuity in times of transition is important for health outcomes [4, 5]. While much of the research in the ED literature has focused on how identities can maintain disordered behaviours, McNamara et al. demonstrated that a shared sense of identity with others in an online support group can reduce ED symptoms [6]. However, there is limited understanding of the role that other important identities may play. Thus, drawing on work in the 'social cure' tradition [3], we argue the importance of understanding how meaningful everyday connections, supported by affiliative identities, impact people's ED symptoms in the face of a life transition.

The social identity approach, which incorporates social identity theory [7] and self-categorisation theory [8], offers a rich framework for understanding how identity processes might work for young people who are at risk of exacerbating ED symptoms. Tajfel defined social identity as the sense of self derived from meaningful connections [9]. Depending on the context, social identities can act as a benefit or a burden to people's health [3]. To date, social identity researchers have focused their efforts on understanding how identification with therapy and support groups can influence ED symptoms [6, 10]. However, we argue different types of identity, such as identification with those who are an important part of our everyday lives, must also be considered to facilitate understanding of the relation between identity and ED symptoms. Billig's conceptualisation of the banality has been used to refer to social identities that are unexpressed, but nevertheless present and available when required [11]. In other words, banal identities refers to "background identities" which are often unnoticed and taken for granted. They are linked to group memberships that are so inherent to who we are that they are often unremarkable, unworthy of comment, banal. These banal identities give rise to affiliative identities: connections made up of groups, such as family and friend networks, that are the assumed backdrop to everyday life [12]. These affiliative identities hinge on feelings of belongingness and while they may not be within our conscious awareness, they are ready to be mobilised during periods of adjustment.

Prior research suggests that pre-existing identities play an important role during the university adjustment period as they have shown to act as a basis for forming new identities [1]. Iyer and colleagues also found that people who have a history of successful meaningful connections are more likely to develop new connections [1]. In the context of this research, affiliative identities represent potentially important connections that have existed prior to university transition and should be present during the university adjustment period [4]. These can provide a sense of identity continuity to people with EDs and ED symptoms, which not only assists in a successful adjustment, but also has the potential to optimise their health. Thus, we argue affiliative identities are important for understanding ED symptoms as they can play an important role in adjusting to change [12], associated with university transition.

Affiliative identity makes social support possible, and thereby the receipt of support is implicated in the health-protecting benefits of identities [13]. The basic premise of the social identity approach is that belonging to a group provides people with a definition of who they are. If a person feels that being a group member is important to them, they are more likely to construe the support they receive more positively [14]. While there is strong evidence that social support is likely to be a critical mediator of the relation between identity and health [15], the role that this plays in promoting fewer ED symptoms during university adjustment remains to be tested. However, significant contributions have been offered suggesting that the perception of poor social support from meaningful connections can be considered as a risk factor for the development of ED symptoms [16]. Given that young people with EDs and ED symptoms are at significant risk of increases in ED behaviours during university adjustment [2], there is an imperative to understand how affiliative identities can provide support to protect their health.

Researchers in the social identity literature have also argued the importance of norms for understanding eating behaviour [17]. Norms are a broad concept with diverse meanings, and therefore researchers must consider the types of norms important for understanding specific behaviours. Descriptive norms examine what other group members do. Injunctive norms examine the perception of what group members endorse as appropriate and emerge through everyday connections. Both types of norms have shown to predict health-related outcomes

[18]. However, we argue that injunctive norms are most important for ED symptoms, as they have shown to be useful for understanding social dimensions of eating behaviour [17]. Hence, the present research focuses on injunctive norms around disordered eating behaviours.

Prior research suggests that norms have an effect on eating behaviours. For instance, researchers have demonstrated that in a college environment, norms around healthy eating and exercise habits were associated with healthier eating behaviours [19]. Cruwys et al. also showed that normative change during an ED group program predicted improvements in dieting intentions and body dissatisfaction [18]. On the other hand, people who strongly identify as students, and perceived unhealthy eating as normative of student populations, were more likely to report unhealthy eating intentions [20]. Similarly, Neumark-Sztainer et al. showed the importance of dieting norms in determining the frequency of disordered eating in adolescents [21]. Based on these findings, it appears that the norms associated with a particular group have the potential to promote healthy or unhealthy eating behaviours. We propose that the impact of both affiliative identity and social support on ED symptoms may be contingent on whether injunctive norms promote healthy or disordered eating behaviours. Therefore, we argue the need to consider a combination of identity, social support and norms in order to generate a more accurate representation of the processes influencing ED symptoms.

Despite recognition of the importance of identity and social support for ED symptoms, at present the precise nature of these relations remain unclear. Researchers in the clinical ED field suggest that ED symptoms can be reduced through the support and understanding of people in therapy groups [6, 22]. Contrarily, ED groups may also contribute to the maintenance of disordered eating behaviours through identity-based support [23, 24]. While there have been numerous studies conducted which examine these variables separately, only a small number have considered how social support may underlie the relation between identity and ED symptoms. However, Leonidas et al. argued the need to move away from a reliance on ED therapy groups as a main source of support, to include significant connections, such as family and friends [25]. This is where the present research has particular value as we focus on social support derived from affiliative identities.

A body of evidence also points towards the interactive impact of identity and norms, such that people only conform to a norm when they strongly identify with its source [26]. For example, Stevenson et al. found that people are more likely to engage in certain eating behaviours, in part, because these behaviours are seen as normative of a group to which they affiliate [27]. Likewise, researchers in the addiction literature have shown that people who identified strongly with an addiction therapy group, whose norms endorsed lower substance use, showed greater abstinence behaviours [28, 29]. Given the associations between identity, norms and health behaviours, we argue that injunctive norms may also help explain the association between affiliative identity and ED symptoms.

Taking the available research together, it is evident that identity, social support and norms have important implications for ED symptoms. However, while studies have often examined the direct relations between these variables, no study as of yet has tested the interactive impact that these identity processes have on ED symptoms. Recent research by Cullum et al. showed when perceived social support derived from identification with peer groups is low, student drinking behaviours were strongly influenced by peer norms compared to when social support was high [30]. From these findings, Cullum and colleagues highlighted the benefits of considering the relation between perceived social support and norms for health behaviours [30]. And so, we argue that these feelings of social support drawn from affiliative groups may play a role in influencing people's endorsement of disordered eating norms associated with the group. More specifically, we propose that affiliative identities can have benefits for ED symptoms because they afford opportunities to make meaningful contributions through the provision of social support and injunctive norms.

The present study

The aim of the present research was to investigate and attempt to advance understanding of reciprocal processes between affiliative identity, social support, injunctive norms, and ED symptoms amongst a cohort of first year university students with an ED or concerns about ED symptoms. Given the challenges faced by young people with ED symptoms [2], it is important that we understand how they manage adjustment to university, so as to protect their health. The social identity approach has so far explored the role of therapy groups in ED symptomatology during periods of transition but has paid less attention as to how affiliative identities impact ED symptoms. Therefore, in light of previous research, we test a hypothetical model, which explores whether perceived social support and injunctive norms sequentially mediate the proposed relation between affiliative identity and ED symptoms.

Methods

Participants

First year students at an Irish university were recruited through email. Notably, participants were required to have concerns about ED symptoms or a diagnosed ED to take part. Two hundred eighty-one people (44 men and 237 women; $M_{age} = 20.24$, $SD = 5.05$, range 18–56 years) with either an ED or ED symptoms, took part in this study during the first month of their university transition. Twenty three people reported an ED diagnosis. These included anorexia nervosa ($n = 14$), bulimia nervosa ($n = 5$), binge-eating disorder ($n = 3$), muscle dysmorphia ($n = 1$), and other specified feeding or eating disorder ($n = 2$). Participants also indicated the types of disordered eating behaviours they engaged in: frequent dieting ($n = 68$); become anxious about specific foods ($n = 102$); meal skipping ($n = 168$); have a rigid routine surrounding exercise ($n = 39$); use exercise, food restriction, fasting or purging to make up for food consumed ($n = 73$); have a preoccupation with food, weight, and/or body image ($n = 189$); feel a loss of control around food ($n = 122$). Participants could choose more than one type of disordered eating behavior, if it applied to them. Only 36 out of the 281 participants reported seeking help for their concerns about disordered eating.

Based on the final sample size ($n = 281$), an alpha value of .05, and 80% power, sensitivity analysis using G*Power [31] indicated sensitivity to detect small effects ($f = .028$).

Materials and procedure

The study had a cross-sectional and correlational design. Notably, the present study is part of a larger longitudinal study. Ethical approval was granted by the University of Limerick Faculty of Education and Health Sciences research ethics committee (ref: 2019_06_20_EHS). On receiving the recruitment email, potential participants were invited to click on the link provided to take part in online survey hosted using Qualtrics. The study complied with the ethical standards of the Declaration of Helsinki, including notifying participants that the study was voluntary, that they were free to withdraw at any time, and that they would indicate their informed consent by selecting the "agree to take part" button to start the survey. Participants first responded to demographic variables regarding their age, gender, type of disordered eating behaviours or ED diagnosis, duration of disordered eating concerns and whether help had been sought for these concerns.

Predictor variable

Affiliative identity

Ashmore et al. argue the importance of self-categorisation and suggest that researchers should allow people to answer open-ended questions about their group memberships [32]. Consequently, self-categorised affiliative identity was measured in the present study with the question, "Which group of people you belong to is most important to who you are?" See Table 1 for a list of affiliative identities elicited from participants.

Identity strength, in relation to one's most important identity, was measured using the four-item Group Identification Scale (Sani et al. [33]; e.g., I feel a bond with my [group], 1 = *strongly disagree*, 7 = *strongly agree*, Cronbach's $\alpha = .92$). This global scale examines one's sense of belonging to the previously chosen group and one's sense of commonality with in-group members. Each participant's mean score on the four items was calculated, with higher mean scores equating to stronger affiliative identity.

Mediator variables

Social support

The 19-item Medical Outcomes Study Social Support Survey (Sherbourne et al. [34]; e.g., Someone to listen to you when you need to talk, 1 = *none of the time*, 5 = *all of the time*, Cronbach's $\alpha = .94$) was used to measure perceived functional support. The questionnaire contains subsets of functional support including emotional/informational support, tangible support, affectionate support and positive social interaction. Items were averaged to compute mean scores, with higher mean score indicating greater perceived social support. This questionnaire is suited for application in the context of mental health disorders, as it is distinct from structural measures of social support (e.g. number of close friends).

Injunctive norms

Injunctive norms around disordered eating behaviours were established using four-items (Cronbach's $\alpha = .70$; adapted from Åstrosm et al. [35]; Smith et al. [36]; White et al. [37]: "Members of this group think that dieting is a good idea"(1 = *strongly disagree*, 7 = *strongly agree*), "If I were to lose weight, members of the group

Table 1 Affiliative Identities Elicited from Participants

Family	155
School friends	108
College friends	3
Church friends	1
Hometown friends	1
Work friends	2
Partner/family	1
Sports team	4
Rugby team	2
Football team	1
Swim club	1
Scouts	2
Total	281

would ..." (1 = *disapprove*, 7 = *approve*), "Members of this group think I ..." (1 = *should not lose weight*, 7 = *should lose weight*), and "How many members of this group would think that being thin is a good thing?" (1 = *none of them*, 7 = *all of them*). Items were averaged to compute mean score, with higher score indicating greater perceived endorsement of disordered eating behaviours. This measure has also been used by Cruwys et al. [18] to examine injunctive norms in relation to eating behaviours.

Outcome variable

Eating disorder symptoms

The 28-item Eating Disorder Examination Questionnaire (Fairburn et al. [38]; e.g., On how many of the past 28 days have you been deliberately trying to limit the amount of food you eat to influence your shape or weight, Cronbach's $\alpha = .94$) was utilised to measure self-reported ED symptomatology, including: restraint, weight concern, shape concern and eating concern. The 4 subscales capture the eating pathology spectrum, ranging from problems of undereating (i.e., anorexia nervosa) through to problems of overeating (i.e., binge-eating), with body dissatisfaction and bulimia nervosa falling in the middle. Participants were instructed that the questions were to be answered in relation to the 28 days prior to answering the survey. Items were averaged to compute mean scores, with higher mean scores indicating greater severity of ED symptoms.

Approach to analysis

All data were exported from Qualtrics to SPSS 25 for analysis. Preliminary analyses indicated that the variables of interest were not normally distributed. So, non-parametric tests were used for correlation analysis to evaluate the strength and direction of association between non normally distributed variables. First, we examined bivariate correlations between strength of affiliative identity, injunctive norms, social support, self-reported ED symptoms, age and gender (Table 2). Second, we used PROCESS serial mediation analysis (model 6) to test the relationship between affiliative identity (predictor variable) and self-reported ED symptoms (outcome variable) as well as the indirect effect of social support and injunctive norms (mediator variables). In Fig. 1, we illustrate this model. The effect of affiliative identity on ED symptoms is the product of the relation between affiliative identity and social support (labelled a_1), social support and injunctive norms (labelled b_1) and injunctive norms and ED symptoms (labelled c_1). When examining indirect effects in this way, the mediators are hypothesized as a causal chain. However, given this was cross sectional data, following the suggestion of Hayes [39], we also tested alternative explanations that might fit the data (i.e. injunctive norms – social support – affiliative identity – ED symptoms). Age and gender were included in the model as covariates – as these correlated with self-reported ED symptoms in the preliminary analysis. The model was computed for each of the 10,000 bootstrapped re-samples, using bias-corrected 95% confidence intervals, and therefore can deal with non-normal distribution [39].

Results

Indirect effect of Affiliative identity on ED symptoms

The serial mediation analysis conducted demonstrated that affiliative identity affects self-reported ED symptoms via perceived social support and injunctive norms (Fig. 1). As hypothesised, the results indicated that the effect of affiliative identity on self-reported ED symptoms was via perceived social support and injunctive norms, and though small, it was reliable with $b = -.01$, $SE = .01$, 95% CI [−.021, −.001]. The effect of affiliative identity on perceived social support was statistically significant, indicating that affiliative identity was associated with greater perceived social support. The effect of social support on injunctive norms, while controlling for affiliative identity, was also statistically significant, indicating that feelings of support were associated with lower perceived endorsement of disordered eating norms. Finally, the effect of norms on ED symptoms, while controlling for social support and affiliative identity, was also statistically significant. This indicated that those who perceived group disapproval of disordered eating report had lower ED symptoms. The relation between social support and ED symptoms, while controlling for affiliative identity, was significant, indicating that feelings of support were associated with lower ED symptoms. However, the relation between affiliative identity on injunctive norms was not significant. Consistent with our hypothesis that the

Table 2 Means, Standard Deviations and Bivariate Correlations of all Variables of Interest

	M (SD)	1	2	3	4	Age	Gender
1. Affiliative identity	6.00 (1.35)	–	.41**	−.10	−.04		
2. Social support	3.81 (.79)		–	−.16**	−.11		
3. Injunctive norms	3.84 (1.28)			–	.21**		
4. ED symptoms	3.66 (1.34)				–	−.13*	.27**

Note: * $p < .01$; ** $p < .001$

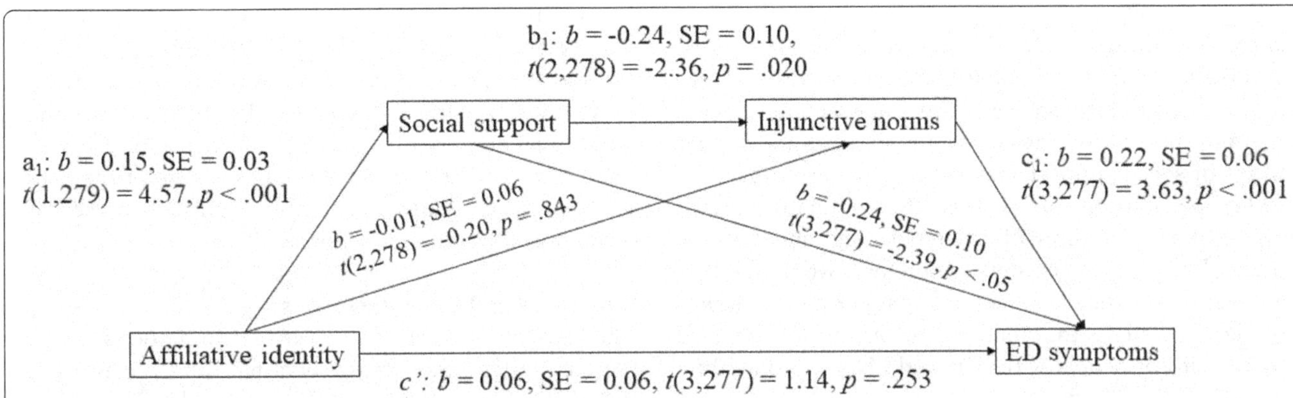

Fig. 1 Serial mediation of the effect of affiliative identity on self-reported ED symptoms via social support and injunctive norms

relation between affiliative identity and self-reported ED symptoms is best understood with due attention to our mediators (social support and injunctive norms), there was no significant direct effect (see path labelled "c'" in Fig. 1). Overall, these findings indicate that affiliative identities have a positive impact on ED symptoms during university adjustment, because the social support linked to affiliative identity is associated with how people perceive norms around disordered eating.

Given that Cruwys et al. argue the predictive utility of norms for eating behaviours [40], a model of an alternative causal explanation (i.e., that injunctive norms had a significant indirect relation with self-reported ED symptoms via social support and affiliative identity as mediators) was also tested. This model was not significant: $b = -.002$, $SE = .003$, 95% CI [−.009, .002].

Discussion

The present research explored the impact that identity processes have on ED symptoms, in a cohort of first year university students with a diagnosed ED or ED symptoms. In line with our hypothesis, we show that affiliative identity predicts lower self-reported ED symptoms, because of its relation with social support and injunctive norms. Consistent with the idea that social identity can be the basis of a social cure [3], we show that the social support derived from affiliative identity has positive implications for how people perceive norms around disordered eating, which subsequently predicts fewer self-reported ED symptoms. The present findings indicate that in the context of EDs, identity processes are not only important for understanding ED symptoms but may also predict fewer ED symptoms during periods of adjustment.

Notably, the present results do not indicate a direct relation between affiliative identity and self-reported ED symptoms. Instead, we show the relation between affiliative identity and ED symptoms, rests in a wider causal chain that includes perceived social support and injunctive norms. Research examining direct effects of social identity on ED symptoms have shown that identification with therapy groups can have both positive and negative implications for ED symptoms [10, 22]. This has parallels to social representations of use and misuse of substances, whereby dis-identification with a group oriented towards addictive behaviours alongside identification with an addiction therapy group can have implications for abstinence behaviours [28, 29]. However, Best et al. argued the extent to which social identities contribute to health behaviours depends on identity-related factors such as social support and the associated norms of the group [28] – highlighting the importance of examining indirect effects for gaining a greater understanding of how or why a relation occurs. In the present research, affiliative identity seems to be necessary but not sufficient for reducing ED symptoms. Our findings suggest that the association between affiliative identity, social support and injunctive norms, are identity processes that may play a role in reducing ED symptoms. Crucially, in examining this indirect effect, our research reveals an effect which would otherwise remain hidden.

The findings make an important contribution to our understanding of people with EDs and disordered eating who are at risk of exacerbating ED symptoms during university adjustment. The study shows that, as expected, injunctive norms are associated with ED symptoms [18, 19]. However, we again caution that this relation is associated with the extent to which people feel supported by their affiliative group. This is consistent with the hypothesis that belonging to a group (affiliative identity) makes social support possible [13, 15]. Our findings also support Cullum and colleagues' suggestion that the level of social support one receives from their peer group may be an important factor in adherence to group norms around drinking [30]. In considering the indirect effect of social support and injunctive norms, the findings demonstrate how the interactive impact of these identity processes may act as a social cure for those at risk of ED symptoms. This supports recent qualitative findings by McNamara et al. which suggest that identification with online support groups can reduce ED behaviours because of the endorsement of positive group norms [6]. However, our findings imply that feelings of social support may have a positive impact on people's perceptions of whether their affiliative group endorses norms around disordered eating, and thereby predicts lower ED symptoms. Therefore, we argue that meaningful everyday connections, supported by affiliative identities, have the potential to play a positive role in the health of people with EDs and ED symptoms during periods of adjustment.

Implications

The present study represents an important addition to the literature within the social identity approach, as it shows how everyday identity processes matter for ED symptoms. We found that social support and injunctive norms are important explanatory factors in the relation between affiliative identity and ED symptoms. This indirect effect allows us to better understand the process underlying the relation between affiliative identity and ED symptoms, rather than a direct effect which would simply portray if affiliative identity predicted ED symptoms. As such, our findings provide evidence which may be used to improve interventions aimed at reducing ED symptoms. For example, group-based interventions that use affiliative identity as a platform for generating healthy norms around eating and access to functional social support, might be especially important to reducing ED symptoms. The present research offers an alternative conceptualisation of ED symptomatology as a social process, which is partially influenced by identity processes. Foran et al. argued the importance of examining social-psychological processes, which are likely to be significant in the context of ED psychopathology [41]. Our findings support this claim and show how moving away from individual level pathology offers prospects for group-based interventions that include identity processes that reduce ED symptomatology.

The present research also has important implications for health professionals working with people with EDs. First year college students are not only a high-risk population for ED symptoms, but are also at a life stage where sources of support are naturally changing in the transition to university, thus, increasing their risk. Given that the data were collected during the first 4 weeks of the transition to university, we argue our findings speak to the benefits of incorporating identities that are important to each person during periods of adjustment or life change. Indeed, family-based treatment has highlighted the important role of family in the treatment of children and adolescents with EDs. Our findings support the focus in treatment on group-based therapies that create a sense of belonging, to address a concern common to all members of the group. Importantly, the present study contributes to the ED field in suggesting that affiliative identities may be beneficial for ED symptoms during periods of adjustment because of the nature of these meaningful connections – through perceptions of support and injunctive norms.

Limitations and future directions

The present research is not without limitations. The research design was cross-sectional and correlational. PROCESS Model 6 [39] was utilised in the present study as it was designed to establish the order of serial mediators in a causal pathway between predictor and outcome variables. Therefore, while the model cannot establish causation, in line with Hayes [39], we argue that this analysis approach does facilitate informed consideration of the potential causal pathways between the variables of interest. Also, as Cruwys et al. argue the predictive utility of group norms in understanding eating behaviours [40], we also explored an alternative model (i.e. that injunctive norms had a significant indirect relation with self-reported ED symptoms via social support and affiliative identity), which we found to be non-significant. While this approach cannot establish the direction of causal flow exactly, it rules out the possibility for an alternative causal order. Nevertheless, a longitudinal design should be employed to examine the role of identity processes on ED symptoms over time.

The present study also focuses on one type of health outcome important for people with EDs: ED symptomatology. This outcome was selected because to date, ED health outcomes have mainly been focused on physiological measures such as BMI and/or weight [42]. Research on identity processes that facilitate understanding of ED symptoms is important, as recent research suggests that the estimated prevalence of EDs is increasing [43]. Given that EDs are complex psychological disorders that affect every aspect of a person's functioning, it is imperative that we consider a range of health outcomes in ED research. Social identity researchers have suggested a link between identity and a variety of psychological and social health outcomes, such as well-being and social functioning [3, 13]. Considering this, further research is needed to understand to what extent identity processes have implications for psychological and social functioning, in individuals with EDs and ED symptoms.

Conclusion

Adjustment to university is a major challenge as it often involves a natural change in meaningful connections. Our findings show that affiliative identity predicts fewer self-reported ED symptoms because of its relation with social support and injunctive norms. We propose that affiliative identities may provide important psychological resources necessary for predicting fewer ED symptoms during the university adjustment period. This presents the possibility of identity processes being a social cure for those at risk of ED symptoms. In applying the social identity approach, our study offers an alternative approach to understanding ED symptoms, by framing these behaviours as a social process. Not only are our findings important for theoretical reasons but they also have the potential to inform practical interventions – in pointing to the importance of harnessing identity processes for ED health outcomes.

Abbreviation

EDs: Eating disorders

Authors' contributions

AMF, OM and AOD designed the study. AMF conducted the data collection and analysis. AMF wrote the manuscript, with critical revisions from OM and AOD. All authors read and approved the final manuscript prior to submission.

Competing interests

The authors declare that there are no potential conflicts of interest with respect to the research, authorship, and/or publication of this article.

References

1. Iyer A, Jetten J, Tsivrikos D, Postmes T, Haslam SA. The more (and the more compatible) the merrier: multiple group memberships and identity compatibility as predictors of adjustment after life transitions. Br J Soc Psychol. 2009;48(4):707–33. https://doi.org/10.1348/014466608X397628.
2. Bodywhys. Annual report [Internet]. Dublin 2017 [Available from: https://www.bodywhys.ie/wp-content/uploads/2018/07/BW-AR-210x280mm-2017-final2.pdf.
3. Jetten J, Haslam C, Alexander SH. The social cure: identity, health and well-being: Psychology Press; 2012. https://doi.org/10.4324/9780203813195.
4. Haslam C, Holme A, Haslam SA, Iyer A, Jetten J, Williams WH. Maintaining group memberships: social identity continuity predicts well-being after stroke. Neuropsychol Rehabil. 2008;18(5–6):671–91. https://doi.org/10.1080/09602010701643449.
5. Walsh RS, Muldoon OT, Fortune DG, Gallagher S. A longitudinal study of relationships between identity continuity and anxiety following brain injury. Front Psychol. 2017;8:648. https://doi.org/10.3389/fpsyg.2017.00648.
6. McNamara N, Parsons H. 'Everyone here wants everyone else to get better': the role of social identity in eating disorder recovery. Br J Soc Psychol. 2016; 55(4):662–80. https://doi.org/10.1111/bjso.12161.
7. Tajfel H, Turner JC, Austin WG, Worchel S. An integrative theory of intergroup conflict. Organ Identity Reader. 1979;56(65):9780203505984–16.
8. Turner JC, Hogg MA, Oakes PJ, Reicher SD, Wetherell MS. Rediscovering the social group: a self-categorization theory: Basil Blackwell; 1987.
9. Tajfel H. Social psychology of intergroup relations. Annu Rev Psychol. 1982; 33(1):1–39. https://doi.org/10.1146/annurev.ps.33.020182.000245.
10. Vandereycken W. Can eating disorders become 'contagious' in group therapy and specialized inpatient care? Eur Eat Disord Rev. 2011;19(4):289–95. https://doi.org/10.1002/erv.1087.
11. Billig M. Banal nationalism: sage; 1995.
12. Stevenson C, Muldoon OT. Socio-political context and accounts of national identity in adolescence. Br J Soc Psychol. 2010;49(3):583–99. https://doi.org/10.1348/014466609X475972
13. Walsh RS, Muldoon OT, Gallagher S, Fortune DG. Affiliative and "self-as-doer" identities: relationships between social identity, social support, and emotional status amongst survivors of acquired brain injury (ABI). Neuropsychol Rehabil. 2015;25(4):555–73. https://doi.org/10.1080/09602011.2014.993658.
14. Jetten J, Haslam SA, Cruwys T, Greenaway KH, Haslam C, Steffens NK. Advancing the social identity approach to health and well-being: progressing the social cure research agenda. Eur J Soc Psychol. 2017;47(7): 789–802. https://doi.org/10.1002/ejsp.2333.
15. Jetten J, Haslam C, Haslam SA, Dingle G, Jones JM. How groups affect our health and well-being: the path from theory to policy. Soc Issues Policy Rev. 2014;8(1):103–30. https://doi.org/10.1111/sipr.12003.
16. Limbert C. Perceptions of social support and eating disorder characteristics. Health Care Women Int. 2010;31(2):170–8. https://doi.org/10.1080/07399330902893846.
17. Cruwys T, Platow MJ, Rieger E, Byrne DG, Haslam SA. The social psychology of disordered eating: the situated identity enactment model. Eur Rev Soc Psychol. 2016;27(1):160–95. https://doi.org/10.1080/10463283.2016.1229891.
18. Cruwys T, Haslam SA, Fox NE, McMahon H. "That's not what we do": evidence that normative change is a mechanism of action in group interventions. Behav Res Ther. 2015;65:11–7. https://doi.org/10.1016/j.brat.2014.12.003.
19. Gruber KJ. Social support for exercise and dietary habits among college students. Adolescence. 2008;43(171):557–75.
20. Louis W, Davies S, Smith J, Terry D. Pizza and pop and the student identity: the role of referent group norms in healthy and unhealthy eating. J Soc Psychol. 2007;147(1):57–74. https://doi.org/10.3200/SOCP.147.1.57-74.
21. Neumark-Sztainer D, Paxton SJ, Hannan PJ, Haines J, Story M. Does body satisfaction matter? Five-year longitudinal associations between body satisfaction and health behaviors in adolescent females and males. J Adolesc Health. 2006;39(2):244–51. https://doi.org/10.1016/j.jadohealth.2005.12.001.
22. Ransom DC, La Guardia JG, Woody EZ, Boyd JL. Interpersonal interactions on online forums addressing eating concerns. Int J Eat Disord. 2010;43(2): 161–70. https://doi.org/10.1002/eat.20629.
23. Haas SM, Irr ME, Jennings NA, Wagner LM. Communicating thin: a grounded model of online negative enabling support groups in the pro-anorexia movement. New Media & Society. 2011;13(1):40–57. https://doi.org/10.1177/1461444810363910.
24. Williams C, Riley S. Finding support and negotiating identity. An analysis of the structure and content of newbie posts and their elicited replies on five pro-eating disorder websites. RESET. 2013;2(1):1–15. https://doi.org/10.4000/reset.117.
25. Leonidas C, Dos Santos MA. Social support networks and eating disorders: an integrative review of the literature. Neuropsychiatr Dis Treat. 2014;10:915.
26. Dingle GA, Cruwys T, Frings D. Social identities as pathways into and out of addiction. Front Psychol. 2015;6:1795.
27. Stevenson C, Doherty G, Barnett J, Muldoon OT, Trew K. Adolescents' views of food and eating: identifying barriers to healthy eating. J Adolesc. 2007; 30(3):417–34. https://doi.org/10.1016/j.adolescence.2006.04.005.
28. Best D, Beckwith M, Haslam C, Haslam SA, Jetten J, Mawson E, et al. Overcoming alcohol and other drug addiction as a process of social identity transition: the social identity model of recovery (SIMOR). Addict Res Theory. 2016;24(2):111–23. https://doi.org/10.3109/16066359.2015.1075980.
29. Buckingham SA, Frings D, Albery IP. Group membership and social identity in addiction recovery. Psychol Addict Behav. 2013;27(4):1132–40. https://doi.org/10.1037/a0032480.
30. Cullum J, O'Grady M, Sandoval P, Armeli S, Tennen H. Ignoring norms with a little help from my friends: social support reduces normative influence on drinking behavior. J Soc Clin Psychol. 2013;32(1):17–33. https://doi.org/10.1521/jscp.2013.32.1.17.
31. Faul F, Erdfelder E, Lang A-G, Buchner A. G*power 3: a flexible statistical power analysis program for the social, behavioral, and biomedical sciences. Behav Res Methods. 2007;39(2):175–91. https://doi.org/10.3758/BF03193146.
32. Ashmore RD, Deaux K, McLaughlin-Volpe T. An organizing framework for collective identity: articulation and significance of multidimensionality. Psychol Bull. 2004;130(1):80–114. https://doi.org/10.1037/0033-2909.130.1.80.
33. Sani F, Madhok V, Norbury M, Dugard P, Wakefield JR. Greater number of

group identifications is associated with healthier behaviour: evidence from a Scottish community sample. Br J Health Psychol. 2015;20(3):466–81. https://doi.org/10.1111/bjhp.12119.

34. Sherbourne CD, Stewart AL. The MOS social support survey. Soc Sci Med. 1991;32(6):705–14. https://doi.org/10.1016/0277-9536(91)90150-B.
35. Åstrosm AN, Rise J. Young adults' intention to eat healthy food: extending the theory of planned behaviour. Psychol Health. 2001;16(2):223–37. https://doi.org/10.1080/08870440108405501.
36. Smith JR, Louis WR. Do as we say and as we do: the interplay of descriptive and injunctive group norms in the attitude–behaviour relationship. Br J Soc Psychol. 2008;47(4):647–66. https://doi.org/10.1348/014466607X269748.
37. White KM, Smith JR, Terry DJ, Greenslade JH, McKimmie BM. Social influence in the theory of planned behaviour: the role of descriptive, injunctive, and in-group norms. Br J Soc Psychol. 2009;48(1):135–58. https://doi.org/10.1348/014466608X295207.
38. Fairburn CG, Beglin SJ. Assessment of eating disorders: interview or self-report questionnaire? Int J Eat Disord. 1994;16(4):363–70.
39. Hayes AF. Introduction to mediation, moderation, and conditional process analysis: a regression-based approach: Guilford Publications; 2017.
40. Cruwys T, Bevelander KE, Hermans RC. Social modeling of eating: a review of when and why social influence affects food intake and choice. Appetite. 2015;86:3–18. https://doi.org/10.1016/j.appet.2014.08.035.
41. Foran AM, O'Donnell AT, Muldoon OT. Stigma of eating disorders and recovery-related outcomes: a systematic review. Eur Eat Disord Rev. 2020; 28(4):385–97. https://doi.org/10.1002/erv.2735.
42. Bardone-Cone AM, Harney MB, Maldonado CR, Lawson MA, Robinson DP, Smith R, et al. Defining recovery from an eating disorder: conceptualization, validation, and examination of psychosocial functioning and psychiatric comorbidity. Behav Res Ther. 2010;48(3):194–202. https://doi.org/10.1016/j.brat.2009.11.001.
43. Galmiche M, Déchelotte P, Lambert G, Tavolacci MP. Prevalence of eating disorders over the 2000–2018 period: a systematic literature review. Am J Clin Nutr. 2019;109(5):1402–13. https://doi.org/10.1093/ajcn/nqy342.

21

Blind versus open weighing from an eating disorder patient perspective

Franzisca V. Froreich[1*], Sarah E. Ratcliffe[2] and Lenny R. Vartanian[1]

Abstract

Background: Weighing is a key component in the treatment of eating disorders. Most treatment protocols advocate for open weighing, however, many clinicians choose to use blind weighing, especially during the early phase of treatment. Despite considerable debate about this issue in the literature, there is no empirical evidence supporting the superiority of one weighing approach over the other. In addition, little is known about patients' perspectives of open and blind weighing and which weighing practice they view as more acceptable and/or beneficial for their treatment.

Methods: Semi-structured qualitative interviews were conducted with 41 women with a current or past diagnosis of Anorexia or Bulimia Nervosa: 26 were undergoing specialist inpatient treatment ($n = 13$ being blind weighed; $n = 13$ being open weighed) and 15 were community members who have recovered from an eating disorder. Interviews were audiotaped, transcribed verbatim and analysed thematically using framework methods. Participant demographics, clinical characteristics, weighing anxiety and weight concerns were also assessed.

Results: Qualitative analyses yielded five themes: *(1) therapy engagement and progress; (2) Control and tolerance of weight uncertainty; (3) treatment team relationships and autonomy; (4) life outside of treatment*; and *(5) weighing practice preferences and rationale.* Participants stated that blind weighing decreased anxiety and eating disorder psychopathology (e.g., weight preoccupation) and increased treatment responsivity. For many, relinquishing control over their weight facilitated body trust and was a necessary step towards recovery. Participants found that not knowing their exact weight helped challenge their overconcern with weight. Lack of support post-discharge was identified as a major difficulty of blind weighing. Overall, the majority of participants preferred blind weighing, particularly at the early, acute stage of treatment, whereas open weighing was viewed as more suitable at later stages of recovery. Quantitative analyses found current blind-weighed patients felt significantly less anxiety around being weighed and had greater tolerance of weight uncertainty than current open-weighed patients.

Conclusions: This study provided in-depth patient insights into open versus blind weighing practices. The next step for future research will be to supplement these insights with treatment outcomes gained from randomised controlled trials comparing the two weighing practices.

Keywords: Eating disorders, Open weighing, Blind weighing, Patient preferences, Qualitative

* Correspondence: franzisca.froreich@gmail.com
[1]School of Psychology, UNSW Sydney, Sydney 2052, Australia
Full list of author information is available at the end of the article

Plain English summary

Weighing is a key component in the treatment of eating disorders, but the particulars of how patients should be weighed (i.e., open vs. blind weighed) is a point of debate in the field. This study explored how current and recovered eating disorder patients ($N = 41$) view and have experienced open weighing and blind weighing in treatment. Analysis of interview data found that the majority of participants preferred blind weighing, particularly at the acute stage of treatment, whereas open weighing was viewed to be most suitable at lager stages of recovery. Participants thought that blind weighing decreased anxiety and eating disorder symptoms and as a result, increased their ability to effectively engage in their treatment. Survey data confirmed that current blind-weighed patients felt significantly less anxiety around being weighed and were more comfortable not knowing their weight than current open-weighed patients. The results of this study provide important insights into eating disorder patients' experiences with open and blind weighing practices and offer options for future research.

Background

In-session weighing is a prominent feature of eating disorder treatments, partly because of the need to monitor the physical safety of some patients [1]. There are two main approaches to weighing, "open weighing" and "blind weighing". Open weighing involves in-session weighing whereby the therapist and the patient check the patient's weight together. The number on the scale is read out loud to prevent avoidance of knowledge of weight. The weight is then plotted and interpreted on an individualised weight graph [2, 3]. Open weighing is grounded in the belief that repeated exposure to one's weight reduces patients' fear of being weighed and/or knowing their weight, and that open weighing provides an opportunity to modify the "broken cognition" many eating disorder patients have that consuming calorie-dense foods leads to exponential and uncontrollable weight gain [1, 4]. Conversely, blind weighing involves the therapist not sharing the patients' weight with her or him. When patients are blind weighed, they are usually asked to step on the scale backwards and the weight is not explicitly discussed [3]. The rationale for blind weighing includes the desire to minimise anxiety and distress that may result from patients seeing their weight (especially when it increases), reduce the patients' focus on the specific number on the scale, and expose patients to weight uncertainty [3, 5].

Two of the most widely established therapies for eating disorders, cognitive-behaviour therapy (CBT) and family-based treatment (FBT), both advocate for open weighing [1], yet specific and compelling evidence demonstrating that open weighing is preferable for patient outcomes is lacking. Moreover, weighing practices by eating disorder professionals, even those who endorse a CBT or FBT orientation, is far from unanimous: only about half of eating disorder clinicians subscribe to open weighing whereas the other half report using blind weighing procedures [3]. Forbush and colleagues [3] failed to find a significant association between endorsement of CBT or FBT and use of open weighing. Instead, their findings suggested that clinicians' decision to practice open or blind weighing depended on patient diagnosis and stage of treatment. Specifically, clinicians were more likely to practice blind weighing if patients were in the acute stages of treatment (and thus perhaps less stable or less committed to treatment) and/or if patients' cognitive or emotional functioning appeared to be impaired from malnourishment [3].

In addition to a lack of empirical evidence supporting the superiority of one weighing approach over the other, little is known about patients' perspectives of open and blind weighing and which weighing practices they view as more acceptable and/or beneficial for their treatment. Poor treatment engagement and premature termination of treatment are particularly common problems for eating disorder patients, with dropout rates ranging between 20 and 51% and 29–73% in inpatient and outpatient settings, respectively [6]. Given that weighing can be experienced as an anxiety-provoking event, it could conceivably contribute to difficulty engaging with the treatment. Thus, understanding patients' perspectives about weighing practices, and integrating their views into current treatments, could help improve client engagement and retention and, as a consequence, treatment outcomes in this population.

The present study used qualitative methodology to explore how current and recovered eating disorder patients view and have experienced open weighing and blind weighing in treatment. Eating disorder inpatients were chosen because they are weighed at a greater frequency than are outpatients (daily to twice weekly, compared to weekly, respectively) [7] and thus are most affected by weighing practices. To complement inpatient views, recovered community members were included to provide post-treatment perspectives that are less affected by the ambivalence which characterises eating disorders as well as to improve understanding of the long-term effects of open and blind weighing. The overall aims of this study were to elucidate: (1) patients' acceptance of open weighing and blind weighing; (2) the factors that shape patients' preferences for a particular approach to weighing; and (3) the impact that open weighing and blind weighing may have on therapy engagement and treatment outcomes including weighing anxiety, dysfunctional beliefs about weight, and intolerance of weight uncertainty.

Method

Participants

Current patients

Current female patients were recruited from two specialised eating disorder inpatient units: one which routinely blind weighs patients (blind weighing group; $n = 14$), and one which routinely open weighs patients (open weighing group; $n = 13$). To be eligible for this study, participants had to be at least 18 years old, diagnosed by the treating psychiatrist with anorexia nervosa (AN), bulimia nervosa (BN), or other specified feeding or eating disorders (OSFED), and have completed two or more weeks of inpatient treatment and hence be familiar with the weighing protocol. All inpatients (100%) approached by the study coordinator (FF) agreed to participate. One blind weighed patient was excluded from analysis because she felt unwell and terminated the interview early.

Recovered participants

Recovered female community members ($n = 22$) were recruited via expression of interest flyers posted on the social media platform of national eating disorders support organisations, the university's social media pages, the National Eating Disorder Collaboration's website, and dissemination via clinician emailing-lists. The study's advertisement indicated that the researchers were looking for women previously diagnosed with an eating disorder who were currently recovered. In this study, "recovered" was defined as no longer meeting the Diagnostic and Statistical Manual of Mental Disorder, Fifth Edition (DSM-5) [8] diagnostic criteria for an eating disorder. To screen for potential threshold or subthreshold eating disorder diagnoses, all recovered participants who expressed interest in the study were assessed using the Eating Disorder Diagnostic Scale – DSM-5 version (EDDS) [9]. Some respondents indicated not knowing their weight (EDDS item 19). For these cases a conservative approach was taken by treating them as if they met the weight criterion for diagnosis of AN; that is, it was assumed that they had a BMI ≤ 18.5. Six recovered participants were excluded because they met EDDS criteria for atypical AN ($n = 1$) and BN ($n = 1$) or did not respond to subsequent contact from FF ($n = 4$), resulting in 16 (72.7%) interviews. In addition, one participant was excluded after completing the interview because of incoherent and incongruent responses.

Recruitment continued until data saturation (i.e., no new information after three consecutive interviews) [10]. Ethical approval for all aspects of the study was obtained by the university's and the two hospitals' ethics committees.

Procedure

At the initial screening stage, FF who had no pre-existing relationship with any of the participants, introduced the nature and purpose of the study to interested participants. After obtaining written informed consent, a one-off face-to-face interview was conducted with participants in the inpatient units. For recovered participants, the interview was conducted over the telephone. The mean duration of current patients' and recovered participants' interviews were 10.69 min ($SD = 2.45$) and 26.86 min ($SD = 8.93$), respectively. Following the interview, participants were asked to complete a short survey online. Participants were debriefed by FF and reimbursed $10 for their participation.

Qualitative data collection

A semi-structured interview protocol (see Additional files 1 and 2) was purposely designed for this study in consultation with an experienced qualitative psychology researcher. The questions were guided by the study's research aims and existing hypotheses from the literature about the benefits and drawbacks of open and blind weighing. Parallel interview protocols were developed for current patients (open weighing and blind weighing) and recovered participants. During the interview, participants were asked about their experience with weighing in the context of the treatment for their eating disorder and any particular benefits and drawbacks they identified. Specifically, questions focused on if and how the weighing practice that they had experienced had affected their progress in treatment, motivation with treatment, ability to comply with meal plan, preoccupation with weight, anxiety around being weighed, and eating disorder symptomatology.

Quantitative measures

Eating disorder pathology in recovered participants was assessed using the 23-item EDDS which captures general eating disorder symptoms, as described in the DSM-5 [8]. Adequate criterion, predictive, and convergent validity, internal consistency, sensitivity, and test-retest reliability were documented for the version of the EDDS developed for DSM-IV [11, 12]. Although validation of the EDDS DSM-5 version is still underway, preliminary data regarding suggest high agreement of EDDS diagnoses with interview measures [13].

Participants' current weight concerns were assessed with five items developed for this study: Intolerance of weight uncertainty (1 item; "I need to know how much I weigh"), weight preoccupation (1 item; "I am preoccupied with my weight"), and weight importance (3 items; e.g., "My weight is very important to me"). Items were rated on a six-point scale from 1 (*Never*) to 6 (*Always*). Weight importance items were averaged, with higher scores indicating greater perceived importance of weight. Cronbach's alpha for the weight importance subscale was .94. In addition, a global weight concern score was calculated by averaging all five items. Cronbach's alpha for the global score was .96.

Weighing anxiety was measured using a visual analogue scale from 0 (*Not at all anxious*) to 100 (*Extremely anxious*). Current patients were asked to rate how anxious they felt being weighed in the context of treatment.

Recovered participants were asked to rate how anxious they would feel if they were weighed right now.

All participants reported their age and ethnicity. Recovered participants also reported their height and weight (if known), which were used to calculate their body mass index (BMI [kg/m^2]). For current patients, height and weight was retrieved from their medical records.

Table 1 Participant Demographic Characteristics

	BW M (SD)	OW M (SD)	Recovered M (SD)	Total M
N	13	13	15	41
Age	30.08 (10.60)	20.62 (2.59)	29.27 (10.21)	26.65
BMI	19.93 (3.56)	15.57 (3.30)	19.8 (3.54)	18.43
	n (%)	n (%)	n (%)	n (%)
Diagnosis				
AN	12 (92.3%)	12 (92.3%)	11 (73.3%)	35 (85.4%)
BN	1 (7.7%)	–	2 (13.3%)	3 (7.3%)
OSFED	–	1 (7.7%)	2 (13.3%)	3 (7.3%)
Treatment Exposure				
Open Weighing	–	5 (38.5%)	3 (20.0%)	8 (19.5%)
Blind Weighing	4 (30.8%)	–	2 (13.3%)	6 (14.6%)
Both	9 (69.2%)	8 (61.5%)	8 (53.3%)	25 (61.0%)
Other	–	–	2 (13.3%)	2 (4.9%)
Preference				
Open Weighing	1 (7.7%)	11 (84.6%)	3 (20.0%)	15 (36.6%)
Blind Weighing	12 (92.3%)	1 (7.7%)	11 (73.3%)	24 (58.5%)
Undetermined	0 (0%)	1 (7.7%)	1 (6.6%)	2 (4.9%)

Note. BW Blind weighing, *OW* Open weighing, *BMI* Body mass index, *AN* Anorexia nervosa, *BN* Bulimia nervosa, *OSFED* Other specified feeding or eating disorder

Data analyses

Questionnaire data were analysed with SPSS version 24.0. Audio-recorded interviews were transcribed verbatim and NVivo 11 was used for thematic analysis [14]. Thematic analysis followed the five main steps of Spencer and Ritchie's [15] framework method: (1) *Familiarisation with the data:* FF conducted all interviews, cross checked each transcript with the audio-recording and read each transcript several times; (2) *Creating a thematic framework:* a preliminary framework was based on independent analyses of 20% of transcripts by FF and a co-author with qualitative expertise (SR). Data were independently organised using themes and subthemes. Differences in interpretations of data were discussed until consensus was reached. (3) *Indexing:* adhering to the thematic framework, FF and SR independently coded all transcripts using NVivo11. Any new themes or questions that emerged during this process were collaboratively discussed and revisions made correspondingly. To ensure methodological rigour, all transcripts were then independently cross-coded by FF and SR and discrepancies discussed and resolved with input from LV. (4) *Charting:* themes and supporting quotes from each transcript were entered into a framework matrix. The matrix was composed using Microsoft Excel as a computerised qualitative data analysis tool [16], with participants as rows and themes as column. (5) *Mapping and Interpretation*: the framework matrix was analysed within and across themes and participants to identify patterns and relationships.

Results

Descriptive statistics

Table 1 presents the demographic and clinical characteristics for all three samples. Blind weighed patients and recovered participants did not differ in their mean age or BMI, but open weighed patients were significantly younger and had lower BMIs than did both blind weighed patients and recovered participants.

Qualitative findings

Qualitative analyses yielded five inter-related themes: (1) therapy engagement and progress; (2) control and tolerance of weight uncertainty; (3) treatment team relationships and autonomy; (4) life outside of treatment; and (5) weighing practice preferences and rationale. Themes found were represented among all three groups, with blind weighed patients and recovered participants expressing concordant views toward weighing practices (i.e., a preference for blind weighing), whereas open weighed patients expressed stronger preference for open weighing than blind weighing. Illustrative quotes are presented in Tables 2, 3, 4, 5 and 6. Because the majority of participants (61.0%; $n = 25$) had been exposed to both open and blind weighing across their treatment history, their responses were grouped together and are described with respect to the particular weighing practice that was being discussed rather than presenting the results separately by participant groups.

Theme 1: therapy engagement and progress

Within this theme, three subthemes were identified.

Weighing experience Participants' experience of being weighed differed depending on whether they saw or did not see their weight when stepping on the scale. When open weighed, participants described weighing days as anxiety-, fear-, and stress-ridden. Negative emotions and thoughts about being weighed often started the day prior to being weighed, impacting participants' sleep and triggering urges to engage in compensatory and self-harm behaviours. Similarly, following open weighing, participants reported experiencing distress, low mood, rumination, and worry which did not improve until the end of the day. In contrast, blind weighing was described as quick and routine-like. Leading up to weighing, participants

Table 2 Illustrative Participant Quotations for Theme 1: Therapy Engagement and Progress

Subtheme		Illustrative participant quotations
1.1 Weighing experience	BW	*"There is a lot less anxiety around [being weighed] ... I just kind of get it over and done with. Because I'm not, dreading it really, since I'm not seeing it. I don't love it, but I'm not dreading it the same way I was."* (Reduced anxiety, BW109) *"I feel a bit anxious for a bit, but then I'm like, 'whatever', and just go do something."* (Reduced anxiety, OW112) *"[BW] was quick and painless, you just kind of get up, get weighed go back to bed"* (Reduced anxiety, R315)
	OW	*"I'm more stressed before weighing days, and then the day I'm being weighed, thinking about it more probably … I get anxious, tossing and turning, I think about it, I catastrophise like 'oh my god it's gone up 10 kg it's probably gone up this much, it's gonna [sic] be this weight. If it's up this high I'll do such and such, if it's below this I'll do such and such."* (Increased anxiety, OW211) *"Yeah I think that weighing days were definitely the worst ones … you'd wake up and you'd know that you have to be weighed and it was, you know when you get that pit in your stomach where you kind of want to throw up, it was like that."* (Increased anxiety, R315)
1.2 Therapy engagement	BW	*"I think sometimes [BW] can exaggerate or catastrophise what your thoughts are because you don't have any evidence, like you can eat something you are scared of and think 'Oh my god it's going to make me gain 5 kg' and then you don't really have any way of proving it wrong? Which I think can be hard. But obviously, I know like if I said that, my treatment team would happily provide me evidence that it didn't make me gain a ridiculous amount of weight. But I think that can be hard."* (Distorted cognitions about weight gain, BW113) *"Not knowing [my weight helps me comply with my meal plan], because then I'm not kind of obsessed about a number all the time and I'm just doing what I have to do really."* (Increased meal plan compliance, BW102) *"I was like well I don't know my weight. Yes it's terrifying but at the same time it meant that I focused on getting through my meal and focused on my psychology sessions and the group therapy that we did instead of 'oh my weight was this today' … I guess it was just one less thing that I had to deal with."* (Increased therapy engagement, R315) *"The more you check something the more it might be on your mind and by not checking my weight it was something that became less and less pronounced in my day to day [routine]."* (Reduced weight preoccupation, R310)
	OW	*"The longer I get into the admission and the more weight I gain, I get more preoccupied with it [my weight] and I get more anxious.* (Increased weight preoccupation, OW212) *"Obviously if it's gone up more than I'm comfortable with I'm less likely to comply [with my meal plan]. The other week I only drank supplements for the whole day, and refused to get out of the bed other than for meals because of the number jumping up"* (Increased resistance to meal plan, OW211) *"Being open weighed definitely impacted on my motivation and ability to stick to meal plan. It made me work "against" therapy and made it harder to comply."* (Increased resistance to meal plan and reduced motivation, R311)
1.3. Progress	BW	*"Initially, it was worse...not knowing, predicting the worst, I guess. But then after a couple of weeks, you kind of got used to it and now it's a bit more peaceful."* (Early adjustment difficulties, OW213) *"[BW] keeps your mind on track of the end result which is getting better. It doesn't leave you with all these preoccupations and distractions."* (Reduced preoccupation, OW110) *"[BW] was in many ways the only way that I had to learn to not put all the emphasis into my own weight. That, by not knowing my weight, I had to learn to be comfortable not knowing it, and therefore not emphasizing it."* (Reduced weight importance, R306)
	OW	*"If it [my weight] goes up I tend to get very anxious and tend not to want to do the right things in my treatment, and I want to go home."* (Treatment resistance, OW212) *"I think like weighing for me was the thing that probably kept me back the most when I decided to recover."* (Barrier to recovery, R315) *"I think it's important for us to see the weight go up because it's what's needed, and it will help rationalise those thoughts that if you eat something, you're not going to magically gain 10 kg, like most of us think."* (Challenging of distorted weight beliefs, OW209)

Note. BW: Quotes relating to blind weighing; OW: Quotes relating to open weighing; BW# blind weighed inpatient; OW#, open weighed inpatient; R#, recovered participant

expressed little to no negative thoughts about their weight. Although anxiety was experienced by many immediately before stepping on the scale, participants appeared to be able to recover quickly and refocus on their treatment.

Therapy engagement Participants noted that weighing practices influenced their motivation, meal plan compliance, compensatory behaviour engagement, rumination, and therapy engagement, especially on weighing days. Open weighing was said to decrease motivation ($n = 14$), increase resistance to meal plan compliance ($n = 23$), and increase engagement in compensatory behaviours ($n = 22$). Open weighing was further thought to trigger increased rumination and preoccupation with weight ($n = 22$) which was reported to negatively impact on therapy engagement immediately following weighing. In contrast, blind weighing was reported to maintain motivation towards recovery and treatment ($n = 5$), improve meal plan compliance ($n = 15$), and reduce urges to engage in compensatory behaviours ($n = 10$). However, not knowing one's exact weight in blind weighing was noted to lead to catastrophic cognitions about possible weight gain because of the lack of evidence to disconfirm one's distorted beliefs ($n = 11$).

Treatment progress The majority of participants identified open weighing as a hindrance to recovery. Being exposed to one's weight was said to increase anxiety ($n =$

Table 3 Illustrative Participant Quotations for Theme 2: Control and Tolerance of Weight Uncertainty

Subtheme		Illustrative participant quotations
2.1 Need of control	BW	*"Especially because once you're in here [treatment], you have no control … and sometimes you just want to hold onto one thing. And not just another thing that you lose."* (Need for control, BW111)
	OW	*"I would never be blind weighed. … what I care about is numbers. If I don't know the number, then I don't feel in control … It's like the one thing you can control … you don't have control over how much petrol is going to be, if there's going to be red lights or green lights, you don't have control if there's going to be crashes. So, the one constant thing I can control is what I put in my body and what my weight will be."* (Need for control, OW211) *"If you knew the number, there was a kind of disorder mindset where it had to keep going down and if it wasn't, then that wasn't okay."* (Need for control over weight, R310) *"[If I had been OW], I don't think I could've been able to keep going once I saw that I had hit a certain number."* (Acceptable number, R316)
2.2 Tolerance of Weight Uncertainty	BW	*"[BW] is definitely good that you don't have that preoccupation around the number, but still there's a worry that obviously you constantly have about how much you are weighing and how much weight you are gaining doing this program."* (Intolerance of weight uncertainty, BW110) *"I've been in other clinics where I have had to see my weight every week and it's been traumatising, and it sucks. And like, I find ignorance is bliss."* (Reduced weight-related anxiety, BW113) *"I think it's just one less thing to worry about... I think that it's very easy to fixate on individual numbers and figures whereas what I think is most important in here is the overall trend... and I just find it less stressful not having another number to deal with in my head, as long as I know that my weight is going up, that's all I really need to know."* (Reduced weight-related anxiety, BW107) *"For me personally, there is a bit less fear around weight change at the moment because I'm not going to see the weight change. Like, I just kind of have to accept whatever's happening and just roll with it, since I can't see it."* (Reduced weight-related anxiety, BW109) *"I don't think normal people would like, would weigh themselves like every day. It's not something they think about, they might just do it.... I would, probably like to just never have to weigh myself again, and not care about it. And just be healthy."* (Normalising lack of control over weight, BW106) *"Having to relinquish that control [over my weight] was terrifying but was also a huge relief and it really helped me to learn to be at peace with my body and to trust [my body]."* (Increased body trust, R310) *"When I think about what I want my life to be in recovery, I don't want to know, and I want to be okay not knowing, because to me, that sounds like a more free life to me, than one where I have to know."* (Tolerance of weight uncertainty, R316) *"I think it [BW] kind of sets the platform for you to then be able to then take the focus off the weight when you go back into the real world and to be able to go 'actually it [not knowing my weight] hasn't killed me, it's not the worst thing in the world, and it's okay."* (Tolerance of weight uncertainty, R315) *"I don't weigh myself now. I am happy knowing that I look and feel healthy.* "(Tolerance of weight uncertainty, R304)
	OW	*"I couldn't cope [not seeing the number]."* (Inability to cope with weight uncertainty, OW211)
2.3 ED-Self vs. Healthy-Self	BW	*It annoys me [not seeing my weight], but at the same time, that's my eating disorder that it annoys, but like, for my healthy self, it's good."* (Need for control is ED-driven, BW101) *"[BW] takes control away from the eating disorder rather than the person."* (Need for control is ED-driven, BW109) *"I feel like my eating disorder was very much like control, and about controlling... just my life. And it was, as soon as I let go of the control of the scales … it was easier to just let that part of me go. So that control... that inner voice that had control over me just went away."* (Need for control is ED-driven, R302) *"I do know of other people … that did see their number … they would feel really shit about it but still maintain 'oh no it's important that I see it because I know where my weight is' and I was like 'is it important for you or is it important for your eating disorder?'"* (Need for control is ED-driven, R310) *"As soon as I stopped looking at the scales, I had to stop thinking about the number, and it stopped controlling me … then I learnt how to eat better...and treat my body well, and it wasn't about losing weight or gaining weight because I just let it go."* (Increased body trust, R311)
2.4 Food-Weight Associations	BW	*"I guess because it's over the week, and we have three weigh-ins. I don't know when I gained the most weight or anything. I just know the overall trend so that means I can't pinpoint to 'oh my god that was that meal!' BW helps not associating certain weight gains with certain meals."* (Challenged food-weight associations, BW105)
	OW	*"I just think it [OW] would be so much harder to like complete meals or like keep going forward because the thoughts in your head, it's saying like 'Oh, if I eat this I'm going to gain weight" and then you're actually seeing it happen, it's like reinforcing it all.'* (Maintenance of food-weight associations, BW113) *One part of me wants to know [my weight] I guess so I can micromanage things, and be like, 'Okay, what do you think would have tipped it over?'"* (Maintenance of food-weight associations, OW213) *"If numbers had been there and it had been tracked closely I think for me personally it would have been really hard to separate those really intertwined concepts of food and weight."* (Maintenance of food-weight associations, R310)

Note. BW: Quotes relating to blind weighing; OW: Quotes relating to open weighing; BW# blind weighed inpatient; OW#, open weighed inpatient; R#, recovered participant

16), trigger eating disorder behaviours in an attempt to control one's weight ($n = 17$), and maintain both the patient's and treatment team's focus on weight ($n = 7$). Further, participants found that exposure to their weight fuelled their ambivalence towards recovery and increased resistance towards treatment ($n = 11$). Although

Table 4 Illustrative Participant Quotations for Theme 3: Treatment Team Relationships and Autonomy

Subtheme		Illustrative participant quotations
3.1 Treatment autonomy	BW	*"I found it [BW] very like punitive in some ways. Like I don't know I'm an adult and I just felt like I was a child being like weighed backwards and then kind of like in trouble if it wasn't the outcome that was hoped for or something like that."* (Lack of treatment autonomy, R316)
	OW	*"You can see how your weight is going up steadily, and your meal plan's working. Whereas if they were to just increase your meal plan and you're like, 'why?', it kind of answers some of those questions."* (Treatment progress feedback, NW213) *"I feel like knowing the number includes you in the conversation with the treatment team."* (Inclusion in treatment conversations, NW207) *"I can't see any benefits [to OW] other than feeling a little more autonomous and "normal"."* (Increased treatment autonomy, R304) *"It was good to feel like I had some autonomy and was allowed to see it although I guess I could equally be autonomous choosing not to see the weight right?"* (Role of autonomy in treatment, R304)
3.2 Trust in treatment team	BW	*"I like that they are in control of my weight and I can't know it. They just showed you what your [weight trend] was doing and I liked that, if you did it with someone you trusted."* (Importance of trust in treatment, N101) *"In the beginning I hated it … I always used to think like, 'oh no, they're lying, they're lying, they're lying, they're lying' … but I think after coming to [BW facility] now for a year, and I know now that my relationship with [psychiatrist and psychologist], I know that I can trust them, like a 100%. Now it's kind of nice as well to give the control over to someone else."* (Importance of trust in treatment, N112) *"I think those are the two things you really lose sight off when you're unwell you, there's so much control and so little trust and [BW] kind of just turns it on its head."* (Importance of trust, R310) *"I previously had a psychologist that completely lied to me about my weight so it got -- like, a really long time and just, it's made me petrified. She used to say, 'No I won't let you look.' And I would say, 'Well, is it below this number?' And she would say, 'Yes.' And then one day I found out that she had been lying all that time."* (Need for honesty, NW209)
3.3 Strategies for Enhancing Autonomy and Trust	u/s	*"I wish we had the ability to kind of… Talk to somebody about it [best weighing practice], without being shut down."* (Involvement in treatment decision-making, N108) *"I feel that the way they do it here is quite good with giving you a choice…challenging 'Hey do you want to try and see your number and have therapy around that while you're here?"* (Choice, NW213) *"During therapy, I knew my weight at some stages and then I didn't know it at others. It depended in what the therapist thought was best. I sometimes felt like I wasn't being asked, I wasn't being treated like a "normal person" who could be trusted and could take responsibility of it. Perhaps it would have been good to have that discussion with me and see if it was a "recovery day" where I felt capable of seeing it or not."* (Involvement in treatment decision-making, R304)

Note. BW: Quotes relating to blind weighing; OW: Quotes relating to open weighing; BW# blind weighed inpatient; OW#, open weighed inpatient; R#, recovered participant

Table 5 Illustrative Participant Quotations for Theme 4: Life Outside of Treatment

Subtheme		Illustrative participant quotations
4.1 Weighing, weight exposure, and discharge support	BW	*"While being here it's better not to know but then I'm going to go home and I'm going to find out the number and then, like, what are we going to do?"* (Lack of support post-discharge, BW103) *"[BW] didn't help you deal… with weight… They'd just let you out and you'd go home and you'd be a higher weight and you'd have to deal with it."* (Lack of support post-discharge, OW205) *"I feel like sometimes you're faced with it … unexpectedly like at a doctor's appointment … Then it's like such a big difference from what you last saw. And then it's just like… It ruins everything."* (Weighing is inevitable, BW108)
	OW	*"I prefer to know, so that I can get help dealing with it. Because when I'm at home, if I get weighed, I have to so often get weighed, I need to know how to deal with it."* (Support dealing with weight exposure, OW205)
4.2 Weight change awareness	BW	*"Not knowing my weight doesn't mean that like, I'm not, like conscious, that I'm not aware that it's changing.* (Weight change awareness without numbers, BW101) *"Even if you can't see [your weight] like you know it's still happening, and you can be told that you weight is trending upwards or it's going in the right direction or whatever but, it doesn't reinforce [the food-weigh associations] as much in your head."* (Weight change awareness without numbers, BW113) *"I'm aware I'm gaining weight without seeing the number …. I guess when you leave, if you did weigh yourself, it could be a bit of a shock. But to be honest, they give us enough feedback I kinda [sic] know where I would sit."* (Weight change awareness without numbers, BW105)

Note. BW: Quotes relating to blind weighing; OW: Quotes relating to open weighing; BW# blind weighed inpatient; OW#, open weighed inpatient; R#, recovered participant

Table 6 Illustrative Participant Quotations for Theme 5: Weighing Practice Preferences

Subtheme		Illustrative participant quotations
5.1 Open Weighing	OW	*"I like to see the number … Like I can't sit comfortably if I don't know."* (Need for Control, OW201) *"I think it's a way I can see progress, and it gives a sense of comfort I guess, in terms of just knowing what your body is doing."* (Progress feedback, OW207) *"I'm finding it [OW] more useful because then I can kind of rationalise that you know that you know I gained like 2 or 3 k in a week when that's not the truth. So, it kind of helps me challenge the eating disorder a bit by knowing that you're wrong, because I only gained this much. But I always prefer to know."* (Cognitive challenging, OW210) *"Blind weighing was the worst because it gave me that panicky feeling of not knowing."* (Intolerance of weight uncertainty, R309)
5.2 Blind Weighing	BW	*"I think not knowing makes treatment, I think it, sort of takes it away from the weight, and it's just what your body is supposed to be."* (Reduced weight importance, BW106) *"I think it's just one less thing to worry about... I think that it's very easy to fixate on individual numbers and figures whereas what I think is most important in here is the overall trend."* (Reduced anxiety and preoccupation with weight, BW107) *"I think it [BW] kind of sets the platform for you to then be able to then take the focus off the weight when you go back into the real world and to be able to go "actually it hasn't killed me it's not the worst thing in the world and it's okay."* (Exposure to weight uncertainty, R315) *"[not seeing my weight] certainly helps me to make progress and be much healthier on a day to day basis"* (Progress towards recovery, R311)
5.3 Blind weighing adaptations	BW	*"At [BW treatment facility] they had a weight graph … it didn't have numbers, it just showed you what your weight was doing...and I like that … it's … a little bit of exposure."* (Weight Graph, BW101) *"BMI banding gave me some safeguards … I would know where I might be sitting … I think it's kind of exposure [to weight gain] but without exposure to the actual kilo amount. Banding for me gave me leeway of the flexibility of being able to move up and down, so 100 g wouldn't send me into panic, you know, if I moved from, I don't know, 40 kg to 40.1 kg then knowing that would send me spiralling into anxiety … but not seeing those really small incremental changes, I think reduced … the emphasis that I had on my weight, but the bands still meant that I didn't feel like I was out of control."* (BMI Banding, R306)
5.4 Stage of Treatment	BW	*"I think during the weight gain process, [blind weighing] definitely makes things a lot easier. Like obviously it's not completely, stress free... But … if I were continuing to see my weight go up I'd be a lot more stressed out. So... I think it helps a little bit with the motivation to keep following my meal plan, and stuff like that, and comply."* (Acute stage, BW108) *"I would say for girls who have first come in that, perhaps blind weighing is more beneficial … Because the eating disorder voice is so strong, and any upwards movement it doesn't matter if it's 200 g or 2 kg, I think that that would completely freak you out and you'd be a mess for that whole day I'd imagine after weighing. And your head would be screaming at you to not follow the program."* (Acute stage, OW207)
	OW	*"[OW] definitely not early on. Perhaps when you start being on the recovery road you may discuss it with the clinician and together decide what would be best. But even when I thought I was ready later it turned out that I wasn't so maybe patients wouldn't have that insight …? Perhaps when fear of weight change is gone you can start seeing the weight …"* (Best timing for OW, R304)

Note. BW: Quotes relating to blind weighing; OW: Quotes relating to open weighing; BW# blind weighed inpatient; OW#, open weighed inpatient; R#, recovered participant

participants noted these adverse effects of open weighing, many valued being exposed to their weight while in treatment where they had access to support from their treatment team (as opposed to at home post-discharge where they had less support; $n = 6$). Participants also acknowledged that exposure to the number could help disconfirm irrational beliefs about the relationship between food intake and weight gain ($n = 10$), challenge disturbances in self-perceived weight gain (e.g., feeling that one is gaining weight when body weight is stable), and help with weight acceptance ($n = 13$).

Blind weighing was largely seen has having a positive impact on participant's progress towards recovery ($n = 32$). Initially, participants struggled to adjust to the blind weighing protocol, identifying feelings of lack of control, uncertainty over their weight and catastrophic cognitions about possible weight gain to be most challenging ($n = 11$). However, participants also reported that, over time, they experienced reduced preoccupation with weight ($n = 22$). They described being able to "let go" of thoughts about weight more easily because they did not have any evidence to reinforce their fears. Participants also found blind weighing to help challenge the importance placed on weight and the need to control their weight ($n = 22$). Participants explained that blind weighing took the focus away from weight and helped them "direct their attention elsewhere" (BW107),[1] especially towards other aspects of recovery. Participants also commented that not knowing their weight forced them to stop determining their self-worth based on weight. Additionally, blind weighing was seen to promote a recovery mindset supporting movement towards recovery goals instead of eating disorder goals ($n = 10$).

[1]Codes associated with particular responses reflect the following: BW, blind weighed inpatient; OW, open weighed inpatient; R, recovered participant; #, participant number.

Theme 2: control and tolerance of weight uncertainty
Within this theme, four subthemes were identified.

Need for control The need for control was a phenomenon noted in all three samples and raised at various points throughout the interviews. Specifically, not seeing one's weight was linked to not being in control. Participants who endorsed open weighing reasoned that they "don't feel in control" (OW211) unless they are privy to their exact weight information ($n = 8$). Treatment was perceived to threaten participants' sense of control because they were not able to engage in disordered eating behaviours such as dietary restriction, self-induced vomiting, or excessive exercise. In this context, not knowing one's weight was seen as yet another form of losing control. Further, participants felt the need to monitor their weight to ensure that it was lower than or did not exceed what they perceived to be an "acceptable weight" each time they were weighed ($n = 8$).

Tolerance of weight uncertainty When participants were blind weighed, they commonly struggled with weight uncertainty and feelings of lack of control ($n = 16$). For some participants, being kept in the dark regarding their weight while their treating team knew their weight was the most challenging aspect of treatment ($n = 4$). In spite of these challenges, participants saw the benefits of blind weighing in that it relieved some of the anxiety associated with weight change, reduced their preoccupation with weight and, as a result, allowed them to focus on recovery instead of the number on the scale ($n = 16$). Furthermore, tolerance of weight uncertainty was viewed as something worth striving for because it was regarded as a marker of recovery ($n = 10$). In fact, many recovered participants preferred not to weigh themselves post-treatment, commenting that the need to control their weight was associated with their eating disorder ($n = 12$). Instead, recovered participants preferred to rely on non-weight related markers to determine their level of "health" or "well-being," including the fit of their clothing, reflection in the mirror, or food consumed ($n = 8$).

ED-self vs. healthy-self Participants referred to the "Eating Disorder-Self" and "Healthy-Self" as two distinct mindsets which influenced their need for control and knowing their weight ($n = 21$). The Eating Disorder-Self (ED-Self) was described as a separate, disordered self that kept participants trapped in the obsession of controlling their weight. The need to know one's weight (and, therefore, feeling in control of one's weight) was viewed as intrinsically connected to the eating disorder and hence pathological. Thus, when participants identified their ED-Self to be more dominant than their Healthy-Self, there was a preference for open weighing. The Healthy-Self, on the other hand, was described as the side of the self which desires recovery and to "do the right thing," including giving up control over weight. Blind weighing was perceived as an opportunity to practice tolerating weight ambiguity and normalise the lack of control over weight. Amongst recovered participants, there was also specific reflection on how blind weighing helped rebuild body trust. Rather than eating (or not eating) in response to the number on the scale, participants reported increased trust and reliance on their body's natural hunger and fullness signals. Furthermore, participants explained that blind weighing helped change the rationale for food and eating from sources for controlling one's weight and shape to sources for looking after one's body.

Food-weight associations A subset of participants reflected on how different weighing practices affected their beliefs about the relationship between ingestion of specific foods and their weight. When participants saw their weight, they attributed weight changes to specific foods previously consumed ($n = 6$). If, for example, participants had eaten a "feared food" and experienced increased weight, the weight increase would be attributed to the feared food, reinforcing dysfunctional beliefs associated with that particular food. In contrast, blind weighing seemed to help break some of these links by providing limited or no weight information at all ($n = 5$).

Theme 3: treatment autonomy and team relationships
Within this theme, three subthemes were identified.

Treatment autonomy Treatment autonomy was highly valued by participants across groups ($n = 10$). Participants expressed the belief that open weighing satisfies autonomy because it provides them with regular progress feedback (e.g., whether they are reaching their weight goals), evokes a sense of responsibility and ownership over their treatment, includes them in treatment conversations, and helps clarify changes to treatment (e.g., meal plan modifications). Open weighing also made participants feel as though they were "treated like a 'normal person' who could be trusted and could take responsibility" of their own treatment (R304). In comparison, blind weighing was associated with feeling "powerless" (BW107), "like a child" (R316) who could not be given responsibility, and excluded from treatment decisions.

Trust in treatment team Trust in the treatment team was considered key for successful blind weighing ($n = 14$). Participants explained that, after establishing trust in their treating professionals, they were able to relinquish control over their weight. In contrast, when trust was compromised, participants reported continued self-weighing outside of the treatment program and increased treatment resistance.

Strategies for enhancing autonomy and trust Participants highlighted that autonomy could be enhanced by providing a sense of choice over weighing practices. Participants strongly valued participation in treatment decision-making, including consultation about their views and preferences. Further, psychoeducation about the rationale for different treatment strategies (including weighing) and treatment decision-making transparency were viewed as important in facilitating patient cooperation and reducing anxiety. In this context, participants commented that alterations to blind weighing that included some weight feedback without disclosing actual numbers (e.g., whether or not the person had made a significant weight gain or loss of more than 1.5 kg) could help increase trust in the treatment team and explain (otherwise unexpected) changes to treatment (e.g., meal plan increases).

Theme 4: life outside of treatment

Within this theme, two subthemes were identified.

Weighing, weight exposure, and discharge support Participants feared that exposure to their weight post-discharge would be confronting following blind weighing. Some participants deemed weighing to be "inevitable" ($n = 4$; e.g., in the context of a doctor's appointment) and participants were concerned about their ability to cope and about possible relapse following weight confrontation on or post-discharge when they no longer had therapist support ($n = 15$). Continued blind weighing by the outpatient team on discharge from the inpatient program or gradual weight exposure throughout treatment were identified by participants as strategies to manage weight exposure post-discharge.

Weight change awareness Participants reported that the number on the scale was not the only indicator of weight change ($n = 7$). Blind weighing participants expressed that, although they did not see the number when weighed, they were aware of shifts in their body weight based on fit of clothes and appearance in mirrors. Others found nonspecific feedback about their weight during blind weighing to be helpful to gain a sense of their progress (see Theme 5). Participants further elaborated that *nonspecific* weight information helped prevent unnecessary fixation on a *specific* number while providing enough information regarding weight change to prevent overt shock if they were incidentally weighed post-discharge.

Theme 5: weighing practice preferences and rationale

Within this theme, four subthemes were identified.

Preference Weighing practice preferences differed with current treatment condition, although across all samples blind weighing was preferred by 58.5% ($n = 24$) of participants and open weighing by 36.6% ($n = 15$). Among recovered participants, 73.3% ($n = 11$) preferred blind weighing.

Open weighing Participants who preferred open weighing ($n = 15$) expressed a strong "need" to know their weight, mainly to feel in control. Participants imagined or had previously experienced distress regarding "not knowing" their exact weight during blind weighing. Open weighing was reasoned to provide progress feedback, facilitate weight habituation, and help challenge exaggerated weight gain beliefs.

Blind weighing Participants who preferred blind weighing ($n = 23$) thought that it relieves anxiety associated with weight change, shifts therapy from being predominantly weight-centred to focus on other aspects of the disorder and recovery, and facilitates body trust. Participants reported reduced engagement in eating disorder symptoms, less preoccupation with weight, and increased capability to engage in recovery. Further, some participants reported a preference for modified blind weighing ($n = 6$), that is the indication of weight changes without disclosing exact weight. Examples included the use of a numberless *weight graph* (graph depicts the weight trend but no specific numbers), *BMI banding* (patients are told when they move up or down a BMI band when their weight is in the "new band" for three consecutive readings), *significant weight gain or loss* (what is considered "significant" depends on the agreement between therapist and client), *meeting guideline* (confirmation whether a patient has met treatment guidelines regarding weekly weight gain), or *no gram information* (patient sees the kilograms on the scale but not the grams). Having an estimate of one's weight was reported as helpful to challenging distorted cognitions about weight gain and providing a sense of security and control which facilitated trust in the treatment team and tolerance of weight uncertainty.

Stage of treatment Participants' weighing practice preference was related to stage of treatment. Blind weighing was rationalised to be most appropriate in the early, acute stages when the ED-Self is likely to be stronger than the Healthy-Self. Participants argued that blind weighing can shield patients from distress associated with weight change and thus improve therapy engagement and progress. At the same time, participants reflected on the importance of patients understanding the rationale for blind weighing, "being ready," and trusting the treatment team for blind weighing to be effective. Conversely, open weighing was viewed as more suitable

Table 7 Group Mean (SD) Ratings of Quantitative Variables

	OW *M (SD)*	BW *M (SD)*	Recovered *M (SD)*
Weight-Related Anxiety	86.48 (11.67)[a]	57.80 (25.87)[b]	48.97 (29.72)[b]
Weight Concerns	5.25 (0.75)[a]	4.86 (1.04)[a]	2.27 (0.84)[b]
• Intolerance of Weight Uncertainty	5.62 (0.65)[a]	4.31 (1.55)[b]	
• Weight Preoccupation	5.23 (1.09)	5.23 (0.93)	
• Weight Importance	5.13 (0.90)	4.92 (1.06)	

Note. OW: Open Weighing; BW: Blind Weighing. Means within a row with a different superscript are significantly different at $p < .05$. Subscale analyses for differences between current and recovered patients were not conducted

at later stages of recovery when patients are "in a better head space" and cognitive challenging has more potential to be effective.

Quantitative findings

Weighing anxiety and weight concerns

Two separate Analyses of Variance (ANOVAs) were conducted to test for differences among the three samples (i.e., open weighing, blind weighing, recovered) in their reaction to being weighed (i.e., weight-related anxiety) and/or overall concern with weight. Group mean ratings of each variable are presented in Table 7. Results revealed a significant effect of sample on both weighing anxiety, $F\ (2,\ 38) = 9.02$, $p = .001$, $\eta_p^2 = .32$, and overall weight concerns, $F\ (2,\ 38) = 47.77$, $p < .001$, $\eta_p^2 = .72$. Post hoc comparisons using the Tukey HSD test indicated that mean weight-related anxiety for the open weighing group was significantly higher than it was for the blind weighing group ($p = .004$) and the recovered group ($p < .001$). The blind weighing group and the recovered group were not significantly different in weight-related anxiety ($p = .339$). Furthermore, recovered participants scored significantly lower on the weight concern scale than did both the blind weighing group ($p < .001$) and open weighing group ($p < .001$). There was no statistically significant difference on weight concerns between the two current patient groups ($p = .275$).

A follow-up two-tailed independent samples t-test was conducted to examine whether the two current patient samples (open weighing and blind weighing) differed in their scores on any of the three subscales comprising the weight concern scale.[2] The results showed that open weighed patients reported significantly greater intolerance of weight uncertainty compared to blind weighed patients, $t(24) = 2.81$, $p = .002$, $d = 1.10$. Mean scores on the subscales, weight preoccupation and weight importance, were not significantly different.

Discussion

Weighing is an established component of the treatment of eating disorders but there is little available data to indicate whether open or blind weighing is ideal. The current study explored how current and recovered eating disorder patients view and experience blind and open weighing practices. The findings provide insights into the acceptability of weighing practices and their perceived impact on therapy engagement and treatment outcomes.

In this study, most participants preferred blind weighing over open weighing. Consistent with eating disorder clinicians' views [3], participants deemed blind weighing particularly beneficial in the acute stages of treatment when change ambivalence is most prominent. Participants thought that blind weighing decreased anxiety and eating disorder psychopathology (e.g., weight preoccupation, urges to engage in compensatory behaviours) and that blind weighing therefore increased their ability to engage and progress in treatment. In comparison, the majority of participants identified open weighing as a barrier to recovery, particularly throughout weight restoration, when seeing the number on the scale was thought to have negative effects on motivation, anxiety levels, urges to engage in compensatory behaviours, and treatment responsivity. Instead, participants saw merit in exposure to the number on the scale (i.e., open weighing) when in a better headspace during the later stages of recovery because it allowed them to challenge distorted cognitions regarding their weight. Patients' accounts of increased distress when exposed to their weight were supported by quantitative findings in this study in which open weighing was associated with significantly greater weight-related anxiety than blind weighing. Based on the current findings, withholding weight information early in treatment may be beneficial as a means of reducing weight-related anxiety and maximising treatment engagement. Early response to treatment can help prevent premature treatment dropout [17] and is predictive of better outcomes [18]. Thus, at least in the early stages of treatment, it makes

[2]Note that analyses of differences on weight concern subscales were only conducted for current patient groups to determine whether the two weighing practices had a differential effect on these variables. The majority of recovered participants (53.3%) had been both open and blind weighed throughout their treatment and so changes on these variables in the recovered group could not be attributed to a specific weighing practice.

conceptual sense to use a weighing practice that mitigates patients' distress and facilitates treatment responsivity. However, it is conceivable that, at least for some patients, blind weighing represents a safety behaviour which allows patients to avoid some of their fears (e.g., knowing their weight) and interfere with long-term treatment outcomes. Thus, it is important to consider that different approaches to weighing might be suited at different stages of treatment. For example, blind weighing early in treatment might help patients engage more thoroughly in other aspects of the treatment (e.g., adhering to meal plan), but transitioning to open weighing when patients are less acute (e.g., in an outpatient setting) may be preferable in order to challenge the "broken cognition", extinguish the patient's fears of being weighed and help patients cope with being a certain weight.

In reference to weight-related anxiety, the findings of the present study stand in contrast to the habituation effect postulated for open weighing which assumes that patients experience a reduction in weight-related anxiety following repeated exposure to their weight [1]. There may be several possible explanations for the current findings. For example, as alluded to by Forbush and colleagues [3], open weighing is only effective for decreasing weight-related anxiety when all maladaptive coping strategies and responses (e.g., increased eating disorder behaviours following weighing) are blocked. Given that the patient sample in the current study consisted of women who were very acute and therefore required inpatient care, they may not have been able to resist engaging in some eating disorder behaviours during their admission, thereby rendering weight exposure ineffective and potentially explaining the high level of anxiety symptoms in the open weighing group. An alternative explanation for the current findings is that the inclusion criteria used for the patient sample in the current study (i.e., completion of two or more weeks of inpatient treatment) possibly meant that some patients had not been in inpatient treatment for long enough to experience the habituation effect. However, if weight-related anxiety negatively affects treatment retention as suggested by participants in this study, it may be that patients drop out before habituation can occur. Future research is needed to address these issues.

The theme of control and intolerance of uncertainty emerged in most interviews. Participants who had experienced blind weighing described initially having significant difficulties adjusting to weight ambiguity, noting that not knowing their weight was a threat to their sense of control. However, participants viewed this need for control to be pathological (i.e., ED-Self driven) and consequently reasoned that learning to tolerate uncertainty around one's weight is a necessary step towards recovery from an eating disorder and living a normal, healthy life. This is consistent with existing literature recognising that patients' readiness to let go of pathological control is crucial to treatment success [19–21]. Blind weighing was perceived to provide an opportunity to modify the distorted beliefs regarding the need to know and control one's weight. Supporting participants' accounts, quantitative analyses found that blind weighed patients had greater tolerance of weight uncertainty than did open weighed patients. These results suggest that blind weighing could have clinical utility in that it (1) reduces weight-related anxiety and maximises engagement, and (2) successfully exposes patients to uncertainty and lack of control over their weight, facilitating a shift in maladaptive beliefs regarding the dangers of uncertainty or lack of control (e.g., "I must know my exact weight at all times"). An interesting finding was the suggestion of using blind weighing adaptations that provide some level of weight feedback without disclosing "exact" weight information. Participants perceived these alternative approaches to satisfy their need for certainty and control without reinforcing the obsession over the numeric value. These findings suggest that weighing adaptations may be promising in lowering the perceived barrier to blind weighing (i.e., perceived lack of control over weight). Empirical research is required to determine the precise benefits of these adaptations and explore the impact they have on treatment outcomes.

Almost uniformly, participants valued autonomy and involvement in treatment decision-making. Autonomy could be experienced two ways: by retaining control of one's weight or by choosing to let go of that control, as long as the decision was made autonomously by the participant. A trusting and collaborative therapeutic relationship appeared to enable participants to relinquish control over their weight and adhere to the weighing practice guidelines (i.e., not to self-weigh outside of treatment). In contrast, when the therapeutic relationship was precarious, participants reported poorer adherence to blind weighing guidelines (i.e., not weighing themselves outside of treatment), which they thought negatively affected their recovery progress. These findings are consistent with research showing that patients who comprehend the treatment process and feel that their need for autonomy is met by being involved in important treatment choices are less likely to drop out of treatment [22] and also achieve improved treatment motivation, engagement, and outcomes [23, 24] than do patients whose autonomy needs are not supported as strongly. Thus, whatever weighing practice is used, clinicians should ensure that patients are consulted and involved as much as possible.

Finally, participants expressed concerns regarding incidental weight exposure post-discharge after not having seen their weight during their admission. As it stands, research acknowledges that, in eating disorders, the transition from inpatient treatment to home is often problematic and associated with a high risk of relapse [25–27]. To minimise risk of readmission, it is recommended that a continuous stepped care approach, including a post-discharge support system, be provided [26, 28]. This may be particularly important for blind weighed patients who have not been aware of their weight throughout the inpatient admission and thus are at risk of relapsing if exposed to their weight prematurely. To explore the possible link between blind weighing and relapse, longitudinal research comparing patient trajectories after blind versus open weighing is needed. Furthermore, future research may benefit from investigating how patients' transition between different levels of care (e.g., from inpatient to outpatient services) can be improved to be as seamless and supportive as possible.

Limitations of this study include the "opt-in" nature of recruitment and potential for self-selection bias. Thus, findings may reflect the views of people with eating disorders who are more interested in the debate about weighing practices. Second, the current patient group consisted exclusively of female adults with severe eating disorders (i.e., requiring inpatient care), the majority of whom met criteria for AN. Therefore, this study might not be representative of the wider spectrum of eating disorders or those individuals who receive outpatient treatment. The recovered participants, however, included women who had experienced both inpatient and outpatient care thus speaking to the generalisability of the findings. Third, current blind weighed patients and recovered participants differed significantly in age and BMI from current open weighed patients. Furthermore, information regarding duration of illness and time in treatment were not collected. It is conceivable that the groups' experiences and opinions would vary with these factors. Finally, the current study focused on patient perspectives rather than on treatment outcomes. Patient perspectives can help maximise therapy engagement and, consequently, retention (both of which are particularly difficult when treating eating disorder patients), however future randomised controlled trials comparing the two weighing practices are necessary to determine how open and blind weighing influence treatment effectiveness. Ideally these trials would include qualitative assessments of patient's experience so that the direct link between treatment effectiveness and experience can be mapped out.

Conclusions

Qualitative research allows exploration and understanding of lived experience and is ideally suited to expanding the research base on weighing practices in eating disorders. Overall the findings of the current study suggest that both open weighing and blind weighing have clinical utility. Blind weighing appears to be preferred by patients, especially in the acute stages of treatment, because it reduces weight-related anxiety and increases patients' ability to engage in recovery. In addition, blind weighing is viewed to promote tolerance of weight uncertainty. In comparison, open weighing is perceived to be more beneficial in later stages of treatment. Although informative, this was a qualitative study, and clinical practice should not be guided by patients' perspectives alone. Thus, experimental designs comparing the two weighing practices are needed before definitive conclusions can be drawn. The next step for future research will be to connect the patient insights gained from the current study with treatment outcomes gained from randomised controlled trials in order to develop treatment protocols that maximise effectiveness, as well as patient engagement and retention.

Abbreviations

AN: Anorexia nervosa; ANOVA: Analysis of Variance; BMI: Body mass index; BN: Bulimia nervosa; BW: Blind weighing; CBT: Cognitive-behaviour therapy; DSM-5: Diagnostic and Statistical Manual of Mental Disorder, Fifth Edition; EDDS: Eating Disorder Diagnostic Scale – DSM-5 version; ED-Self: Eating disorder-self; FBT: Family-based treatment; OSFED: Other specified feeding or eating disorders; OW: Open weighing

Acknowledgements

The authors would like to thank Dr. Alana Fisher for her helpful comments on this project. We would also like to express our gratitude to the collaborating Northside Clinic and Northside West Clinic, and to the individuals who took part in the study.

Informed consent

Informed consent was obtained from all individual participants included in the study.

Authors' contributions

FVF and LRV were involved in the design of the study; FVF collected the data; FVF and SER analysed the data; and FVF, SER, and LRV drafted and approved the final manuscript.

Competing interests

FVF, SER, and LRV declare that they have no conflict of interest.

Author details

[1]School of Psychology, UNSW Sydney, Sydney 2052, Australia. [2]School of Psychology, University of Sydney, Sydney 2006, Australia.

References

1. Waller G, Mountford VA. Weighing patients within cognitive-behavioural therapy for eating disorders: how, when and why. Behav Res Ther. 2015;70:1–0.
2. Fairburn CG. Cognitive behavior therapy and eating disorders. New York: Guilford Press; 2008.
3. Forbush KT, Richardson JH, Bohrer BK. Clinicians' practices regarding blind versus open weighing among patients with eating disorders. Int J Eat Disord. 2015;48(7):905–11.
4. Murray SB, Loeb KL, Le Grange D. Dissecting the core fear in anorexia nervosa: can we optimize treatment mechanisms? JAMA Psychiatry. 2016; 73(9):891–2.
5. Kesby A, Maguire S, Brownlow R, Grisham JR. Intolerance of uncertainty in eating disorders: an update on the field. Clin Psychol Rev. 2017;56:94–105.
6. Fassino S, Pierò A, Tomba E, Abbate-Daga G. Factors associated with dropout from treatment for eating disorders: a comprehensive literature review. BMC Psychiatry. 2009;9(1):67.

7. Kelly-Weeder S, Kells M, Jennings K, Dunne J, Wolfe B. Procedures and protocols for weight assessment during acute illness in individuals with anorexia nervosa: a National Survey. J Am Psychiatr Nurses Assoc. 2018; 24(3):241–6.
8. American Psychiatric Association. Diagnostic and statistical manual of mental disorders. 5th ed. Washington, DC: American Psychiatric Association; 2013.
9. Stice E. Eating Disorder Diagnostic Scale - DSM-5 version. In: Oregon Research Institute. Available from https://www.ori.org/sticemeasures. .
10. Bowen GA. Document analysis as a qualitative research method. Qual Res J. 2009;9(2):27–40.
11. Stice E, Fisher M, Martinez E. Eating disorder diagnostic scale: additional evidence of reliability and validity. Psychol Assess. 2004;16(1):60–71.
12. Stice E, Telch CF, Rizvi SL. Development and validation of the eating disorder diagnostic scale: a brief self-report measure of anorexia, bulimia, and binge-eating disorder. Psychol Assess. 2000;12(2):123–31.
13. Sysko R, Glasofer DR, Hildebrandt T, Klimek P, Mitchell JE, Berg KC, et al. The eating disorder assessment for DSM-5 (EDA-5): development and validation of a structured interview for feeding and eating disorders. Int J Eat Disord. 2015;48(5):452–63.
14. Braun V, Clarke V. Using thematic analysis in psychology. Qual Res Psychol. 2006;3(2):77–101.
15. Ritchie J, Spencer L. Qualitative data analysis for applied policy research. In: Huberman AM, Miles MB, editors. The qualitative Researcher's companion. Thousand Oaks: Sage Publications; 2002. p. 305–29.
16. Meyer DZ, Avery LM. Excel as a qualitative data analysis tool. Field Methods. 2009;21(1):91–112.
17. De la Rie S, Noordenbos G, Donker M, van Furth E. Evaluating the treatment of eating disorders from the patient's perspective. Int J Eat Disord. 2006; 39(8):667–76.
18. Vall E, Wade TD. Predictors of treatment outcome in individuals with eating disorders: a systematic review and meta-analysis. Int J Eat Disord. 2015;48(7): 946–71.
19. Bruch H. Anorexia nervosa: therapy and theory. Am J Psychiatry. 1982; 139(12):1531–8.
20. Lee S, Lydia Chan YY, Kwok K, George Hsu LK. Relationship between control and the intermediate term outcome of anorexia nervosa in Hong Kong. Aust N Z J Psychiatry. 2005;39(3):141–5.
21. Patching J, Lawler J. Understanding women's experiences of developing an eating disorder and recovering: a life-history approach. Nurs Inq. 2009;16(1): 10–21.
22. Vandereycken W, Vansteenkiste M. Let eating disorder patients decide: providing choice may reduce early drop-out from inpatient treatment. Eur Eat Disord Rev. 2009;17(3):177–83.
23. Sheridan G, McArdle S. Exploring patients' experiences of eating disorder treatment services from a motivational perspective. Qual Health Res. 2016; 26(14):1988–97.
24. van der Kaap-Deeder J, Vansteenkiste M, Soenens B, Verstuyf J, Boone L, Smets J. Fostering self-endorsed motivation to change in patients with an eating disorder: the role of perceived autonomy support and psychological need satisfaction. Int J Eat Disord. 2014;47(6):585–600.
25. Kaye WH, Kaplan AS, Zucker ML. Treating eating-disorder patients in a managed care environment: contemporary American issues and a Canadian response. Psychiatr Clin North Am. 1996;19(4):793–810.
26. Koskina A, Campbell IC, Schmidt U. Exposure therapy in eating disorders revisited. Neurosci Biobehav Rev. 2013;37(2):193–208.
27. Vandereycken W. The place of inpatient care in the treatment of anorexia nervosa: questions to be answered. Int J Eat Disord. 2003;34(4):409–22.
28. Hay P, Chinn D, Forbes D, Madden S, Newton R, Sugenor L, et al. Royal Australian and new Zealand College of Psychiatrists clinical practice guidelines for the treatment of eating disorders. Aust N Z J Psychiatry. 2014; 48(11):977–1008.

Permissions

All chapters in this book were first published by BioMed Central; hereby published with permission under the Creative Commons Attribution License or equivalent. Every chapter published in this book has been scrutinized by our experts. Their significance has been extensively debated. The topics covered herein carry significant findings which will fuel the growth of the discipline. They may even be implemented as practical applications or may be referred to as a beginning point for another development.

The contributors of this book come from diverse backgrounds, making this book a truly international effort. This book will bring forth new frontiers with its revolutionizing research information and detailed analysis of the nascent developments around the world.

We would like to thank all the contributing authors for lending their expertise to make the book truly unique. They have played a crucial role in the development of this book. Without their invaluable contributions this book wouldn't have been possible. They have made vital efforts to compile up to date information on the varied aspects of this subject to make this book a valuable addition to the collection of many professionals and students.

This book was conceptualized with the vision of imparting up-to-date information and advanced data in this field. To ensure the same, a matchless editorial board was set up. Every individual on the board went through rigorous rounds of assessment to prove their worth. After which they invested a large part of their time researching and compiling the most relevant data for our readers.

The editorial board has been involved in producing this book since its inception. They have spent rigorous hours researching and exploring the diverse topics which have resulted in the successful publishing of this book. They have passed on their knowledge of decades through this book. To expedite this challenging task, the publisher supported the team at every step. A small team of assistant editors was also appointed to further simplify the editing procedure and attain best results for the readers.

Apart from the editorial board, the designing team has also invested a significant amount of their time in understanding the subject and creating the most relevant covers. They scrutinized every image to scout for the most suitable representation of the subject and create an appropriate cover for the book.

The publishing team has been an ardent support to the editorial, designing and production team. Their endless efforts to recruit the best for this project, has resulted in the accomplishment of this book. They are a veteran in the field of academics and their pool of knowledge is as vast as their experience in printing. Their expertise and guidance has proved useful at every step. Their uncompromising quality standards have made this book an exceptional effort. Their encouragement from time to time has been an inspiration for everyone.

The publisher and the editorial board hope that this book will prove to be a valuable piece of knowledge for researchers, students, practitioners and scholars across the globe.

List of Contributors

Kara A. Christensen
Department of Psychology, University of Kansas, 1415 Jayhawk Blvd Rm 440, Lawrence, KS 66045, USA

Ann F. Haynos
Department of Psychiatry and Behavioral Sciences, University of Minnesota, 2450 Riverside Ave, F253, Minneapolis, MN 55454, USA

Mohsen Khosravi
Department of Psychiatry and Clinical Psychology, Baharan Psychiatric Hospital, Zahedan University of Medical Sciences, Zahedan, Iran

Paulo P. P. Machado, Ana Pinto-Bastos, Rita Ramos, Tânia F. Rodrigues, Elsa Louro, Sónia Gonçalves and Ana Vaz
Psychotherapy and Psychopathology Research Unit – Psychology Research Centre, University of Minho, School of Psychology, Braga, Portugal

Isabel Brandão
Faculty of Medicine, Psychiatry Department, University Hospital Center of São João, 4200-319 Porto, Portugal

Dawn Branley-Bell and Catherine V. Talbot
Department of Psychology, Northumbria University, Newcastle upon Tyne, England, UK

Kerrie Doyle and Adam Burt
School of Medicine, Western Sydney University, Campbelltown, Australia

Deborah Mitchison
Translational Health Research Institute, School of Medicine, Western Sydney University, Campbelltown, Australia
Centre for Emotional Health, Department of Psychology, Macquarie University, North Ryde, New South Wales, Australia

Phillipa Hay
Translational Health Research Institute, School of Medicine, Western Sydney University, Campbelltown, Australia
Campbelltown Hospital, SWSLHD, Campbelltown, Australia

Rhonda M. Merwin, Ashley A. Moskovich, Lisa K. Honeycutt, Jan Mooney, Sara P. Freeman, Heather Batchelder and Michael Babyak
Department of Psychiatry and Behavioral Sciences, Duke University Medical Center, Durham, NC 27712, USA

Mark Feinglos
Department of Medicine, Division of Endocrinology, Metabolism and Nutrition, Duke University Medical Center, Durham, NC, USA

Devdutta Sangvai
Department of Family Medicine and Community Health, Duke University Medical Center, Durham, NC, USA

Noriko Numata, Akiko Nakagawa and Daisuke Matsuzawa
Research Center for Child Mental Development, Chiba University, 1-8-1 Inohana, Chuo-ku, Chiba 260-8670, Japan

Kazuko Yoshioka
Department for School of Human and Social Sciences, Fukuoka Prefectural University, Fukuoka, Japan

Kayoko Isomura
Centre for Psychiatry Research, Department of Clinical Neuroscience, Karolinska Institutet, Stockholm, Sweden

Eiji Shimizu
Research Center for Child Mental Development, Chiba University, 1-8-1 Inohana, Chuo-ku, Chiba 260-8670, Japan
Department of Cognitive Behavioral Physiology, Graduate School of Medicine, Chiba University, Chiba, Japan

Rikukage Setsu
Department of Cognitive Behavioral Physiology, Graduate School of Medicine, Chiba University, Chiba, Japan
Koutokukai Sato Hospital, Yamagata, Japan

Michiko Nakazato
Department of Psychiatry, Graduate School of Medicine, International University of Health and Welfare, Chiba, Japan
Department of Psychiatry, Graduate School of Medicine, Chiba University, Chiba, Japan

L. Vuillier, M. Greville-Harris, R. Surman and R. L. Moseley
Department of Psychology, Bournemouth University, Poole, UK

L. May
Department of Psychology, Bournemouth University, Poole, UK
Dorset Healthcare University NHS Foundation Trust, Poole, UK

Hannah Shaw
The Eating Disorder Young Person's Service, Alder Hey Children's Hospital Foundation Trust, Liverpool, UK
Royal Holloway University of London, Egham, UK

Sarah Robertson
The Eating Disorder Young Person's Service, Alder Hey Children's Hospital Foundation Trust, Liverpool, UK

Nadia Ranceva
The Eating Disorder Young Person's Service, Alder Hey Children's Hospital Foundation Trust, Liverpool, UK
Vilnius University, Vilnius, Lithuania

Victoria Burmester, Esme Graham and Dasha Nicholls
Division of Psychiatry, Department of Brain Sciences, Imperial College London, Du Cane Road, London W12 0NN, UK

Jordan Andre Martenstyn
Clinical Psychology Unit, School of Psychology, The University of Sydney, Sydney, Australia
InsideOut Institute for Eating Disorders, The Boden Collaboration for Obesity, Nutrition, Exercise and Eating Disorders, The University of Sydney, Sydney, Australia

Stephen Touyz
InsideOut Institute for Eating Disorders, The Boden Collaboration for Obesity, Nutrition, Exercise and Eating Disorders, The University of Sydney, Sydney, Australia

Sarah Maguire
InsideOut Institute for Eating Disorders, The Boden Collaboration for Obesity, Nutrition, Exercise and Eating Disorders, The University of Sydney, Sydney, Australia
Sydney Local Health District, NSW Health, St Leonards, Australia

Jennifer Brunet
School of Human Kinetics, University of Ottawa, 125 University Private, Montpetit Hall, Room 339, Ottawa, Ontario K1N 6N5, Canada
Cancer Therapeutics Program, Ottawa Hospital Research Institute, 1053 Carling Avenue, Ottawa, Ontario K1Y 4E9, Canada
Institut du savoir Montfort, Hôpital Montfort, 713 Montreal Road, Ottawa, Ontario K1K 0T2, Canada

Francis Del Duchetto
School of Human Kinetics, University of Ottawa, 125 University Private, Montpetit Hall, Room 339, Ottawa, Ontario K1N 6N5, Canada
Present address: Université du Québec à Trois-Rivières, 3351 Boulevard des Forges, Trois-Rivières, Québec G8Z 4M3, Canada

Amanda Wurz
Faculty of Kinesiology, University of Calgary, 2500 University Drive, Calgary, Alberta T2N 1N4, Canada

Giuseppe Colella, Vincenzo Santillo and Gianpaolo Tartaro
Multidisciplinary Department of Medical-Surgical and Dental Specialties, Oral and Maxillofacial Surgery Unit, University of Campania "Luigi Vanvitelli", 80138 Naples, Italy

Giorgio Lo Giudice, Roberto De Luca, Antonio Troiano and Carmelo Lo Faro
Department of Neurosciences, Reproductive and Odontostomatological Sciences, Maxillofacial Surgery Unit, University of Naples "Federico II", 80138 Naples, Italy

Yael Doreen Lewis, Rinat Grundman-Shem Tov and Eynat Zubery
Hadarim Eating Disorders Treatment Center, Shalvata Mental Health Center, Hod Hasharon, Israel
Sackler Faculty of Medicine, Tel Aviv University, Tel Aviv, Israel.

Roni Elran-Barak
School of Public Health, University of Haifa, Haifa, Israel

Won Sub Kang and Sang Min Lee
Department of Psychiatry, Kyung Hee University Hospital, Kyung Hee University College of Medicine, 1 Hoegi-Dong, Dongdaemug-Gu, Seoul 130-701, South Korea

Minha Hong
Department of Psychiatry, Myongji Hospital, Hanyang University College of Medicine, 55 Hwasu-ro 14 beon-gil, Deogyang-gu, Goyang 10475, South Korea

Saengryeol Park
Department of Physical Education, College of Education, Chonnam National University, 77 Yongbong-ro, Buk-gu, Gwangju 61186, South Korea

In-Hwan Oh
Department of Preventive Medicine, Kyung Hee University School of Medicine, 1 Hoegi-Dong, Dongdaemug-Gu, Seoul 130-701, South Korea

Nancy A. Uriegas, Allison B. Smith and Toni M. Torres-McGehee
University of South Carolina, Blatt PE Center 212, Columbia, SC 29208, USA

Dawn M. Emerson and Melani R. Kelly
University of Kansas, 1301 Sunnyside Avenue, Robinson 161, Lawrence, KS 66045, USA

Laura Vuillier and Jemma Joseph
Faculty of Science and Technology, Department of Psychology, Bournemouth University, Poole, UK

Matthew P. Somerville and Amy Harrison
UCL Institute of Education, University College London, London, UK

Marko Biberdzic, Josephine Tang and Junhao Tan
School of Psychology, University of Wollongong, Wollongong, NSW 2522, Australia

Martina Isaksson and Mia Ramklint
Department of Neuroscience, Psychiatry, Uppsala University, Entrance 10, Floor 3B, SE-751 85 Uppsala, Sweden

Ata Ghaderi
Division of Psychology, Department of Clinical Neuroscience, Karolinska Institutet, SE-171 77 Stockholm, Sweden
Stockholm Centre for Eating Disorders, Stockholm Health Care Services, Stockholm County Council, SE-171 77 Stockholm, Sweden

Martina Wolf-Arehult
Department of Neuroscience, Psychiatry, Uppsala University, Entrance 10, Floor 3B, SE-751 85 Uppsala, Sweden Psychiatry Northwest, Region Stockholm, Clinical Management, SE-191 22 Sollentuna, Sweden

Aoife-Marie Foran, Orla T. Muldoon and Aisling T. O'Donnell
Centre for Social Issues Research, Department of Psychology, University of Limerick, Castletroy, Limerick, Republic of Ireland

Franzisca V. Froreich and Lenny R. Vartanian
School of Psychology, UNSW Sydney, Sydney 2052, Australia

Index

www.ingramcontent.com/pod-product-compliance
Lightning Source LLC
LaVergne TN
LVHW060552210926
848485LV00005B/1301
* 9 7 8 1 6 3 9 2 7 9 8 9 0 *